The Herbal Henhouse
Nurturing Your Chickens with Nature's Remedies

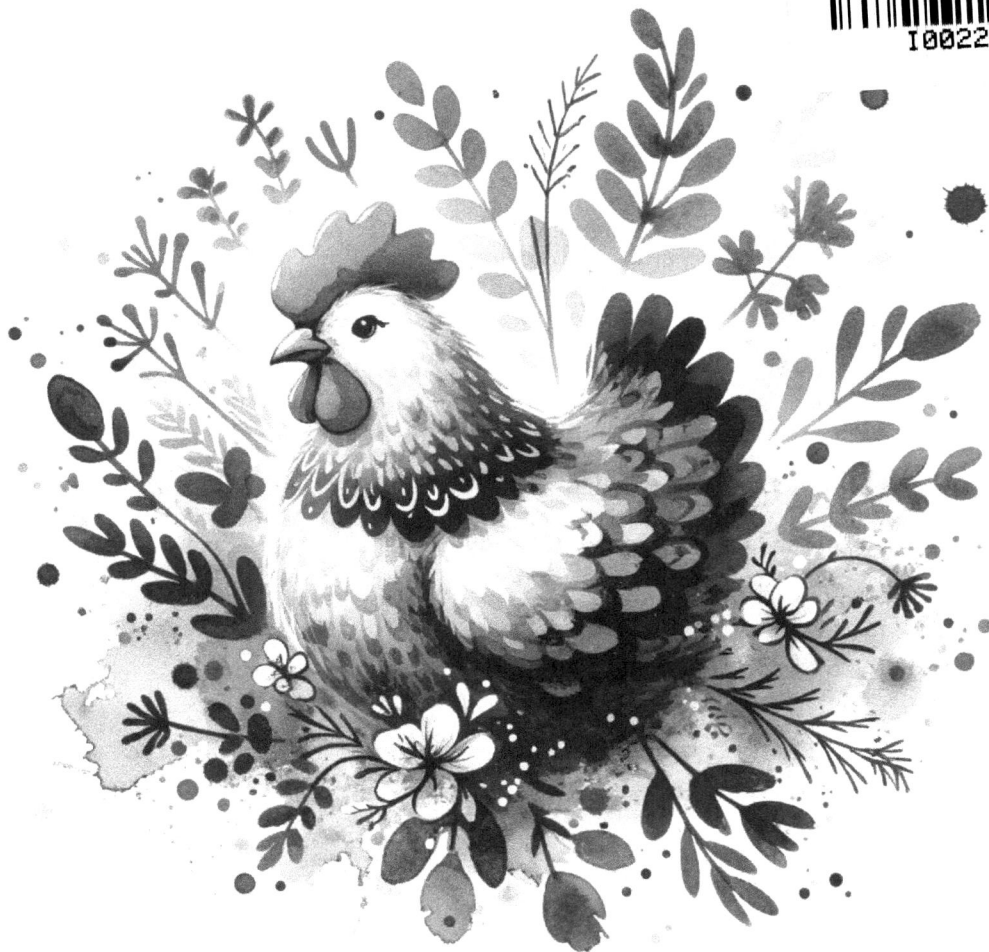

To all the crazy chicken tenders, may your eggs boast yolks of the richest gold, your roosters conduct themselves with noble grace, and may your coop flourish, for in the delightful arithmetic of chicken math, may your numbers joyfully increase!

The Herbal Henhouse: Nurturing Your Chickens with Nature's Remedies

ISBN:
Paperback: 979-8-9903758-0-2
Hardback: 979-8-9903758-2-6
Ebook: 979-8-9903758-1-9

Library of Congress Control Number (LCCN): 2025911011

Printed in The United States of America

Contact Information:
hello@authormarybutler.com

Acknowledgments

I am deeply grateful to my husband, Rico, whose unwavering belief in me, relentless encouragement to pursue excellence, and enduring patience with my passionate avian pursuits have been the bedrock of my journey. His support has been a constant source of strength and inspiration.

I want to express my heartfelt thanks to my parents, who sowed the seeds of diligence, compassion for all, and boundless aspiration in my heart. Their enduring faith in my potential to achieve anything I set my mind to has been a guiding light throughout this endeavor.

The love and support I have received from each of you have been indispensable, enriching this journey beyond measure. You are all truly blessings in my life. Your collective faith and encouragement have been instrumental in the realization of this project, and for that, I am eternally grateful.

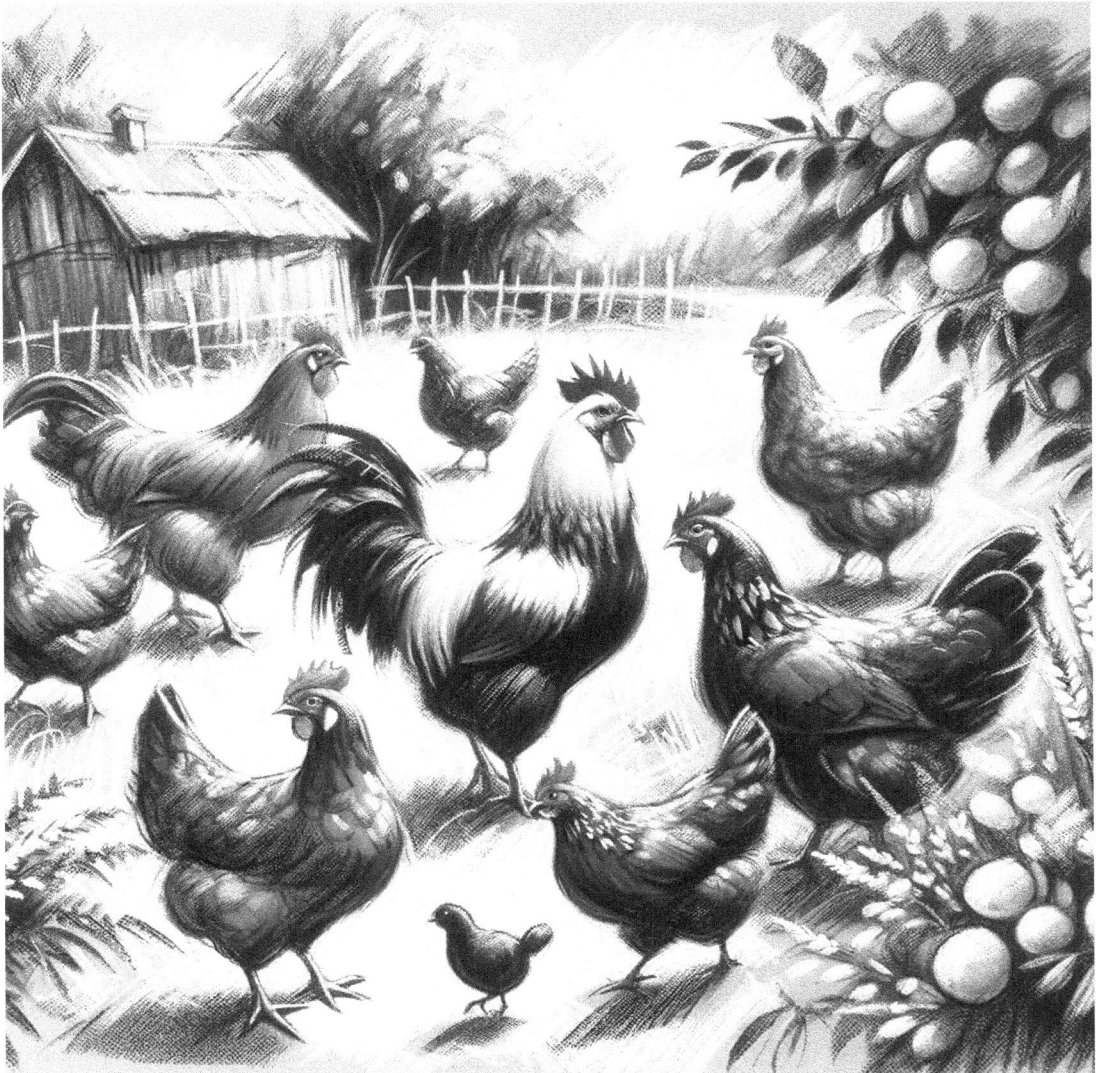

Dear Readers,

Welcome to *The Herbal Henhouse: Nurturing Your Chickens with Nature's Remedies*. I'm thrilled to share my passion for holistic chicken care and the natural healing power of herbs. This book is the culmination of years of hands-on experience, careful research, and a deep love for my flock.

While I am not a veterinarian or licensed herbalist, I've spent countless hours studying herbal practices and applying them with great success in my own coop. I firmly believe that, much like in humans, the regular use of herbs in a chicken's diet can help reduce the occurrence of illness and parasites — a belief backed by experience and observation.

This book is designed to offer you practical insights, tested herbal remedies, and a framework for making informed decisions about your flock's care. As you explore the chapters ahead, I encourage you to keep the following key points in mind:

- **Prevention is powerful**: Herbs work best as daily wellness support, helping the body stay strong and resilient.

- **Consult licensed professionals**: For personalized guidance, reach out to a licensed herbalist or holistic animal health practitioner.

- **Work with a veterinarian**: Always consult a qualified vet for diagnoses and to safely integrate herbal treatments with conventional care.

- **Observe and adapt**: Each chicken is unique. Monitor responses to any new herbal addition and discontinue use if adverse reactions occur.

- **Use herbs with care**: Just like medications, herbs should be used thoughtfully. Follow dosage guidance and consult experts as needed.

- **Own the process**: Ultimately, your flock's well-being rests in your hands. Prioritize safety, ask questions, and trust your instincts.

Throughout the book, you'll find recipes interwoven with guidance and deeper background information. I strongly recommend reading the chapters before jumping into the recipes — this foundation will help you use herbs more effectively and confidently.

I hope *The Herbal Henhouse* becomes a trusted resource on your journey toward holistic chicken care. May your chickens flourish in the natural comfort of herbal wisdom.

With warmth and love,
Miss Mary & my HAPPY Chickens

s

"A hen is only an egg's way of making another egg."
— Samuel Butler

Table Of Contents

"Nature does not hurry, yet everything is accomplished."
— Lao Tzu

Chapter 1: Pecking Around the Herbal Basics

Part I: Understanding Herbs: A Beakful of Knowledge

Herbs—what a delightful word! When you hear it, don't you picture a garden overflowing with green, vibrant plants, sending wafts of delightful aromas into the air? You're not alone! Yet, for all their popularity, what exactly is an herb? Have you ever pondered that?

Well, fear not, for we're about to dig into the roots of this question. Interestingly, there isn't just one universally agreed-upon definition for herbs. Some define herbs based on their culinary applications, others on medicinal usage, and yet some others on their botanic characteristics. Here, we are concerned with the broadest and most inclusive perspective that aligns with our mission of nurturing our beloved feathered friends with nature's remedies. Let's sprout some knowledge, shall we?

At its very basic level, an herb is any plant or plant part that possesses therapeutic properties. This wide-ranging definition includes everything from leafy greens to aromatic flowers and healing roots to nutritious seeds. In the world of chickens, we don't just restrict ourselves to parsley or dill - oh, no! We tap into the myriad of plant forms Mother Nature offers to ensure our hens are pecking their way to the best health.

The term 'herb' comes from the Latin 'herba,' meaning 'grass,' 'green stalks,' or 'blades.' Over time, the definition has stretched to encompass all parts of a plant used for flavoring, food, medicine, or perfume. Now, isn't that just fantastic? A word so humble in its origins now carries such a rich tapestry of meanings.

Now, what sets herbs apart from other plants? It's their unique concentration of potent bioactive compounds. These naturally occurring chemicals, such as essential oils, flavonoids, and alkaloids, are like nature's magic potion. Each herb has its own unique composition, and that's what gives it its unique healing properties. These compounds can enhance immunity, promote digestion, repel pests, and even act as mood uplifters. We just need to know which herb does what, and that's what this book will help you with.

But let's take a step back and appreciate the journey of these fantastic plants. Many of the herbs we use today have been on an extraordinary voyage through time. Imagine: They were first discovered in ancient times, cultivated and treasured in medieval herb gardens, celebrated in Shakespeare's writings, and now find a place in our chicken coops.

Culturally, herbs have deep roots. Almost every civilization recognized and valued the power of herbs. Ancient Egyptians included them in their embalming practices. The Greeks crowned their heroes with dill and marjoram. Chinese traditional medicine, one of the oldest healing systems, stands firmly on a foundation of herbs. Even today, in our world of synthetics and technology, these humble plants continue to hold their own, and rightly so.

In the realm of chicken care, these plant champions are our greatest allies. They support the health of our flock, make them happier, and, as an added bonus, make our coops smell like an enchanted garden. Truly, using herbs is like inviting Mother Nature herself into our backyards to care for our hens.

It is important to remember, though, that while herbs are natural, they are also potent. When used correctly, they can contribute significantly to the health and happiness of your flock. Used indiscriminately, they can cause more harm than good. With knowledge comes confidence, and that's what you will gain from this book - the confidence to harness the power of herbs for your flock's well-being. We have just scratched the surface of the definition of herbs, and now it's time to explore another layer: the lifespan of herbs. By breaking it down to the basics, you'll gain a deeper understanding and be better equipped to choose the best herbs for your chickens' needs.

Let's begin with the annuals. These are the herbs that have a one-year life cycle. They sprout from seeds, bloom, produce seeds, and then gracefully bow out - all in one growing season. These short-lived plants may seem like a lot of work for a little reward, but don't let their fleeting life dissuade you. Annual herbs, like basil, coriander, or dill, are powerhouses of flavor and nutrients. Your hens will be clucking with joy as they peck on these fresh green treats. Plus, their prolific seed production ensures you have a steady supply for the next season. Remember to collect the seeds at the end of the season or let some drop to the ground for a pleasant surprise next year!

Next up, we have biennials. These hardy herbs live for two years. The first year is all about growth as they focus on developing their leafy greens. Come the second year, they switch gears, putting all their energy into flowering and seeding before bidding adieu. Parsley, a popular biennial, provides great nutritional benefits for your flock, particularly for laying hens. Its high calcium content supports strong eggshells, and its rich flavor makes it a hit in the coop. Be patient with your biennials; they may not be as flashy in their first year, but their second-year performance is worth the wait.

Finally, we move on to perennials, the long-livers of the herb world. Perennial herbs, such as rosemary, thyme, and mint, keep going strong year after year. Once established, they require minimal upkeep and offer consistent rewards. Their hardiness makes them a fantastic choice for the coop. Imagine a garden where you plant once and reap the benefits for years. Sounds like a dream, doesn't it? However, keep in mind that perennial herbs do require some care. They need a good pruning from time to time to keep them healthy and productive. Also, be mindful of the spreading habit of some perennials (looking at you, mint!). Without proper control, they can take over your garden.

Understanding the life cycles of herbs will help you plan your herb garden more effectively. Do you want a quick burst of greenery and nutrients? Go for annuals. Do you prefer plants that will hang around for a couple of years? Opt for biennials. Or do you want a steady supply of herbs year after year? Perennials are the answer.

Knowing this will also help you manage your expectations. It's not uncommon for new herb gardeners to get disappointed when their parsley doesn't flower in the first year or their annual herbs die off after a season. Understanding that this is a natural process and that each herb has its own rhythm and pace will make your gardening journey more enjoyable and rewarding.

So, annuals, biennials, perennials - each type of herb brings its own charm to your garden and your coop. They all have unique benefits and uses that can be harnessed for the well-being of your chickens. It's all about knowing what to plant, when to plant, and how to care for them. Equally important, however, is understanding why these plants are so beneficial. To grasp this, we need to delve into the fantastic world of phytonutrients and essential oils, the active components in herbs that make them a powerful ally for the health and well-being of your chickens.

Phytonutrients, often called phytochemicals, are naturally occurring compounds found in plants, including herbs. They're part of the plant's defense mechanism against pests, diseases, and UV radiation, but they also serve as a valuable source of health-boosting properties for our feathered friends and us. Just like they protect plants, phytonutrients can protect our chickens against diseases, boost their immune systems, and even improve their egg production.

Each herb contains a unique combination of these phytonutrients. For instance, the vibrant orange hue of marigold petals comes from lutein, a phytonutrient known for its potent antioxidant properties. It is often added to chicken feed to deepen the color of egg yolks. Similarly, garlic is rich in allicin, a sulfur-containing compound with powerful antimicrobial properties, protecting your flock against various diseases.

Essential oils, another category of active components, are responsible for the wonderful aromas that herbs emit. Essential oils not only make the coop smell pleasant, but they also have a host of health benefits for your chickens. They can serve as natural insect repellants, respiratory health boosters, stress relievers, and much more.

For example, the sharp, refreshing scent of peppermint comes from its essential oil, which contains menthol. This can help deter pests in the coop and, when ingested, support digestive health. Lavender, on the other hand, is known for its calming properties, mainly due to its essential oil, linalool. Adding a sprig of lavender to your hens' nesting boxes can provide a soothing environment, helping to keep your laying hens relaxed.

It's important to note, however, that not all essential oils and phytonutrients are beneficial or safe for chickens. Some can be harmful or even toxic. This underscores the importance of careful research and consultation with a knowledgeable herbalist or avian vet before introducing a new herb to your flock.

One final point worth mentioning is that the levels of phytonutrients and essential oils in herbs can vary based on several factors, such as the growing conditions, the time of harvest, and the method of storage. Sunlight, soil quality, and temperature all play a role in the herb's potency. Harvesting herbs when their essential oil content is at its peak—generally right before flowering—will ensure you get the most out of your herbs. Storing them correctly, typically in a cool, dark, and dry place, will help preserve these beneficial compounds.

Understanding the power that lies within each leaf, stem, and flower of these herbs allows us to harness their full potential for the well-being of our chickens. This knowledge also aids in appreciating the natural wonders that we're integrating into our coops, creating a healthier and more harmonious environment for our flock. Understanding the science behind how herbs affect chickens' health is an important aspect of this journey. Each system within a chicken's body can be influenced, directly or indirectly, by the herbs they consume or interact with, and knowing the specifics can empower you to make the most beneficial choices for your flock.

Starting with the nervous system, several herbs have a substantial impact on the mood and stress levels of your chickens. This is especially relevant since stress in chickens can lead to a drop in egg production and increased vulnerability to illness. Herbs like chamomile and lavender are known for their calming properties, mainly due to the presence of compounds that can interact with the chicken's nervous system, promoting relaxation and reducing stress levels. They work by enhancing the effect of a neurotransmitter called GABA in the brain, which induces calm and relaxation.

Moving onto the digestive system, this is where herbs can really shine. Many herbs have properties that can support a healthy digestive tract and aid in nutrient absorption. For instance, herbs like dill and fennel are known to help soothe the digestive system and relieve problems like gas and bloating. The active compounds in these herbs stimulate the secretion of digestive enzymes, promoting better digestion and nutrient assimilation. Moreover, some herbs, such as oregano and thyme, contain antimicrobial compounds that can help maintain a balanced gut flora, which is essential for a healthy digestive system and overall chicken health.

The respiratory system of your chickens can also benefit from certain herbs. Herbs like eucalyptus and peppermint are rich in compounds that help clear the airways and have antibacterial and antiviral properties. These compounds can help soothe respiratory discomfort and protect against respiratory infections. When used in the coop, these herbs can release their beneficial compounds into the air, providing a natural and safe way to support respiratory health.

Herbs can also provide support for a chicken's immune system. Many herbs, including echinacea and garlic, are known for their immune-boosting properties. These herbs contain compounds that stimulate the immune system's cells, enhancing their ability to fight off pathogens. They also have antimicrobial properties, providing a natural line of defense against potential infections.

Even the circulatory system can be supported by certain herbs. Garlic, for instance, has been known to support heart health by maintaining blood vessel elasticity and promoting good blood circulation. These benefits stem from garlic's rich content of allicin, a compound with potent antioxidant properties that can protect the cardiovascular system.

In understanding the science behind how herbs can affect the various systems within a chicken's body, you're not only gaining knowledge but also developing a deep appreciation for the power and versatility of these natural wonders. Armed with this knowledge, you'll be able to create a coop environment that isn't just healthy but also harmonious, with chickens that are not only surviving but truly thriving.

But remember, knowledge is power. Use it wisely. Always remember to research each herb and if you are uncertain consult with a knowledgeable professional before introducing a new herb to your flock. This will ensure that you're using herbs in the safest and most effective manner for your chickens. While understanding the science behind how herbs affect chicken health is important, it's also fascinating and useful to look at the historical usage of herbs in poultry keeping. Delving into the past allows us to appreciate traditional and indigenous knowledge, which has contributed significantly to modern practices and enriches our understanding of the potency of nature's gifts.

Herbs and other natural substances have been used for thousands of years in the care and treatment of domestic animals, including poultry. Ancient civilizations like the Egyptians, Romans, and Chinese had a profound understanding of herbs, utilizing them not only for human ailments but also for their flocks. They understood that herbs were not just food but also medicine.

In Egypt, for instance, garlic and onions were fed to birds to boost their health and productivity. These pungent herbs are known for their antiviral and antibacterial properties, making them a natural choice for maintaining the health of a flock. This practice is still used today, with many poultry keepers regularly incorporating garlic into their chicken's diet for its immune-boosting benefits.

In ancient Rome, a writer and naturalist named Pliny the Elder described the use of various herbs for poultry care in his writings. He advocated for the use of a diverse range of herbs, including dill, mint, and thyme. He noted that these herbs not only enhanced the flavor of the birds but also contributed to their overall well-being, mirroring our modern understanding of these herbs' benefits.

Chinese culture, with its rich tradition of herbal medicine, also provides insights into the historical use of herbs in poultry keeping. Traditional Chinese Veterinary Medicine (TCVM) involves the use of herbs in the treatment and prevention of various ailments in animals. A key principle of TCVM is the balance of Qi (life force or energy), Yin (cooling energy), and Yang (warming energy). Herbs like ginger, which is warming, and mint, which is cooling, have been used for centuries to maintain this balance and promote good health in chickens.

Indigenous cultures around the world also have a rich history of using herbs for poultry care. Native American tribes, for instance, often used herbs like sage, cedar, and yarrow in their poultry practices. These herbs were believed to have protective and purifying properties and were used to maintain the health of the flock and the cleanliness of the coop.

These historical practices reflect an intuitive understanding of the medicinal properties of herbs and their positive impact on chicken health. Despite the absence of modern scientific knowledge, these early poultry keepers harnessed the power of herbs to boost the well-being and productivity of their flocks. They saw the value in what the earth provided, using nature's pharmacy to care for their animals.

As we continue to explore the world of herbs in the context of chicken keeping, it's worth remembering that our practices are not new but rather an extension and refinement of time-honored traditions. The wisdom of the past continues to guide us, adding depth to our understanding and encouraging us to continue exploring and learning.

Part II: Kitchen Herbs: Not Just for Omelettes

Step into your kitchen, and you're likely to find a treasure trove of herbs that do double duty—delighting your taste buds and boosting your flock's health. That's right, common culinary herbs like basil, rosemary, and thyme are not just for omelets; they offer numerous health benefits for your chickens, too.

Let's start with basil. This fragrant herb is a favorite in kitchens around the world, its aromatic leaves adding flavor to everything from pasta to pesto. For your chickens, basil provides a wealth of health benefits. It's packed with antioxidants that aid in fighting off infections. Moreover, it has anti-inflammatory properties that can help reduce any discomfort your chickens might feel from conditions like arthritis. Basil is also believed to boost the respiratory health of your flock, making it an excellent herb to offer during those cold winter months.

Next up, rosemary. This robust and piney herb is a staple in many meat dishes and potato remedies, but did you know it's also a power-packed addition to your chicken's diet? Rosemary is rich in antioxidants and anti-inflammatory compounds, which help boost the chicken's immune system and improve digestion. Additionally, rosemary has an uplifting effect on the mood, which is beneficial for the overall well-being of your flock. An added bonus is that pests don't particularly enjoy the strong scent of rosemary, so it can help deter them from your coop!

Thyme, with its subtle, earthy flavor, is another culinary gem that holds healthful riches for your chickens. This small-leafed herb is packed with Vitamin C and other antioxidants that help support your chicken's immune system. Plus, thyme has been shown to have antibacterial properties, potentially helping your flock ward off harmful bacteria. It's also known to help with respiratory issues, making it another great choice for maintaining the health of your flock during the chillier months.

Don't forget about oregano, another culinary staple that can do wonders for your chicken's health. Often found in Italian dishes, oregano offers antibacterial, antiviral, and anti-inflammatory properties. Many chicken keepers swear by its ability to naturally combat avian flu, coccidiosis, and other infections. It's like a natural antibiotic that you can grow right in your backyard.

Last but not least, consider parsley. This bright, fresh herb is often used as a garnish, but it offers so much more. For chickens, parsley is an excellent source of vitamins A, C, and K, as well as several B vitamins and trace minerals. It's been known to aid in blood vessel health and boost egg production, making it a beneficial addition to your flock's diet.

The wonderful thing about these herbs is that they're not just healthy for your flock. They're also a joy for them to eat. Chickens love pecking around at flavorful greens, and these herbs offer them both a tasty treat and a variety of health benefits. Plus, they're easy to grow, either in your garden or in pots, meaning you can have a constant supply of fresh, healthy herbs for your chickens to enjoy. Now, let's discuss ways to incorporate these fantastic kitchen herbs into your chicken's diet.

When it comes to feeding your flock, variety is key. Imagine if you had to eat the same thing every day – it would get pretty monotonous, wouldn't it? Chickens feel the same way. Supplementing their regular feed with fresh herbs not only provides a change of pace but also adds nutritional benefits. Herbs can be chopped and mixed directly into the feed. This can be particularly beneficial during molting periods when hens need extra nutrients. For instance, adding basil to their feed gives them a tasty treat and provides a boost of antioxidants, which help during this stressful time.

Incorporating herbs into your flock's water is another fantastic way to enhance their health. Herbal waters, sometimes known as "tea" for chickens, can give their immune systems a boost and keep them hydrated. To make herbal water, simply steep a handful of fresh or dried herbs in a pot of boiling water. Allow it to cool, then strain out the herbs. You can offer this nutrient-packed, flavored water to your chickens as a special treat. Oregano, for example, works great for this due to its natural antibiotic properties.

Free-ranging your chickens in an herb garden is like a buffet of health. Not only do they get the joy of pecking and scratching around, but they also get to consume the herbs they need or prefer. A chicken's instinct will guide them to the herbs they require for their health. It's important, though, to ensure that all plants in their range are safe for chicken consumption.

Creating a "pick-your-own" herb station in the chicken coop is a fun and beneficial addition. Hang bunches of fresh herbs, like rosemary or thyme, from the coop ceiling. Your chickens can peck at them, which not only gives them access to these beneficial plants but also provides an activity to keep them busy. This can also help with coop boredom, which can lead to pecking order problems.

Sprouting herbs for your chickens is another method that provides a fresh, nutrient-dense supplement to their diet. Sprouting amplifies the nutrient content of seeds, making them an even more potent health booster. Parsley seeds, for example, are quick to sprout and are rich in vitamins A, C, and K, which are beneficial to your flock's health.

Another interesting way to include herbs is in the nesting boxes. Herbs like lavender and mint can promote a calm environment for your hens to lay their eggs. Plus, they help to keep the coop smelling fresh! Some chicken keepers swear by the practice of adding herbs to nesting boxes to deter pests and promote the overall health and well-being of their hens.

With a little creativity, you can easily provide your chickens with these potent plants and help enhance their health and happiness. So whether it's in their feed, water, or nesting box, don't be shy about giving your chickens a little herbal boost. They'll thank you for it! Now, we dive into another related topic: Can chickens eat kitchen scraps of these herbs? Well, the short answer is yes, but with some caution. We want our feathered friends to benefit from our herbal kitchen endeavors, not harm them. So let's get into the do's and don'ts of feeding chickens herb scraps.

When you're cooking and find yourself with leftover herbs, it might be tempting to toss all your scraps to the chickens. For the most part, chickens can handle a lot of variety in their diet, and most kitchen scraps are safe for them. As we've discussed, herbs provide many health benefits to chickens. Parsley can support organ health, rosemary can help with respiratory health, and basil may help mellow out an overly aggressive hen.

However, not all food and herb scraps are created equal. While many herbs are beneficial, others can be harmful. For instance, foxglove and hemlock, although they may technically be considered herbs, are highly toxic to chickens. Even commonly used herbs like chives, garlic, and onions should be given sparingly as they can taint the taste of eggs if consumed in large quantities.

Certain cooking residues can also be harmful. If your herb scraps are coated in salt, oil, or heavy spices, you might want to think twice about sharing them with your flock. These additives aren't good for chickens and can cause health problems over time.

Moreover, the condition of your scraps matters, too. Fresh or dried herbs are generally safe for chickens. But if your scraps are moldy or overly wilted, it's best to compost them instead of feeding them to your flock. Chickens can be susceptible to certain molds and bacteria that grow on decomposing food..

Now let's talk about the do's. When you're preparing a meal and find you've got leftover herbs, why not make a little side dish for your flock? Fresh or dried thyme, for example, can be scattered on the ground or mixed into their feed. They'll enjoy the new flavors and the health benefits that come with them.

Remember, even when it comes to good things, too much of anything can throw off a balanced diet. The kitchen scraps you share with your chickens should supplement their diet, not replace their regular chicken feed.

Don't forget about water! Infusing your chicken's drinking water with herb scraps can be a beneficial and refreshing treat. A little rosemary or a couple of basil leaves can give them a nice change of pace and promote overall health.

Kitchen scraps can also be a great tool for enrichment. Throwing a mixed pile of safe scraps into the run can provide entertainment as your chickens peck, scratch, and sort through the pile. These foraging activities are fun for the flock. The health benefits, behavioral improvements, and aesthetic enhancements brought about by these humble herbs are quite remarkable.

Remember, the most important thing is to understand your flock's individual needs. As you gain confidence and experience, you'll find that integrating herbs into your chicken-keeping practices can open up a world of possibilities. If you're thinking about going the extra mile by planting an herb garden specifically for your flock, you're embarking on an exciting journey. Planning an herb garden for chickens is a unique project that requires thoughtful consideration. The factors you'll need to take into account will determine the success of your endeavor.

First, the location of your herb garden is a primary concern. The spot should have adequate sunlight, as most herbs thrive under full to partial sun. It should also have good soil drainage to prevent waterlogged roots. The proximity to your chicken coop is another key factor. While having the garden close can provide your flock with easy access to the herbs, remember that chickens are natural foragers and might overindulge or damage tender plants. Some keepers find success in planting an herb garden just outside the chicken run where the flock can access fallen leaves and seeds, but the main plants are protected from overenthusiastic beaks.

The next thing to consider is what herbs to plant. As we've discussed, many kitchen herbs are beneficial to chickens. Still, there are countless other varieties of herbs that your chickens might enjoy. Herbs like lavender and chamomile can have a calming effect, while others like wormwood and peppermint can help keep parasites at bay. When choosing herbs, consider your flock's needs, your climate, and the individual growing requirements of each plant. It's important to include a mixture of perennials, which will come back year after year, and annuals, which you can switch out according to the season or your flock's changing needs.

Think about the layout of your garden, too. It can be as simple or as complex as you like. Some chicken keepers go for a basic row layout, while others prefer to arrange their plants in circles, squares, or even intricate knot garden designs. Whichever layout you choose, make sure your chickens can access the herbs without trampling everything in sight.

You might also want to think about companion planting. This is the practice of planting certain plants together for mutual benefit. Some plants repel pests that prey on their neighbors, others attract beneficial insects, and some can even enhance the growth and flavor of other plants. For instance, planting basil alongside tomatoes is said to make the tomatoes taste better. In a chicken herb garden, you could plant calendula amongst your herbs; not only will it add a pop of color, but it will also attract pollinators to your garden. Plus, as we learned from Maria's case, calendula can be a great addition to your chickens' diet.

Don't forget about maintenance. Just like any garden, an herb garden for your chickens will need care. You'll need to water, weed, and harvest regularly. Depending on the size of your garden and the number of herbs you plant, this could be a significant commitment. But remember, this is not just any garden; it's a living supplement provider, a natural pharmacy, a playground, and a haven for your chickens.

Lastly, be patient and open to learning. Gardening is a process of trial and error. Some herbs might be a hit with your chickens while others get ignored. Certain plants may thrive in your garden, while others might struggle. Take note, adjust, and remember that you're gaining valuable knowledge with each season that passes.

Planning an herb garden for your chickens is an investment of time, energy, and resources. However, the payoff can be immense. Not only will you have a beautiful garden to admire, but you'll also have a natural, sustainable way to support your flock's health and happiness. As you delve into the world of herb gardening, a fundamental question to answer is how to grow these botanical wonders. Let's delve into the specifics - from seeds versus transplants to sunlight needs and watering, we've got it covered.

First off, let's tackle the seeds versus transplants debate. Starting herbs from seeds can be a more economical approach, as seed packets often come with a generous amount of seeds at a relatively low cost. Moreover, growing from seeds may offer a wider variety of herb options, as many specialty or heirloom varieties may not be available as transplants in your local garden center. However, this method requires more time and patience, as you'll need to wait for the seeds to germinate and grow to a size suitable for transplanting.

On the other hand, using transplants or seedlings can give your garden a jump-start. These are young plants that have already been started from seeds and nurtured to a certain size. With transplants, you can have herbs ready for your chickens to enjoy in a shorter amount of time. This is particularly handy if you're starting your garden late in the season. The downside is that transplants can be more expensive and the selection may be limited.

Next, consider the sunlight needs of your herbs. As a general rule, most herbs enjoy full sun, which means they need at least six hours of direct sunlight each day. Some herbs, like rosemary and thyme, are sun-loving and thrive in bright, sunny locations. Others, like mint and chives, can tolerate partial shade. Understanding the sunlight needs of each herb will help you plan the layout of your garden and ensure each plant is positioned for optimal growth.

Now, onto watering. Each herb has its own watering needs, and understanding these can mean the difference between a thriving plant and a wilting one. Mediterranean herbs like oregano, rosemary, and lavender prefer drier conditions and well-drained soil. Overwatering can lead to root rot and other diseases in these herbs. On the other hand, herbs like parsley and cilantro prefer consistently moist soil. A good rule of thumb is to water when the top inch of soil feels dry to the touch. Remember, it's better to give a thorough watering less frequently than to give small amounts of water more often.

You may also need to consider soil conditions. While most herbs are not overly fussy about the soil they grow in, they generally prefer well-draining soil rich in organic matter. If you're planting directly into the ground, consider having your soil tested to understand its structure and nutrient content. You can then amend it as needed with organic matter like compost or well-rotted manure to improve its fertility and drainage.

Pest control is another crucial aspect of growing herbs. While chickens can help control many garden pests, you may need additional measures to protect your herbs. Consider natural pest control methods such as introducing beneficial insects or using organic sprays to keep your herbs healthy without introducing harmful chemicals to your chickens' environment.

Growing herbs for your chickens is an exercise in patience and observation. You'll need to monitor your garden closely, adjusting your care routine as you learn more about what each plant needs. With time, you'll find your stride and understand what works best in your unique setting. Don't be disheartened if things don't go perfectly at first. Remember, every gardener, no matter how experienced, learns through trial and error. Embrace the process, and enjoy the rewards of your efforts as your flock thrives amidst the green abundance you've created. This flourishing oasis isn't just visually stunning but a robust source of health for your chickens. With the right approach to maintaining your herb garden - pest control, harvesting, and winter care- you can keep this green haven thriving.

Pest control in your herb garden is as essential as feeding your flock. Insects and other pests can hinder your plants' growth and reduce their health benefits. While it's tempting to reach for a commercial pesticide, remember that these can be harmful to your chickens. Luckily, there are organic pest control methods that can keep your garden flourishing without causing harm.

Introduce beneficial insects like ladybugs, lacewings, or praying mantises that feed on common pests. Planting a variety of herbs also helps, as some plants naturally repel certain pests. Marigold, for instance, is known to deter a variety of insects. And remember that your chickens can also be excellent pest controllers, foraging for insects that they relish as part of their diet.

Next, let's talk about harvesting. Most herbs can be harvested as soon as they have enough foliage to maintain growth. By cutting off the tops of the plants, you encourage bushier growth.

For some herbs, you'll want to harvest before they flower for the best flavor and nutritional content. But keep in mind that some flowering herbs, like lavender and echinacea, can provide additional benefits for your flock, not to mention adding beauty to your garden.

Harvest in the morning after the dew has dried but before the heat of the day. This is when the oils that give herbs their flavor and medicinal properties are at their peak. Always leave enough foliage on the plant to promote continued growth.

Winter care varies depending on your climate and the types of herbs you're growing. Some herbs are annuals, which means they complete their lifecycle in a single growing season. These herbs will die back in the winter, but you can collect their seeds to replant in the spring.

Perennial herbs, on the other hand, live for several years. Many will go dormant in the winter and return in the spring. These plants may benefit from some winter protection, such as a layer of mulch to protect their roots from freezing temperatures.

Some Mediterranean herbs, like rosemary and sage, are evergreen, which means they retain their leaves throughout the year. These herbs may need to be brought indoors or given extra protection in colder climates, as they can be sensitive to freezing temperatures.

In the end, maintaining your herb garden is a process of constant learning and adjustment. Not every herb will thrive in every condition, and some trial and error may be necessary. But with careful observation and a willingness to adapt, you can cultivate a verdant garden that meets your flock's needs and brings you joy.

By managing pests organically, harvesting wisely, and preparing for winter, your herb garden can become a sustainable, year-round resource. Imagine the satisfaction of seeing your chickens scratch and peck around the herb garden and the peace of mind that comes with knowing that you're providing a natural, healthful environment for them. That's the power of a well-maintained herb garden. However, if you want to ensure that your chickens benefit from the garden without entirely decimating it, some thoughtful design considerations can come in handy.

First and foremost, let's discuss the raised beds. Elevated from the ground, these structures provide several advantages. They protect your herbs from overly enthusiastic scratching and digging, keeping the root systems intact. They also offer better drainage, a vital factor for many herbs that prefer well-draining soil. Furthermore, raised beds can ease the stress on your back, making your gardening chores less strenuous.

When constructing raised beds, aim for a height of at least two feet to deter most chickens. Some, however, might still be tempted to fly over. A removable net or light mesh can dissuade adventurous fliers while allowing you easy access for maintenance.

Next, fencing. While chickens can be great at pest control, left unchecked, they can be a bit too efficient and strip your herb garden bare. A sturdy fence around the herb garden, therefore, could be your best bet. Chicken wire or hardware cloth with small openings, not larger than an inch, is an excellent choice. Keep in mind, it should be high enough to prevent them from flying over and dug a foot into the ground to stop them from tunneling underneath.

A gate that provides you easy access for planting, weeding, and harvesting is also essential. It could be as simple as a gap in the fence that you can close with a removable section of chicken wire or a more elaborate gate, depending on your preference.

Consider the idea of rotation - a system of moving your chickens between different areas. By rotating access to various parts of the garden, you give plants time to recover before they're visited again. This can be done by dividing the garden into sections and only allowing access to one section at a time. As chickens naturally forage, fertilize, and control pests, rotation provides benefits to both your flock and your garden.

While designing your garden, think about including dust baths. Chickens love to dust bathe—it helps them control parasites. You could create dedicated spaces filled with a mix of soil, sand, and diatomaceous earth. Encourage use by planting herbs like lavender and rosemary nearby, which chickens will use in their dust bath naturally, enhancing the pest-repelling properties of the dust bath.

Lastly, consider shelter and shade in your garden design. Plant taller herbs and plants like sunflowers or amaranth. They not only add structure and interest to your garden but also provide much-needed shade on hot days, contributing to your flock's comfort.

A well-designed chicken-friendly herb garden takes into account both the needs of your chickens and your herbs. It isn't just about the herbs you plant but how you set up and manage the space. With these design tips in mind, you'll be well on your way to creating an enticing, enriching space that's beneficial for your flock and gratifying for you. Still, despite all our efforts, there may be moments when challenges arise, and your chickens may get a bit too enthusiastic about the buffet of herbs laid out before them. In this segment, we'll tackle how to troubleshoot common issues, such as when your chickens eat all the herbs.

So, you've stepped out to your herb garden, basket in hand, ready to gather some fresh sprigs of rosemary and thyme. But to your surprise, the herbs are all but gone, and a flock of very content chickens are lounging in the sun. What to do now?

First, don't panic. Chickens are natural foragers, and a new garden full of interesting plants can be very tempting. It's important to remember that the herbs in your garden are there for your chickens' benefit as much as your own, so don't be too discouraged if they get a bit carried away initially.

Now, the first line of defense is prevention. If you're planning a new garden, consider including deterrents from the get-go. As we've previously discussed, raised beds, fences, and rotating access to different garden areas can all help control your chickens' impact on the garden.

But if it's too late for that, or if your current measures aren't quite cutting it, there are still steps you can take. One of these is reinforcing physical barriers. If your chickens are making it over or through your existing fences or netting, it may be time to reassess. Make sure the fence is high enough and dug deep enough into the ground to prevent both flying over and tunneling under.

Another option is to provide a decoy. Planting a separate patch of chicken-friendly plants just for them could divert their attention away from your main herb garden. Consider sacrificial plants that grow quickly and are hardy enough to recover from a chicken feast. Fast-growing greens like clover, alfalfa, or even grass can make a great decoy patch.

Training can also be an effective tool. Just as dogs can learn not to dig in the garden, chickens can learn which areas are off-limits. Using a combination of treats and deterrents can help establish boundaries. For instance, reward your chickens for staying in their designated area and use safe, natural deterrents like citrus peels or vinegar to discourage them from entering the herb garden.

It might also be helpful to reassess your chickens' diet. If your flock is excessively foraging in the garden, they may not be getting all the nutrients they need from their feed. Making sure they have a balanced diet that meets all their nutritional needs could reduce their interest in the herb garden.

Last but not least, remember that patience is key. It might take some time for your chickens to adjust to the rules of the herb garden, but with a little persistence, they'll get the hang of it.

If your chickens seem to be eating all the herbs, there are plenty of solutions to try. From prevention and physical barriers to training and diet adjustments, it's all about finding what works best for you and your flock. And remember, the goal is harmony - a balance where your chickens can enjoy and benefit from the herbs without leaving your garden bare. So, as you face these challenges, take heart in knowing that each one brings you one step closer to creating that perfect, chicken-friendly herb garden.

Part III: Safe and Toxic Herbs: Know your Cluckin' Greens

We've spent a good amount of time discussing how beneficial herbs can be for your chickens, from enriching their diet to enhancing their environment. But it's equally important to understand that not all herbs are created equal when it comes to chicken health and safety. Just as there are plants and herbs that can support their well-being, there are also those that can cause harm. In this part, we're focusing on the green light category — a comprehensive list of safe herbs that your chickens can freely nibble on.

Let's start with some of the most common herbs you'll find in a kitchen garden. We've talked about these before, but they're worth mentioning again. Basil, rosemary, and thyme are all fantastic options for your chickens. They're safe to eat and have numerous health benefits. Basil, for instance, is a good source of protein and vitamins, and it can help repel insects. Rosemary has antibacterial properties and can improve circulation, while thyme can boost the immune system and help with respiratory health.

Next, there's parsley, another herb that's safe and beneficial for chickens. It's rich in vitamins and minerals, and it can support kidney function. Then there's oregano, which has been shown to act as a natural antibiotic, helping to fight off diseases. And let's not forget about mint, which can cool chickens down on hot days and help control pests.

But don't limit yourself to just these herbs. There are many others that your chickens can safely enjoy. For instance, lavender can calm and soothe, while comfrey can support bone health. Lemon balm can repel insects and has calming properties, while dill can aid digestion and is a good source of antioxidants.

Other safe herbs include echinacea, which can support the immune system; fennel, which can boost egg production; and marjoram, which can also help with egg laying. Sage can support general health and well-being, while wormwood can be used sparingly to help control parasites.

This is by no means an exhaustive list, but it gives you a good starting point when planning your chicken-friendly herb garden. Please refer to the appendix in the back of this book for a more detailed list. However, please note that even though these herbs are safe for chickens, it doesn't mean they should make up the majority of their diet. They should be considered supplements to a balanced poultry diet, not replacements for a complete poultry feed.

Remember, if your chickens are eating all the herbs in your garden, consider the strategies we discussed earlier, like implementing physical barriers, providing a decoy patch, adjusting their diet, or training them to respect certain boundaries.

Always observe your flock when introducing a new herb. Chickens are usually good at avoiding plants that aren't good for them, but it's always best to monitor their behavior and health. If you notice any adverse reactions, remove the new herb immediately.

Understanding the herbal world in relation to your chickens is an ongoing journey filled with trial and error, observation, and adaptation. It's an immensely rewarding experience that deepens your connection with your flock and the earth. So, as you introduce your chickens to these safe herbs, know that you're doing your part in providing them with a diverse, engaging, and healthy environment. However, it's equally important to know what not to feed your chickens or what to keep out of their pecking reach. This is all about maintaining that balance of exploration and safety for your flock. Let's dive into a comprehensive list of toxic herbs and plants that can cause harm to your chickens.

First up is foxglove. This beautiful plant is often a favorite in ornamental gardens, but it contains a potent toxin that can harm your chickens. The same goes for rhubarb leaves. While the stalks are safe to eat for humans, the leaves contain high levels of oxalic acid, which is toxic to chickens.

Nightshade family plants, including tomatoes, potatoes, and eggplants, are tricky. While the ripe fruits are safe for chickens to eat, the leaves, stems, and green fruits contain solanine, a compound that's toxic to chickens. It's best to keep your chickens away from these plants unless you can ensure they'll only eat the ripe fruits.

Some common garden flowers, such as tulips and daffodils, can also be toxic to chickens. This includes all parts of the plants, from the flowers to the bulbs. The same goes for lily of the valley, which is toxic in its entirety.

Certain trees and shrubs can also pose a risk. The leaves of cherry and peach trees, for example, contain cyanide, which can be lethal to chickens if ingested in large quantities. Similarly, the leaves and berries of yew and holly can also be toxic.

Then there are herbs like pennyroyal and tansy, which can be harmful if consumed in large quantities. While they can repel insects and may have some medicinal uses, they should be used sparingly and under close observation, if at all.

Many of these plants and herbs only pose a risk if your chickens ingest them in large amounts. Nonetheless, it's best to avoid these plants or to take measures to keep your chickens away from them.

But what do you do if you find your chickens munching on something they shouldn't? First, don't panic. Chickens are hardy animals, and a few nibbles of a toxic plant may not cause harm. However, if you notice any signs of distress or illness — such as a change in behavior, difficulty breathing, or a decrease in egg production — it's essential to seek veterinary care immediately.

Next, identify the plant in question and remove any remnants from your chicken's reach. Then, take steps to prevent future access to the plant. This might involve placing a fence around the plant, moving your chicken's enclosure, or removing the plant entirely.

It's a lot to consider, but don't let this intimidate you. Most chickens are naturally cautious about what they eat and often avoid toxic plants. Your role is to provide them with a safe, diverse environment where they can exercise their natural behaviors without harm. The result? Happier, healthier chickens and peace of mind for you. The journey may require some vigilance and adaptation, but trust me, it's well worth it. Keeping chickens safe and healthy often involves knowing what to look for in terms of signs and symptoms, especially if you suspect herb toxicity. Though it might seem daunting, understanding the potential symptoms of toxicity in chickens can equip you with the information needed to take swift action, if necessary.

Chickens are surprisingly robust creatures, and they have a natural instinct to avoid harmful substances. But in situations where they ingest harmful or toxic herbs, they may exhibit symptoms that are out of the ordinary for their normal behavior. It's important to be aware of these symptoms so that you can take action immediately.

Firstly, let's address changes in behavior. Chickens with toxicity issues may display signs of lethargy or weakness, seem disoriented, or lose their balance. They might separate themselves from the rest of the flock, display unusual aggression, or show a significant decrease in their normal activity level.

You might also notice changes in their physical appearance or condition. Chickens affected by toxic substances might have ruffled feathers, a dull look in their eyes, or a change in comb or wattle color. Their skin might look discolored, they may have difficulty breathing, or their crop might feel unusually full or empty.

Another key symptom to keep an eye out for is a change in their droppings. This can be anything from unusual colors, the presence of undigested food, or an unusual consistency. If the toxic substance has affected their digestive system, you may also notice a decreased appetite or excessive thirst.

A drop in egg production can be another sign of toxicity in laying hens. While egg production can vary based on many factors, a sudden drop, especially if combined with other symptoms, can indicate a problem.

Lastly, seizures or convulsions are a severe sign of toxicity. In such cases, immediate veterinary attention is necessary.

Prevention is the best cure. A little knowledge and vigilance can go a long way in keeping your flock healthy and happy. By being aware of the potential hazards in your chickens' environment and keeping a close eye on their behavior and appearance, you'll be well-equipped to nip any potential problems in the bud. But let's take it a step further and consider what to do if you encounter the situation of suspected herb poisoning in your chickens. The first few moments after discovery can be crucial, so it's beneficial to have an understanding of the immediate steps to take.

First and foremost, you must remain calm. Chickens are highly perceptive creatures and can sense stress in their human caregivers. Your composed presence can help keep the flock calm as you proceed with the necessary steps.

Immediately separate the affected bird or birds from the rest of the flock. It's crucial to prevent any further consumption of the toxic herb and also avoid causing panic within the flock. Having a designated quarantine space prepared can save you precious time in such scenarios.

Next, try to identify the potential toxin. If you have recently introduced a new herb or plant into their environment, start there. Check the plants in their vicinity, and remember, some plants can be toxic only in specific parts, like the roots or leaves. Knowledge of your garden or the birds' ranging area can be incredibly beneficial here.

Contact a veterinarian or a local animal poison control center as soon as possible. These professionals can provide guidance based on the herb in question and your chickens' symptoms. Make sure to share all the relevant information with them – the herb you suspect, the amount you believe was consumed, the size and age of the chicken, and any symptoms you've noticed.

While waiting for professional guidance, you can initiate some general supportive measures. Hydration can help dilute the toxicity and support the chicken's body in flushing it out. Provide the chicken with fresh water, but don't force it to drink. Chickens can inhale water into their lungs if they are not drinking voluntarily.

Keep the chicken warm and comfortable. Stress can worsen the condition, so ensuring a quiet, comfortable space can help the chicken rest and recover.

If advised by a professional, you might need to administer activated charcoal. This substance can bind with many toxins, reducing their absorption by the body. Keep in mind that it's essential to receive guidance on the correct dosage and administration process.

Depending on the herb and the severity of the poisoning, your chicken might need further veterinary care. This could include fluid therapy, supportive nutrition, or specific antidotes if available. The veterinarian can guide you best on this.

Finally, once the immediate crisis is over, consider it a learning opportunity. Identify how the chicken accessed the toxic plant and take steps to prevent future occurrences. Whether this involves better fencing, changing free-ranging areas, or learning more about local plants, taking steps to prevent a repeat of the situation is the silver lining in such a crisis.

Remember, even the most vigilant chicken keepers can face unexpected situations. It's the readiness to act and the willingness to learn that makes the difference. The safety of our flock is paramount, so continue gaining knowledge and applying it for a happier, healthier chicken environment. But it's essential to keep one crucial concept in mind: balance. As with most things in life, balance is key, especially when it comes to your chickens' herb diet.

Sure, herbs offer numerous health benefits, from boosting immune function to deterring pests, and they can serve as exciting additions to your chickens' environment. But they shouldn't replace a balanced, complete chicken feed, which is carefully formulated to meet all of the nutritional requirements of your birds. You can consider herbs as dietary supplements and enriching elements of their environment.

An herb-rich diet for chickens is like a well-varied diet for humans. Eating a variety of foods from different food groups ensures that we get a wide range of nutrients, and the same principle applies to chickens. By offering a variety of herbs, you provide a spectrum of flavors, textures, and health benefits, contributing to the overall well-being of your flock.

Varying the herbs you give your chickens also helps in preventing overconsumption of any one herb. Even beneficial herbs, when consumed in excess, can cause issues. For example, while oregano has known antibacterial properties, too much of it can lead to digestive issues. It's all about moderation.

Plan your chicken herb garden with diversity in mind. Opt for a mix of culinary herbs, like rosemary, thyme, and basil, and medicinal ones, like echinacea and calendula. Include different types of plants, such as leafy ones, flowering ones, and root herbs, to offer your chickens a variety of pecking and foraging experiences.

Also, consider seasonal variety. Some herbs thrive in specific seasons. Having a mix of spring herbs, summer herbs, and hardy ones that last through the colder months ensures a year-round supply of greenery for your chickens.

When introducing a new herb to your chickens, do so gradually and monitor their reactions. Chickens are often hesitant about new foods and may take time to warm up to a new herb. Also, gradual introduction helps you observe any adverse reactions, which, while rare, can occur due to individual sensitivities.

While we've discussed the benefits of individual herbs, keep in mind that their overall impact is much more significant when they're part of a varied herb diet. Different herbs have different nutrient profiles and health benefits, so a variety offers comprehensive support to your chickens' health.

Ultimately, incorporating herbs into your chickens' diet and environment is an art that marries knowledge and observation. Understanding the properties of different herbs equips you with the tools to support your flock's health. Simultaneously, closely observing your flock's behavior and health helps tailor your approach, creating a unique, beneficial herb experience for your chickens.

So, whether you're tossing some parsley into the coop for some pecking fun, planting comfrey for its medicinal properties, or hanging bunches of mint to deter pests, remember that balance and variety are your allies. They're the keys to creating a vibrant, healthful, and enriching herb environment for your flock.

As we delve deeper into the world of herbs and chickens, keep these concepts in mind. They will guide you towards a harmonious, natural way of caring for your flock, enhancing their health, happiness, and your satisfaction as a chicken keeper.

Chapter 2: Herbs for Healthy Hens

Part I: Dill-ightful Boosters: Immune-Supporting Herbs

Immunity, in its most basic sense, is the body's defense mechanism against disease. It's an intricate and dynamic system composed of various cells, tissues, and organs working in harmony to protect the body from harmful invaders like bacteria, viruses, and parasites.

Immunity matters for every living being, and chickens are no exception. Think of your chicken's immune system as an invisible shield, constantly at work to protect your feathered friends from harmful agents in their environment. Without a robust immune system, your chickens would be much more susceptible to a wide range of illnesses, which can impact everything from their egg-laying capacity to their overall lifespan.

The importance of a strong immune system in chickens becomes particularly evident when you consider their lifestyle. Chickens are naturally curious creatures who love to peck, scratch, and explore their environment. This behavior, while part of their charm, also means they come into contact with a vast array of microbes every day.

The earth they scratch in, the bugs they peck at, and even the air they breathe are teeming with potential pathogens. Without a competent immune system to neutralize these threats, they would quickly become overwhelmed, leading to illness and disease.

Beyond their exposure to environmental pathogens, chickens also live in relatively close quarters with each other, especially in backyard or commercial settings. This proximity means that if one bird gets sick, the others are at a higher risk of contracting the illness as well. A robust immune system is key to preventing the spread of disease within the flock.

On a broader scale, immune health in chickens plays a significant role in poultry production worldwide. An outbreak of disease in a chicken farm can lead to massive losses, both in terms of the flock's health and the economic cost to the farmer. Maintaining strong immunity in chickens, therefore, is also of great importance from a food security perspective.

A robust immune system is also instrumental in ensuring your chickens are at their healthiest and happiest. Healthy chickens are more active, show natural behaviors like foraging and dust bathing, and generally exhibit signs of contentment. They also tend to have shinier feathers, clearer eyes, and a greater appetite – all indicators of good health.

Moreover, a well-functioning immune system contributes to better egg production. Healthy chickens lay eggs regularly and with fewer issues, ensuring a steady supply for your breakfast table.

So, how can you support your chickens' immune system? One of the most effective ways is through nutrition. A balanced diet that meets all their nutritional needs is the first step in promoting good immune health. In addition to a quality chicken feed, adding immune-boosting herbs to their diet can provide an extra layer of protection.

Herbs have been used for centuries in traditional medicine systems worldwide for their healing properties. Many of these herbs have been scientifically studied and shown to boost immunity in a variety of ways, from increasing the activity of immune cells to providing anti-inflammatory and antimicrobial benefits.

As we dive into the fascinating world of herbs for chicken health, we'll explore some of these immune-boosting herbs in detail. We'll look at their properties, how they can be incorporated into your chickens' environment, and how they contribute to a vibrant, healthy flock. Your chicken coop will soon be buzzing with vitality, thanks to these green allies!

It's important to keep in mind that the immune system is a complex entity that thrives on balance and variety, much like your herb garden. Providing a diverse array of immune-supporting herbs will ensure your chickens are well-equipped to fend off any potential threats, keeping them healthy, happy, and productive. Each herb possesses unique properties that bolster immunity in different ways. Let's explore some of these herbs.

First, we have Echinacea, a long-time favorite in the world of herbal remedies. This vibrant purple flower, also known as purple coneflower, is known for its immune-enhancing abilities. It increases the number and activity of immune cells, making it easier for the body to fight off infection. Including Echinacea in your chicken's environment can stimulate their immune response, fortifying their defense against potential pathogens.

Garlic is another superfood that's not just for warding off vampires. Allicin, the active component in garlic, has potent antimicrobial properties. It can kill a wide range of bacteria and viruses, effectively preventing them from causing harm. Adding crushed garlic to your chickens' feed or water not only enhances the taste but also strengthens their immunity. Plus, it serves as a natural wormer, making it a multi-purpose addition to their diet.

Astragalus is a lesser-known herb but an impressive immune booster. Used extensively in traditional Chinese medicine, Astragalus stimulates the production of immune cells and promotes their activity. This herb is typically given to chickens during times of stress or illness to bolster their immune response and promote a speedy recovery. You can add dried Astragalus root to your chicken's feed or steep it in their water.

Oregano is more than just a pizza topping. This aromatic herb is packed with antioxidants and has antimicrobial properties that can help to ward off infection. Carvacrol and thymol, two of the active compounds in oregano, are particularly effective against certain bacteria, including those that can cause respiratory infections in chickens. You can sprinkle dried oregano in your chicken's feed or add fresh leaves to their nesting boxes for an immune-boosting treat.

Thyme is another aromatic herb with similar benefits. It's known for its antibacterial and antifungal properties, making it an excellent tool in the fight against a variety of pathogens. Thyme can be particularly useful in managing respiratory health in chickens, thanks to its antiseptic properties. Like oregano, you can add thyme to your chicken's feed or nesting boxes. Alternatively, you can make a thyme-infused vinegar to add to their water.

Elderberry is a berry-producing shrub with immune-boosting properties. Elderberries are rich in vitamins and antioxidants that help support the immune system. The berries can be given to chickens as a treat, or you can make an elderberry syrup or tincture to mix into their feed. Just be sure to cook the berries first, as raw elderberries can be toxic.

Lemon balm, a member of the mint family, is a calming herb that can also enhance immune function. It has antiviral properties and can help to reduce stress, which is beneficial for immune health. Chickens tend to love the taste of lemon balm, so it can be a great addition to their diet.

Speaking of the mint family, another herb to consider is peppermint. Peppermint is a potent aromatic that is not just refreshing but also serves as a natural insecticide. It can ward off pesky bugs that bother your chickens. More importantly, it's packed with vitamins A and C, which are key players in immune function. It helps stimulate the production of white blood cells - the immune system's first line of defense against pathogens.

Next up is parsley. This curly-leafed herb does more than garnish plates. It is packed with vitamins A, C, and K, and contains more vitamin C per volume than an orange! This super herb can support the overall wellness of your chickens, providing an immune boost and promoting healthier and thicker eggshells.

Turmeric, a vibrant yellow spice, is worth mentioning. This powerful anti-inflammatory herb, thanks to its active compound curcumin, has been proven to boost the immune system. Incorporating turmeric into the diet of your chickens can help keep their immune system in top shape. You can easily mix turmeric powder in their feed or water.

Another plant you wouldn't want to miss is aloe vera. This succulent plant has been used for centuries for its healing properties. It's excellent for external uses on your chickens like wounds or skin irritations. Internally, aloe vera can boost the immune system due to its antiviral and antibacterial properties. The gel from the aloe leaves can be added directly to their water or food.

Cinnamon, known for its warm, sweet flavor, isn't just a baking staple. It's full of antioxidants that can help defend the body against damage from free radicals. Chickens, too, can benefit from this aromatic spice. Cinnamon has antimicrobial properties and may help to regulate blood sugar levels in your flock. A sprinkle of cinnamon over their food is all it takes.

Let's not forget about lavender. This beautiful, aromatic herb is a calming agent for both humans and chickens. The scent of lavender can reduce stress and increase the feeling of contentment in chickens. But more than just a mood enhancer, it's also an effective anti-bacterial and increases blood circulation, all contributing to an optimized immune system.

Last but certainly not least, let's talk about rosemary. This sturdy herb is as beneficial as it is fragrant. Its active ingredient, rosmarinic acid, has anti-inflammatory, antibacterial, and antioxidant effects. It's a great aid in digestion for chickens and serves as a potent booster for their immune system.

Growing these herbs for your chickens does not require a green thumb. Most herbs are hardy and require minimal care, especially once established. By dedicating a section of your garden to these immune-boosting herbs, your chickens will not only have an all-natural health booster, but they'll also have a beautiful, fragrant space to explore and enjoy. It's a win-win situation, for sure!

It's important to keep in mind that these herbs can assist in boosting your chicken's immune system, they are not a substitute for good husbandry and a balanced diet. Keep your chicken's environment clean, provide them with plenty of space to roam and forage, and feed them a nutritionally complete diet. This, combined with The immune-boosting power of herbs can help to ensure your flock stays in the best possible health. The key to their health is in your hands, and in their coop! A garden filled with these immune-boosting herbs will not only be a sanctuary for you but a fortress of health for your feathered friends. With all these elements, you're setting the stage for a flock of healthy, happy chickens.

But knowing the herbs isn't enough, it's also crucial to understand how best to administer these herbal wonders to your flock. Here are some of the most effective ways:

The first and simplest method is through their regular feed. This can be as simple as sprinkling dried, crushed herbs over their daily rations, or mixing it into homemade feed. If you're using herbs like turmeric or cinnamon, remember they are potent. A little goes a long way, so start with small amounts and adjust as needed based on their acceptance.

Next is the water method. Some herbs, like aloe vera or echinacea, can be infused in the water that your chickens drink. For aloe vera, you can squeeze the gel directly into their water container. For herbs like echinacea, you can make a strong tea, let it cool, and then add it to their water.

Free-range grazing is another excellent way to introduce these herbs. Plant the herbs around areas where your chickens like to peck and scratch. They'll benefit from the fresh leaves and seeds of these plants. Be sure to fence off young plants though, as chickens are notorious for digging up fresh sprouts before they have a chance to establish!

You can also create 'bouquets' of fresh herbs that can be hung in the coop. This not only provides a flavorful snack for the chickens but can also help keep the coop smelling fresh and deter pests. Lavender and mint are particularly good for this purpose.

For external use, like aloe vera for wounds or skin irritations, apply the gel directly to the affected area. Similarly, lavender can be used as a rub for a calming effect.

One creative method is to use herbs in nesting boxes. Herbs like lavender, mint, and lemon balm can create a calming and aromatic environment for your hens, promoting a positive laying experience. The essential oils in these herbs can also help deter pests.

Now, in colder seasons, a warm mash can be a comforting treat for chickens, and it's an excellent vehicle for herbs. Adding herbs to a warm grain and vegetable mash is another effective way to introduce these immune-boosting herbs.

Another tip is to freeze herbs in ice cube trays with water during the summer. These herby ice cubes can then be added to their water on hot days, providing both a refreshing treat and a healthy boost.

Please remember that the introduction of herbs should be gradual.. Start with small quantities and observe. Chickens have a great way of knowing what's good for them. If they don't take to a particular herb, don't force it. Try different herbs and methods until you find what works best for your flock.

It's always a joy to see chickens pecking at a leaf of peppermint or a sprig of rosemary. It's an even greater joy knowing that these little actions are helping to keep them healthy, boosting their immune system, and setting them up for a long, productive life. Health, like many things in life, begins at home. In this case, it starts in their coop and in your garden. With the right herbs and methods of administration, you can provide a veritable health fortress for your feathered friends. So, let's create some magic with immune-boosting herbal blends for your chickens. You will find more remedies in the appendix at the back of this book.

First up, we have the "Flock Fortifier" blend. This combines several powerhouse herbs known for their immune-boosting properties. It's simple but potent. For this blend, you'll need:

- 2 parts dried echinacea
- 2 parts dried astragalus
- 1 part dried oregano
- 1 part dried turmeric

Combine all these herbs in a bowl and store them in an airtight container. Sprinkle this blend over your chickens' daily feed. These herbs are potent so a sprinkle or two is all you need.

Next is the "Free-Range Feast" blend, perfect for those who allow their chickens to free-range graze. For this, you need:

- Lemon balm plants
- Echinacea plants
- Garlic (plant cloves around the yard)

Plant these herbs throughout your yard. Your chickens will enjoy pecking at them, and they'll be none the wiser that they're feasting on immune-boosting herbs!

The third blend is the "Nesting Box Blend". This mix is as much for pest prevention and comfort as it is for immunity. This aromatic blend consists of:

- Lavender (fresh or dried)
- Mint (fresh or dried)
- Lemon balm (fresh or dried)

Combine these in equal parts and scatter them in the nesting boxes. The scent will keep pests away and create a calming environment for your hens, contributing to overall health and wellbeing.

The "Winter Warmth Mash" blend is a comforting remedy for the colder months. For this, you'll need:

- 2 parts warm cooked grains (like oats or rice)
- 1 part chopped fresh or dried rosemary
- 1 part chopped fresh or dried thyme
- A pinch of dried cayenne pepper

Mix the herbs with the warm grains until well combined and serve. The herbs will provide immune support, and the cayenne pepper will help keep them warm!

Lastly, the "Summer Sipper" blend is an ideal way to offer herbs in the hotter months. You'll need:

- Fresh basil leaves
- Fresh mint leaves
- Fresh cucumber slices

Freeze these in ice cube trays filled with water. Once frozen, pop them out and add them to your chickens' water. They'll love pecking at the ice, and it's an excellent way to help them stay cool and hydrated while giving them an immune boost!

These blends are suggestions. Feel free to get creative and experiment with what works best for your flock. Just remember, as with anything new, introduce these blends gradually and watch how your chickens respond.

The beauty of using herbs with your chickens is it's not only about disease prevention. It's also about promoting a thriving environment where chickens can live their happiest, healthiest lives. And that's a win in my book! Now, how can you tell if your efforts are paying off? Well, keeping an eye on your flock and knowing what to look for will provide the answer.

For starters, a healthy chicken is a busy chicken. Hens with robust immune systems are energetic and engaged with their environment. They're interested in their surroundings, actively foraging, dust-bathing, scratching about, and interacting with their coop-mates.

A healthy hen's appearance is another good indicator of a strong immune system. Lustrous feathers free from mites and parasites, bright eyes, a red and erect comb, and a clean vent area are signs of a well-functioning immune system.

Equally telling is a chicken's appetite. Hens with robust health will have a hearty appetite. So if you see them eagerly pecking at their feed and your immune-boosting herbal blends, that's a fantastic sign!

The quality of their eggs can also offer clues. Regularly laying eggs with firm, thick shells is another indication of a healthy hen. Keep in mind, that the occasional soft-shelled or oddly shaped egg can occur even in the healthiest hens. But if they're consistently producing quality eggs, you can bet their immune systems are firing on all cylinders.

Let's not forget about their poop. Yes, poop! It can tell you a lot about a chicken's health. Healthy chicken droppings should be firm with a white cap of urates. Any major changes in color, consistency, or frequency might signal a potential health issue.

And lastly, listen to your chickens. Healthy hens will fill your yard with a symphony of happy clucks, purrs, and gentle squawking. Changes in their vocalizations, such as silent periods or distressed noises, might indicate discomfort or illness.

Remember, no one knows your chickens better than you do. Even subtle changes in behavior, appearance, appetite, egg production, droppings, or vocalization can signal that a chicken's immune system might be under siege.

If you've been applying the immune-boosting herbal knowledge we've covered, you should start noticing these positive signs of health in your flock. If not, remember, adjustments might be needed. Maybe it's changing the type of herb, the method of delivery, or the quantity. And always, always, always, remember that a well-balanced diet is key. Herbs are a fantastic supplement to promote health, but they're not the whole picture.

It's a journey, folks. There's no one-size-fits-all solution. But with attention to detail, patience, and a whole lot of love, you can help your chickens thrive and live their best lives, one immune-boosting herb at a time. And that's something to cluck about!

Part II: Chicks Love Chia: Herbs for Digestive Health

Let's discuss the fascinating world of the chicken's digestive system. You're probably asking, why does understanding the chicken's digestive system matter? Well, by understanding how chickens process their food, we can better provide them with the dietary supplements they need for optimal health, like herbs. In addition, we'll also know why certain herbs benefit them in specific ways.

The journey of a chicken's dinner starts in the beak, equipped with a hard outer layer to peck and collect food. Chickens lack teeth and rely on their beaks to break down food. Interestingly, they also have an exceptional ability to select tiny bits of grit, stones, or sand while they're foraging. You'll soon see why this is important!

From the beak, the food then travels down the esophagus into the crop, a storage pouch where food can be softened and prepped for the journey ahead. This remarkable organ allows chickens to eat quite a bit in a short amount of time and then digest their meal slowly throughout the day, even while they're resting.

The next stop is the proventriculus, also known as the chicken's first stomach. Here, the food is mixed with hydrochloric acid and digestive enzymes that kickstart the breakdown process, especially of proteins.

Then we reach the gizzard, often called the chicken's second stomach, and this is where those tiny bits of grit come into play. The gizzard is a muscular organ that uses the grit to grind down the food, much like how we use our teeth to chew. The processed food is then mixed with more enzymes for further breakdown.

Now, it's onto the small intestine. This is where most nutrient absorption happens. More enzymes are added to the mix to break down the remaining proteins, as well as carbohydrates and fats. The lining of the small intestine is covered in tiny, finger-like projections called villi that increase the surface area for nutrient absorption. This area is a crucial point of health, and many herbs can support a healthy population of good bacteria here.

Up next is the ceca. While the small intestine absorbs most of the nutrients, the ceca takes care of those that are left behind, especially the complex carbohydrates. This is a fermentation vat of sorts where beneficial bacteria further break down food particles.

Finally, we reach the large intestine or the colon. It's relatively short in chickens compared to mammals, but it's essential for absorbing the last bits of nutrients and most of the water left in the food.

At the end of this journey, the waste materials are combined with urates—the chicken equivalent of urine—and are excreted through the vent. And voila! The process is complete.

Now that we've taken a tour of the chicken's digestive system, we can appreciate how complex it is and why it's essential to keep it healthy. Many herbs have properties that can support different aspects of this process, from aiding digestion in the crop to fostering a healthy microbiome in the small intestine and ceca. Armed with this knowledge, we can now explore these herbs and their benefits in more detail.

Let's start with Aloe Vera. It's more than just a beautiful succulent! When we think of Aloe Vera, we usually think of skin health, but it's equally beneficial for the digestive system. The gel inside Aloe Vera leaves is rich in enzymes that help break down food and improve nutrient absorption. Plus, it has a mild laxative effect that can aid in smooth digestion, helpful in keeping the chicken's digestive tract running smoothly.

Next on our list is Peppermint. This fragrant herb is not just a treat for our senses but a potent digestive aid for chickens. Peppermint helps to soothe the muscles of the gastrointestinal tract, which can ease any spasms or discomfort your chickens might be experiencing. Moreover, it's excellent for combating flatulence and aiding in overall digestion. It's also an excellent appetizer, stimulating the chicken's desire to eat and peck around.

Let's not forget Fenugreek. This versatile herb has been used in traditional medicine for ages, and it's a great addition to your chickens' diet. The seeds contain a high amount of mucilage, a sticky substance that forms a protective coating on the lining of the digestive tract. This helps soothe any inflammation and promotes smoother digestion. Moreover, fenugreek has been found to stimulate the appetite, encouraging your chickens to eat more, which is particularly beneficial for underweight chickens or during molting season when they need extra nutrients.

We must also mention Slippery Elm. This herb has a long history of use by Native American cultures and is terrific for digestion. Much like fenugreek, slippery elm contains a good deal of mucilage. When consumed, it forms a slick gel that coats the lining of the digestive tract, reducing inflammation and promoting easy digestion. It also helps maintain a healthy balance of bacteria in the gut, fostering a beneficial microbiome.

Another all-star herb for digestive health is Chamomile. These dainty little flowers pack a punch when it comes to digestive support. Chamomile has antispasmodic properties that can soothe an upset stomach and help alleviate any cramping. Its calming effects also reduce stress, which, in turn, promotes better digestion. Chickens love foraging for these, making it an easy herb to incorporate into their diet.

Finally, let's consider Dandelion. Often considered a weed, dandelion is a powerhouse of nutrition. The leafy greens and roots can stimulate appetite and aid in digestion, plus they serve as a rich source of vitamins A, C, and K, along with calcium and potassium. All of these are essential nutrients that support overall health, including digestive health.

So, now you see, incorporating these herbs into your chicken's diet can help them maintain a healthy and efficient digestive system. Each herb has a unique profile of benefits and uses, and combining them can create a potent mix that boosts not just digestion, but overall well-being. Recognizing when to introduce these herbs into your chickens' diets requires an understanding of their needs, behaviors, and the signs they exhibit when things might be off balance.

As chicken keepers, we aim to ensure that our flock is not only surviving but thriving, and a key component of this lies in prevention. Prevention is about creating an environment that bolsters the health of your chickens before issues arise. For instance, regularly incorporating digestive herbs into your chickens' feed or forage can help maintain their digestive health, reducing the chance of problems down the line.

Aloe Vera, Peppermint, Fenugreek, Slippery Elm, Chamomile, and Dandelion - these herbs, when used consistently, can help optimize digestion, nutrient absorption, and overall gut health. Having these herbs as part of their regular diet means you're establishing a strong foundation, like an insurance policy for their digestive health.

Now, let's shift gears to discuss the usage of herbs to address specific issues. Chickens, like any other living beings, can experience off days or fall under the weather. It's during these times that their behaviors, eating patterns, and physical appearance can give you insights into their health. Loose stools, loss of appetite, reduced egg-laying, lethargy, and changes in their feathers can all be signs of a potential digestive issue.

In such instances, you might consider upping the ante on the usage of certain herbs. For instance, if your chickens are showing signs of reduced appetite, incorporating more fenugreek, known for its appetite-stimulating properties, can be beneficial. Or if they seem to have an upset stomach, peppermint and chamomile can help soothe their discomfort.

Remember, while herbs are a powerful tool, they are not an immediate cure-all. It's crucial to observe your chickens and note any changes after you've introduced these herbs. If issues persist, it may be indicative of a more serious problem requiring veterinary attention.

When it comes to herbs, there is no one-size-fits-all solution. Each flock is unique, and what works for one chicken might not necessarily work for another. That's why it's essential to know your chickens, understand their needs, and observe their behaviors.

Incorporating herbs into your chickens' lifestyle is a process that requires patience and understanding. You're not just giving your chickens a meal; you're providing them a quality life, enriched with nature's best offerings. And to make this task easier and more enjoyable for both you and your flock, let's delve into some tasty and therapeutic remedies that utilize our chosen digestive herbs.

First up, let's create a Herbal Feed Mix. This is a simple way to introduce herbs to your chickens' diet and can be easily adjusted to suit the preferences of your feathered friends. Start with a base of your chickens' regular feed. Then, add in dried herbs, focusing on the ones we've mentioned like peppermint, fenugreek, and aloe vera. You want the herbs to make up around 10-20% of the total mix. For a flock of six, a weekly feed mix could include two cups of dried, crushed peppermint leaves, one cup of fenugreek seeds, and a half cup of dried, edible aloe vera. Mix it all together, and voila! You have a nutrient-packed feed mix ready to boost your chickens' digestive health.

Next is the Digestive Herbal Tea. Chickens love fresh water, and by infusing their drink with digestive herbs, you're serving health in a waterer. For this, you can use a mix of fresh or dried herbs such as dandelion, chamomile, and peppermint. Add a handful of these herbs to a pot of boiling water and let it steep until it cools. You can then strain it and offer it to your chickens as a refreshing and therapeutic drink.

Third, consider creating an Herbal Foraging Area. Chickens naturally love to forage, so why not let them pick their herbal treats? You can designate a part of your yard as a "herb garden," planting it with chicken-friendly herbs like aloe, dandelion, and fennel. Your chickens can forage freely here, choosing the herbs they fancy.

Last, but definitely not least, is the Herbal Digestive Spray. This spray can be used to spritz your chickens' bedding or the herbs in their foraging area. For this, you'll need to create a strong brew of chamomile and peppermint, let it cool, and then transfer it into a spray bottle. Regularly spritzing the chickens' environment with this blend can help to create a soothing environment that supports digestion and overall well-being.

These remedies are starting points, adaptable to your flock's needs and preferences. The key lies in observing your chickens, noting what they enjoy, and adapting as you go along. As with any changes to your chickens' diets or routines, introduce these new elements gradually and monitor for any changes.

The goal here is not just health; it's about enriching the lives of your feathered friends. As chicken keepers, our job isn't just to ensure our flock's survival; it's to enhance their well-being, allowing them to thrive. A critical part of this task involves keeping an eye on signs of good health, especially when it comes to their digestive systems. Let's explore what these signs look like so you can better monitor your flock's health.

The first checkpoint of your flock's digestive health is their appetite. Chickens with good digestive health typically have a consistent, robust appetite. They will be eager to eat their regular meals and should show interest in any treats you provide, especially their favorite ones. If your chickens are happily pecking away at their feed, that's a good sign. However, if you notice a decrease in appetite or interest in food, it might indicate a digestive issue.

Next up, consider their behavior. Chickens with a healthy digestive system are energetic and active. They forage, run around, and interact with their flockmates throughout the day. When they're not eating or active, they should be contentedly perching or resting. If you notice a drop in energy levels or any unusual lethargy, this could be an indication of a digestive problem.

Excrement is another telling sign. The droppings of healthy chickens will be firm and brown, sometimes with a white cap of uric acid. Their feces should not be runny or discolored regularly. However, don't panic if you see an occasional off-looking stool, as diet changes can temporarily affect their droppings. But, if the unusual feces persist, it might be a sign of a digestive problem.

Egg production is an essential indicator of a hen's health, including her digestive health. A healthy hen will have a consistent laying pattern, and her eggs should have firm, clean shells. If you notice any changes in egg production, such as soft-shelled or misshapen eggs, it could be a sign of a health issue, possibly linked to digestion.

Lastly, look at your chicken's physical appearance. Healthy chickens should have bright, clear eyes, a clean vent, and glossy feathers. They should be neither overweight nor underweight. Any changes in their appearance, like dull eyes or ruffled feathers, can be a sign of ill health.

Observing these signs of health is an ongoing task, not a one-time check. By regularly observing your flock, you'll get a sense of what's normal for them. Any changes from their norm might indicate a problem. However, if they're consistently showing these signs of good health, your efforts to enhance their lives, including the addition of digestive herbs, are likely paying off!

Remember, every flock and each chicken is unique. What works wonders for one might not be as effective for another. It's your job as a chicken keeper to adjust and adapt to your flock's needs. Through this, you can ensure not just their survival but their thriving existence.

Part III: Scratchin' Around Stress

Let's talk about stress in chickens. It might not be something you think about often, but chickens can experience stress just like any other living creature. And just like in humans, chronic stress can negatively impact a chicken's overall health and well-being. Recognizing stress in your flock and understanding its causes and effects can help you manage it effectively.

Stress in chickens can be triggered by several factors. Changes in the environment, such as sudden temperature fluctuations, can cause stress. Even something as seemingly simple as a coop clean-up or rearrangement might unsettle your chickens. New additions to the flock or the loss of a flock member can also create stress. Chickens are social creatures, and disruptions in their social structure can unsettle them.

Predators are a significant source of stress for chickens. Whether they've had a direct encounter with a predator or merely sensed one nearby, this can induce high levels of stress. Even the perceived threat of a predator, like a shadow overhead or a strange noise, can be a stress trigger.

Dietary changes can also lead to stress. Chickens thrive on routine, and sudden changes in their diet can cause stress. This includes changing the type of feed or feeding times. Likewise, nutritional deficiencies can cause stress and, if not addressed, can lead to further health complications.

Health problems are an obvious source of stress. Illness, injury, and parasites can cause not just physical discomfort but also stress. Overcrowding in the coop or run can lead to stress due to lack of personal space and increased competition for resources.

What signs should you look for in a stressed chicken? Changes in behavior are often the most noticeable signs. A stressed chicken may be less active, isolate itself from the rest of the flock, or show changes in eating and drinking habits. You might also notice an increase in aggressive behavior.

Stress can impact egg production in hens. You may see a reduction in the number of eggs laid, or the eggs might be of lower quality, with thin or irregular shells. In severe cases, hens might stop laying altogether.

Physical signs can also indicate stress. Feathers might lose their shine, or the chicken might start losing feathers outside of their regular molting period. You might also see changes in their droppings, which can become loose or discolored.

Chronic stress can weaken a chicken's immune system, making them more susceptible to diseases and infections. It can also slow down their growth and, in severe cases, can lead to death.

The effects of stress on your flock are why it's crucial to maintain a calm, stable environment for your chickens. This includes providing them with a safe, comfortable living space, a consistent, nutritious diet, and, importantly, adding calming herbs into their routine.

As we progress further into this section, we'll explore the wonderful calming herbs at our disposal. These herbs, added in the right amounts and at the right times, can help ensure that our feathered friends lead lives that are not just free of stress but enriched with health, happiness, and contentment. It's a chicken keeper's duty to ensure this, and it's a journey I'm excited to continue with you.

Let's kick things off with a fan favorite: chamomile. This delightful little flower is well-known for its soothing properties. The compounds found in chamomile have been linked to reduced stress and improved sleep quality in animals. The aroma alone can help create a serene environment for your hens. Chamomile can be added to your chickens' feed, scattered in their bedding, or used as a calming tea that can be added to their water supply.

Next up, we have lavender. The scent of lavender has long been associated with relaxation and stress relief. Its beautiful purple flowers can be used fresh or dried to create a calming ambiance in the chicken coop. The dried flowers can also be added to your flock's feed as a stress-relieving supplement.

Lemon balm is another potent calming herb for chickens. A relative of mint, this herb has a lovely lemony scent that chickens seem to enjoy. It's known to have calming effects, and adding fresh lemon balm to their coop can provide your chickens with a relaxing environment while also repelling pesky insects.

Passionflower, though not as commonly used as some of the other herbs we've mentioned, has potent calming effects. It's often used in humans to reduce anxiety and improve sleep, and it can serve similar purposes in chickens. You can use dried passionflower in your flock's bedding or mix it into their feed for a soothing treat.

Valerian is another herb with significant calming properties. Valerian root is often used as a sleep aid in humans, and its calming effects can also benefit your chickens. Its strong scent might not be everyone's favorite, but your chickens are likely to appreciate it. You can scatter dried valerian root in their coop or mix it into their feed.

Lastly, let's talk about ashwagandha, an ancient medicinal herb that's gaining popularity in the modern world. It's known for its stress-reducing properties, and while it's not traditionally used with chickens, some keepers swear by its benefits. The dried root can be added to their feed as a special stress-reducing supplement.

All of these herbs can be grown in your garden, providing you with a readily available supply of natural, calming supplements for your chickens. You can use them individually or create a calming blend to add to their feed, water, or bedding.

While these herbs can help manage stress in your flock, they should be used alongside other stress-management strategies. A comfortable coop, a balanced diet, and regular health checks are crucial for your flock's well-being. A calm, healthy flock is a joy to keep, and with these herbs in your chicken care toolkit, you're well on your way to creating a haven of calm for your feathered friends.

Let's start with the nest boxes. Chickens naturally want a secure, quiet place to lay their eggs, and making their nest boxes a relaxing oasis can help with that. Try adding dried herbs such as chamomile, lavender, or lemon balm directly to the nesting material. The aroma of these herbs will create a soothing environment, which may help reduce stress levels and encourage more frequent laying.

You can also make herbal sprays to mist in the chicken coop. An easy method is to steep your chosen herbs, much like you would tea, strain out the plant matter, and add the cooled herbal infusion to a spray bottle. Spraying this around the coop can create a calming atmosphere. Lavender, with its naturally relaxing properties, is a particularly good choice for this.

A great way to incorporate calming herbs into your chickens' daily life is by adding them directly to their feed. This can be done with dried herbs like passionflower or valerian. Simply mix a small amount of the dried, crushed herbs in with their regular feed. Introduce this slowly and monitor your flock for any changes.

Another option is to create herbal sachets to hang in the coop. These sachets can be filled with calming herbs and hung around the coop where your chickens can peck at them. It creates a sort of "herbal playground" that your chickens can interact with throughout the day, and the steady release of calming scents can help maintain a relaxed environment.

An interesting approach, though it takes a bit more time and effort, is to create a "chicken garden" with a variety of these calming herbs. Planting herbs such as chamomile, lemon balm, and lavender around the chicken yard allows your flock to forage and interact with these plants directly. It's a wonderful enrichment activity for them, and they benefit from the calming properties of these herbs.

Lastly, herbs like ashwagandha can be used in a more targeted way. If you notice a specific chicken seems more stressed or anxious, this can be added to their feed in small amounts. This may help in reducing individual stress levels.

There are many ways to incorporate calming herbs into your chicken care routine. Whether you add them to their nest boxes, spray them around the coop, mix them into their feed, or even plant them in a chicken-friendly garden, these herbs can greatly contribute to a calm and healthy environment for your flock. But as with any changes in your flock's care, introduce new elements slowly, and always monitor your chickens for any changes. With careful observation and a little herbal help, your coop can be the picture of chicken tranquility. A serene coop provides not just a shelter but a home to your flock, a place where they can thrive. To enhance this tranquility, consider these remedies which incorporate calming herbs into your chicken's everyday environment.

Firstly, let's create an herbal nesting blend, a remedy that is easy to concoop (pun intended!) and promotes a relaxing nesting environment. For this blend, you will need dried lavender, dried chamomile, and dried lemon balm. Mix together equal parts of these three herbs and simply sprinkle this blend in your nest boxes. The aroma of these herbs should create a peaceful atmosphere and help encourage your chickens to lay.

Next, consider an herbal coop spray, which can help to maintain a calm environment, while also keeping your coop smelling fresh. For this, you will need a spray bottle, distilled water, and your chosen herbs. Lavender and chamomile are ideal for their calming effects. Start by steeping about half a cup of dried herbs in two cups of boiling water, like making a strong tea. Once cooled, strain the mixture, add to your spray bottle, and mist around the coop. Not only will this spray contribute to a relaxed ambiance, but it can also help keep the coop smelling good.

Thirdly, there's an herb-infused treat that your chickens will love. This remedy combines calming herbs with a chicken's favorite snacks. You will need dried oats, dried mealworms, and your calming herbs - let's use lavender and chamomile for this one. Mix together two cups of oats, one cup of mealworms, and a half cup each of dried lavender and chamomile. You can feed this mix to your chickens as a special treat to help them relax, especially in potentially stressful times like molting or introducing new flock members.

Lastly, a calm chicken garden might be the best project to undertake if you have a little extra time and space. Plant a variety of calming herbs like lavender, chamomile, and lemon balm. Your chickens can directly interact with these plants, benefiting from their calming properties. If you want to go the extra mile, add some marigolds or nasturtiums. These are not only lovely to look at but also act as natural insect repellents.

All these remedies are meant to promote a calm and serene environment for your chickens. They are part of an overall strategy of creating a harmonious home for your flock. But herbs alone can't do the job. There are a variety of other factors to consider when seeking to reduce stress in your chickens, such as environmental conditions and handling practices. So, let's get into that, shall we?

The environment in which your chickens live plays a huge role in their stress levels. A coop that's too small, for instance, can lead to overcrowding, and this could trigger aggressive behavior among your hens. As a chicken keeper, you want to ensure each bird has at least 3-4 square feet inside the coop and 10 square feet in the run. This allows them ample space to scratch, peck, and carry out their normal behaviors without feeling threatened or cramped.

Lighting is another key aspect of the coop environment. Chickens need a balance of light and darkness for optimal health. Natural light helps to regulate their internal clock, affecting behaviors like laying and roosting. Install windows in your coop to allow natural light during the day and make sure there's a way to cover them at night to provide darkness for restful sleep.

Temperature control is also essential. Chickens, like us, can get uncomfortable in extreme weather conditions. Providing proper ventilation in the coop can help keep temperatures down in the summer, while insulating the coop can help keep your flock warm during winter.

Moving onto another crucial part, handling practices. Just like any other pet, chickens need gentle and considerate handling. Rapid movements, loud noises, and abrupt handling can startle and stress chickens. Always move slowly and talk quietly around your chickens. When you need to pick up a chicken, move slowly, hold them gently but firmly, and always support their feet.

Food and water security is another factor that plays into stress. Chickens need to know that they will consistently have access to food and water. Inconsistent feeding can cause anxiety and competitive behavior among the flock. Make sure your chickens always have access to fresh, clean water and a balanced diet, and try to keep feeding times consistent.

Predator protection also cannot be understated. Nothing stresses a chicken out more than a potential predator. Ensure your coop is secure from common predators such as raccoons, foxes, and birds of prey. This could mean installing a secure chicken wire fence, securing the coop at night, or even getting a livestock guardian animal if predator presence is high in your area.

Provide opportunities for natural behavior. Chickens love to scratch, peck and dust bathe. Providing them with a dirt bath, enough space to forage, and perches to roost can make a significant difference in their stress levels. Similarly, introducing beneficial herbs into their routine can also have a remarkable impact on their skin and feather health. With that said, let's explore some of the best herbs for lustrous feathers and healthy skin: Calendula, Comfrey, and Yarrow.

Calendula, often known as marigold, is a strikingly beautiful plant with a host of benefits. These flowers aren't just for show. They are packed with antioxidants and anti-inflammatory compounds. When chickens consume calendula, the pigments in the petals, mainly xanthophylls, can help deepen the yellow-orange hues of their yolks. Topically, it's commonly used in ointments, salves, and washes to soothe irritated skin. It's a natural antiseptic and can aid in wound healing. For chickens, adding dried calendula petals to their dust bath is a fantastic way to introduce this herb.

Comfrey is another powerful herb to consider. This plant has long been used in traditional medicine for wound healing thanks to its high allantoin content, a compound known to speed up wound repair by stimulating cell growth. It also has anti-inflammatory properties that can help soothe irritated skin. If a chicken has lost feathers due to pecking or mites, a topical application of comfrey can soothe the skin and encourage feather regrowth. Remember, though, comfrey is for external use only and should not be ingested due to its high concentration of certain alkaloids.

Next up is Yarrow, a plant that holds a place in many a herbalist's heart. It's not only attractive to beneficial insects in your garden, but it's also a potent healer for your chickens. Yarrow is known for its astringent and antimicrobial properties. It can tighten and dry the skin, helping to heal minor wounds or cuts. In addition, it's a natural insect repellent, so a yarrow-strewn dust bath can help keep pesky parasites at bay.

These are just a few examples. There are many herbs out there with beneficial properties. Other notable mentions include lavender, with its soothing properties and a scent that's relaxing for both chickens and humans; and rosemary, a herb known for its antibacterial properties and a strong, pleasant scent that can help repel insects.

Incorporating these herbs into your chicken care routine can help enhance feather vibrancy and maintain skin health. They can be added to the chickens' dust bath, used in herbal sprays for the coop, or sprinkled in nesting boxes. Just remember, introducing new elements into your flock's environment should be done gradually, and always monitor your chickens for any signs of adverse reactions.

Maintaining the health of your flock's skin and feathers isn't merely about aesthetics. It's a vital part of keeping your chickens in top form. In the upcoming section, we'll go further into how to use these herbs effectively, offering some remedies and methods for your coop. It's all part of the fulfilling journey of raising happy, healthy hens.

It's no secret that chickens love their dust baths. It's their own unique version of a spa day. This is where they roll, fluff, and shake in the dust to keep their feathers clean and free from parasites. Adding beneficial herbs to their dust bath can enhance this natural behavior, providing additional skin and feather health benefits. So, what might an herbal dust bath include?

For starters, consider dried calendula flowers. Not only will these brighten up the dust bath, but they'll also offer their anti-inflammatory and antiseptic properties, helping to soothe any skin irritations. Additionally, you can add dried yarrow. With its insect-repelling qualities, yarrow helps in keeping those bothersome mites and lice away.

Next, let's think about topical applications, especially useful when dealing with skin injuries or irritated patches of skin. Comfrey, for instance, is excellent for this. A poultice made from comfrey leaves can be applied directly to the affected area, supporting the healing process. It's crucial to remember, however, that comfrey should only be used externally, as it contains compounds that can be harmful if ingested.

Herbs can also be used in nesting boxes, providing a calming scent and promoting a peaceful environment. Lavender and rosemary, for instance, are perfect candidates. Both these herbs have pleasant scents known to be calming and repel insects. A few sprigs in each nesting box can go a long way in creating a relaxing environment for your hens.

Moreover, you can create an herbal spray to mist your chickens lightly. A simple spray can be made by steeping herbs in hot water, much like making tea, then allowing it to cool. Spray this mixture lightly on your chickens or in the coop to deter pests and promote skin health.

Let's not forget about feed. Adding herbs to your flock's diet can also be beneficial. While calendula petals can enrich the color of egg yolks, herbs like nettle can provide a nutritional boost. Nettle is high in vitamins and minerals and can support feather health. To feed nettle or other herbs, they can be dried and crushed into a powder, then mixed into the chickens' feed.

Now, we're going to delve into how to prepare some herbal remedies that can boost your chickens' skin and feather health. So let's turn on the chicken charm and create some soothing herbal remedies that your hens will cluck with joy!

First up is an enriching dust bath mix. In a large container, combine one part wood ash, one part sand, and one part dry soil. To this, add a handful each of dried calendula flowers and dried yarrow. Give it a good mix until everything is well combined. This dust bath will not only help keep your hens clean but also offer them the therapeutic benefits of these herbs.

For topical applications, a comfrey salve is easy to make and can be quite handy for treating skin irritations or minor wounds. To make this, simmer fresh comfrey leaves in a cup of coconut oil until the leaves are crispy. Strain the oil, discard the leaves, and allow the oil to cool. Once cooled, it can be stored in a jar and applied as needed to soothe and heal the skin.

Creating an herbal nesting box mix can also help promote a calm and insect-free laying environment. Mix dried lavender and rosemary in equal parts and add to the nesting boxes. The scent of these herbs has a calming effect and can deter pests.

Herbal sprays can also help keep your flock's skin in good condition. Steep a mixture of herbs such as chamomile, calendula, and lavender in hot water. Once cooled, strain the mixture and pour into a spray bottle. Use this to mist the coop or your hens, offering a refreshing and beneficial herbal boost.

A nourishing feed supplement can be made by combining dried, crushed nettle, and calendula petals. Simply mix a small amount of this herbal blend into their regular feed to give their diet a nutritional boost and promote healthier skin and feathers.

Now, I want to emphasize the importance of monitoring your hens' skin and feather health. Regular observation and understanding the signs of healthy and unhealthy feathers and skin are essential components of maintaining a healthy flock.

Let's start with healthy feathers. You want to look for feathers that are smooth and shiny, with no visible breaks. The feathers should lay flat against the body, and there should be no bald spots or uneven feather loss. Healthy chicken skin should be clean and free from sores, lumps, or any signs of irritation. The skin should also be flexible, with a smooth texture.

Now, let's talk about the warning signs. Changes in your chickens' feathers can often be a sign of underlying health issues. Feather loss, for example, is normal during molting, but uneven feather loss can be a sign of mites, lice, or other parasites. Broken, frayed, or otherwise damaged feathers can indicate a nutritional deficiency or stress.

If the skin is red, swollen, or has sores, these are clear signs of trouble. Parasites such as mites can cause intense itching, leading to skin damage. Other skin conditions can be a result of bacterial or fungal infections.

You should also pay attention to your hens' behavior. Chickens that preen excessively, seem unusually restless or lose feathers outside of the molting season could indicate that they are uncomfortable, stressed, or even sick.

Your chickens can't tell you when they feel unwell, so it's up to you to be observant and proactive. A small issue can quickly become a big one if left unattended, but with regular checks and early intervention, you can keep your flock looking fabulous and feeling even better.

Incorporating herbs into your chicken care routine can be a game-changer. With the knowledge you've gained from this chapter, you're now equipped to use these powerful plants to their full potential. But remember, herbs are a tool, not a magic bullet. They should be used in conjunction with proper housing, nutrition, and veterinary care to maintain your flock's health.

I hope you're feeling more confident in using herbs to promote your chickens' health. There's a sense of satisfaction in knowing you're providing your flock with the best care possible, bolstered by the power of nature. And the joy of seeing your chickens thrive? Well, that's simply unbeatable.

Chapter 3: The All-Season Herbal Coop

Part I: Spring Greening: Herbs for a Lively Coop

Spring is like a wake-up call for chickens after the long winter months. It's a period when they'll shake off their winter sluggishness and embrace the buzz of activity. Longer daylight hours trigger a host of physiological changes in chickens, including the onset of molting for some, a surge in energy levels, and for many, the commencement of the breeding season.

Let's first talk about molting. This is a natural process where chickens shed their old, worn-out feathers and grow new ones. While this is most common in the fall, it can happen any time of the year, especially during changes in season. It's a taxing process for chickens, both physically and mentally. The energy that is normally used for egg production is redirected towards growing new feathers. This often results in chickens ceasing to lay eggs for the duration of the molt.

During spring molt, you may notice that your chickens are more sensitive to touch due to the growing pin feathers. These new feathers are rich in blood supply and can cause discomfort when handled. As a chicken keeper, it's essential to be gentle with your birds during this time.

Now, spring's warmer weather and increased daylight also spur a rise in the chickens' activity levels. Hens may lay more frequently, and both hens and roosters are likely to display more social behaviors, including mating behaviors. This uptick in energy is good, promoting exercise and foraging, but it can also bring about issues like pecking order disputes or, in some cases, bullying.

Speaking of egg laying, spring is commonly the start of the breeding season for chickens. Hens are often at their peak fertility during this period. If you're looking to expand your flock naturally, now is the time. However, the increased egg production can also strain the hens' bodies, making it critical to ensure they're receiving ample nutrition.

So, how does one ensure that their flock navigates these changes smoothly? The answer lies in herbs! Yes, those garden miracles have a lot to offer our feathered friends during this vibrant season.

Herbs can be especially beneficial during molting. High-protein herbs like alfalfa can support feather growth, while calming herbs like chamomile can help ease the stress associated with this period. Additionally, herbs rich in calcium like dandelion can provide the extra nutrients hens need for increased egg production.

It's not just the physical health of your chickens that herbs can aid in. They also play a significant role in keeping the coop environment enriched and pleasant. As the activity levels in your coop increase, so can the chances of squabbles. Sprinkling calming herbs like lavender and lemon balm around the coop can help keep the peace.

Moreover, the spring thaw might lead to dampness in the coop, creating a perfect breeding ground for mold and bacteria. This is where herbs with strong antimicrobial properties, such as garlic and oregano, can come to the rescue.

Garlic, though not a herb in the botanical sense, has been used for centuries due to its potent antibacterial properties. Including garlic in your flock's diet can help to keep those pesky bacteria at bay, ensuring a healthier environment for your chickens. Garlic can be added to your chicken's water supply, but remember moderation is key. Too much garlic can lead to strong-flavored eggs that might not be to your liking.

Oregano is another fantastic herb that springs to mind when we talk about antibacterial properties. Often referred to as nature's antibiotic, oregano can also be an effective deterrent for parasites, making it a powerhouse herb for your flock. Sprinkling dried oregano in your coop bedding can help reduce bacterial load, while feeding it to your chickens can boost their immune system, better preparing them to fight off infections.

Moving on, let's talk about the real stars of the spring season, the herbs that truly shine during this time. First up, we have nettles. Nettles are rich in minerals like iron, calcium, and magnesium, as well as being a great source of vitamin A and C. This makes them excellent for supporting overall health, promoting eggshell quality, and aiding in feather growth, especially useful during the molting season. The sting of nettles can be neutralized by drying or cooking, making them safe to feed to your chickens.

Dandelion is another prolific spring herb that your chickens are sure to love. The entire plant, from the roots to the flower, is edible and packed full of nutrients. High in calcium and vitamin A, dandelion can be an excellent herb for laying hens. Its leaves can be fed fresh, or they can be dried and stored for later use.

Then we have comfrey, a herb that's known for its high protein content and rapid growth. Comfrey is packed with vitamin B12, a vitamin not commonly found in plants but essential for egg production. This makes comfrey an ideal spring herb for your laying hens. Just remember, comfrey should be fed in moderation due to its high levels of certain compounds that can be harmful in large amounts.

Calendula, with its bright orange flowers, is a herb that can add a pop of color to your spring garden and your egg yolks! Yes, feeding calendula petals to your hens can result in yolks with a richer, deeper orange color. Besides its color-enhancing properties, calendula also has antiseptic properties that can be beneficial for your flock.

Herbs are truly a gift from nature. With their varied nutritional profiles and unique properties, they can play an essential role in maintaining the health of your chickens, especially during a lively spring season. So, go ahead, add some garlic to your coop bedding, sprinkle some oregano in their feed, or let them forage on fresh dandelions and nettles. After all, a healthy chicken is a happy chicken!

The role of herbs, however, extends beyond nutrition and into the realms of cleanliness and hygiene. And spring, a time of renewal and fresh starts, is the perfect time to give the chicken coop a deep clean. Herbal disinfectants and deodorizers can be useful tools in your arsenal for this task.

For instance, lavender and mint have strong deodorizing properties. They can be scattered in nesting boxes and the coop floor to help neutralize odors. Not only will the coop smell fresher, but these aromatic herbs can also have a calming effect on your flock. Mint, in addition, is a deterrent for rodents and insects, offering a dual role as a pest control agent.

Thyme is another excellent herb for coop cleaning. With powerful antibacterial and antiviral properties, thyme tea can be used to scrub the coop, ensuring a clean environment for your chickens to thrive.

Eucalyptus and tea tree, while not traditional garden herbs, offer powerful antibacterial and antifungal properties. A few drops of these essential oils in your cleaning water can add an extra layer of protection against pathogens. Just make sure to let the coop air out properly before reintroducing your flock to prevent respiratory discomfort caused by the strong aroma of these oils.

Lemongrass, with its fresh, uplifting scent and strong antibacterial properties, is another excellent choice. Lemongrass essential oil can be added to your cleaning water or sprayed around the coop after cleaning to keep it smelling fresh and clean.

Vinegar, while not an herb, is an essential natural cleaning agent that you'll want to have on hand. It's great for cleaning feeders, drinkers, and other chicken accessories. You can make it even more effective by infusing it with antibacterial herbs like rosemary and sage. Simply let the herbs steep in the vinegar for a few weeks, strain, and use for cleaning.

And of course, you can't overlook the power of sunshine, nature's best disinfectant. After cleaning the coop, leave it open to air out and let the sun in. This can help to kill any remaining bacteria, ensuring your coop is as clean as can be.

As the saying goes, an ounce of prevention is worth a pound of cure. By keeping your coop clean, you're helping to prevent diseases and create a healthy, happy home for your chickens. This, coupled with the nutritional boost that herbs provide, makes for a holistic approach to chicken care that aligns perfectly with the natural cycles of the seasons. Spring, with its abundance of fresh herbs, is the ideal time to kick-start this practice, setting the tone for the rest of the year.

So don't shy away from harnessing the power of herbs for your coop cleaning. It's an eco-friendly, effective, and even enjoyable way to take care of your flock. Your chickens will thank you for it! But the use of herbs doesn't stop there. In fact, there are a multitude of ways you can use them to boost your chickens' health, especially after the long, hard winter. And spring, with its surge of fresh growth, is the perfect time to introduce some special herbal blends into your flock's diet.

One of the first herbs that comes to mind when we talk about spring is nettles. This powerhouse plant is packed with nutrients, and it starts growing early in the spring. For an invigorating spring tonic, try a blend of fresh nettle leaves, cleavers, and dandelion greens. These can be chopped finely and added to your flock's daily feed. Your chickens will gobble them up and reap the benefits of the high vitamin and mineral content of these herbs.

Another wonderful spring blend includes the use of garlic and oregano. As we've discussed, garlic has potent antimicrobial properties, and oregano has been studied for its effectiveness against common poultry diseases. Try chopping fresh oregano leaves and mixing them with crushed garlic cloves. This mixture can be added to feed or water and will act as a natural immune booster for your flock as they navigate the transition from winter to spring.

For a more complex blend that taps into the diverse herbal offerings of spring, consider a mix of rosemary, thyme, and lavender buds with a sprinkling of dandelion petals. The rosemary and thyme offer antibacterial benefits, while the lavender has a calming effect. Dandelion petals, besides being a favorite among chickens, offer a slew of vitamins and minerals. Mix these together, let them dry, and then add them to your chickens' nesting boxes. This blend can contribute to a tranquil atmosphere in the coop while also delivering nutritional benefits.

And then there's the all-important task of parasite prevention. Spring often sees a rise in parasitic activity, and some herbs can help fend off these unwanted intruders. Wormwood, for instance, is an effective anti-parasitic herb that can be included in your spring herbal blend. It should be used sparingly, though, as it can be bitter and potent. A pinch of wormwood mixed with more palatable herbs like mint or parsley can make for an effective parasite-preventing blend.

Using herbs in these ways can offer a holistic approach to chicken health. You're not only keeping their living environment clean but also taking steps to boost their immune system, improve their nutrition, and keep them happy and stress-free. As you dive into spring with your chickens, let the abundance of the season guide your choices. The herbs are ready, your chickens are ready, and a season of growth and vitality awaits!

Spring is an amazing time for chickens. As the earth wakes up from its winter slumber, a banquet of fresh greenery appears, providing an exciting opportunity for your flock to forage. Chickens are natural foragers, and this behavior should be encouraged, as it allows them to fulfill their instinctual behaviors and find food that is nutrient-dense and varied.

Foraging encourages chickens to exercise, which contributes to their overall health and well-being. It can also cut down on feed costs and keeps them busy, which reduces stress and potential behavioral problems such as pecking at each other. Foraging can also improve the quality of the eggs they lay due to the rich and varied diet they consume. Therefore, enabling natural foraging in spring is not just about embracing the season's vitality; it's also a practical and beneficial approach to chicken keeping.

One way to encourage foraging is by providing a safe and herb-rich environment for your chickens. If you have space, consider planting a forage garden for your chickens with a diverse mix of herbs, including those we've discussed like nettles, dandelion, and comfrey, as well as other chicken favorites like mint, marjoram, and parsley. Planting a wide variety of herbs will ensure a balanced diet for your flock and will keep them interested.

Safety is another crucial factor. Make sure the foraging area is secure from predators, and ensure the plants your chickens have access to are safe to eat. Always check that the herbs and plants you introduce to your chickens are non-toxic and safe for consumption.

When your chickens are foraging, observe them closely. You will quickly learn which herbs they prefer and which ones they tend to avoid. This information is useful as it can guide you in choosing which herbs to plant more of in the future, and it can help in creating herbal blends for their feed or nest boxes.

Additionally, while chickens are excellent foragers, they may need a little guidance when a new plant is introduced. If your flock is reluctant to try a new herb, you can encourage them by chopping the herb and mixing it with a treat they love, like mealworms or cracked corn. Over time, they will likely become accustomed to the new herb and start eating it on their own.

You can also encourage foraging by regularly moving the chickens to fresh ground, if possible. This practice, known as 'chicken tractor' or 'pastured poultry,' allows chickens to access fresh plants, insects, and seeds, which greatly contributes to their health and happiness.

Encouraging natural foraging is a rewarding activity that contributes significantly to your flock's health. By offering a safe and diverse environment, observing their preferences, and guiding them towards new herbs, you can enhance their springtime experience. Embrace the season's vibrancy and richness with your flock, and let the natural instincts of your chickens lead the way.

Part II: Summer Sizzlers: Cooling Herbs and Dust Baths

As we transition from the vibrant energy of spring into the golden glow of summer, it's essential to consider how the rising temperatures can impact your flock. While chickens are resilient creatures capable of adapting to various climates, the heat of summer can pose specific challenges that require attention and care from you, their dedicated caregiver.

Heat stress in chickens is a genuine concern during the summer months. As the mercury rises, your chickens' bodies work overtime to maintain their optimal body temperature, which ranges between 104°F and 107°F (40-41.7°C). Unlike humans, chickens cannot sweat to cool down. Instead, they rely on panting and holding their wings away from their bodies to dispel heat, which can be an inefficient process in high temperatures.

When chickens become overheated, they may exhibit a range of symptoms, from panting and spread wings to lethargy, loss of appetite, and decreased egg production. In severe cases, heat stress can lead to heat stroke, a potentially fatal condition. Therefore, understanding the effects of heat on chickens is crucial in helping them navigate the summer months in comfort and safety.

Hydration is a primary concern during these hot months. Chickens need access to clean, fresh water at all times, but this becomes even more vital in the summer. Water plays a crucial role in helping them cool down, as they will drink more to compensate for the increased respiratory rate and the resulting moisture loss. Lack of adequate water can rapidly exacerbate the effects of heat stress, leading to severe dehydration and potentially, death.

Egg-laying may also be affected by high temperatures. Chickens lay fewer eggs during extreme heat. This slowdown is a natural response; egg production requires energy and generates metabolic heat, which adds to a chicken's burden in the summer. The reduction in laying is the body's way of conserving energy and keeping cool.

In addition to these direct effects, heat can also indirectly impact chickens through changes in their environment. For instance, parasites such as mites and lice thrive in hot, dry conditions, so infestations can become more prevalent in the summer months. Increased temperatures can also heighten the risk of food spoiling, potentially leading to issues such as mold growth in feed or water supplies.

A significant part of summer chicken care involves recognizing these challenges and taking steps to mitigate them. Providing shade, ventilation, and cool, clean water can go a long way in preventing heat stress in your flock. Observing your chickens closely and responding promptly to signs of distress is also crucial in ensuring their health and happiness.

In addition to these physical measures, using herbs can be an effective and natural way to support your chickens' wellbeing during the hot months. Certain herbs have cooling properties that can help your chickens handle the heat better. Let's delve into a few of these "cooling" herbs.

Mint is a popular choice for summer because of its potent cooling properties. Both peppermint and spearmint have high levels of menthol, which provides a cooling sensation. Besides making a refreshing addition to their water or feed, these herbs can be hung in bunches around the coop for a calming, cooling effect. The strong aroma of mint can also deter some pests, a definite summer bonus!

Lemon Balm, another member of the mint family, is also excellent for summer use. It shares the cooling properties of its mint cousins and adds a lovely lemony scent to the mix. Chickens enjoy its taste, and its calming properties can help reduce stress levels, which can be particularly beneficial in the heat.

Aloe Vera is another excellent herb for summer care. While not necessarily cooling, its moisture-rich leaves can be a treat for chickens on a hot day. Moreover, Aloe Vera's gel is known for its soothing and healing properties. It can be applied topically to help heal any summer sores or skin irritations.

Chickweed, despite its name, is an herb that chickens love, and it can be a great addition to their summer diet. It's a juicy herb that provides much-needed moisture on hot days. Chickweed also has anti-inflammatory properties, which can help soothe any heat-induced discomfort.

Cilantro and parsley are other summer-friendly herbs. Their high water content provides an additional hydration source, and they are packed with vitamins and minerals, ensuring your chickens are getting essential nutrients even if the heat has decreased their appetite.

Remember, while these herbs can contribute to a more comfortable summer for your chickens, they are part of a broader care strategy. Always ensure your chickens have access to plenty of shade and fresh water. Consider the coop ventilation, and make sure to monitor your flock for signs of heat stress regularly.

Growing these herbs can be a delightful aspect of your gardening routine. Seeing your flock relish the fresh greens and knowing the health benefits they're receiving is a reward in itself. A chicken's diet can be greatly varied and enriched with the inclusion of these herbs. And the best part? Many of these herbs are perennials or self-seeding annuals, so once you've planted them, you'll have a supply returning year after year, ready to support your chickens through each hot summer season. Their cooling and health-boosting properties can make a significant difference to your flock during the sweltering summer months. While we've covered herbs that can be added to feed or water or grown around the coop, there's another way to incorporate herbs into your flock's routine that we haven't yet touched upon: dust baths.

Dust bathing is a natural behavior for chickens and plays an essential role in their health and hygiene. Chickens roll and flick dust over their bodies, helping to keep their feathers clean, remove old oils, and deter parasites. You can enhance this natural behavior by adding herbs to their dust bath, creating an aromatic, spa-like experience for your chickens.

One of the most delightful herbs to consider for a dust bath is lavender. The scent of lavender is known to be calming and soothing, a useful trait when dealing with the stress of high temperatures. Plus, lavender's natural oils may deter pests and promote healing of any minor skin irritations.

Another excellent herb to add to the dust bathing area is rosemary. Similar to lavender, rosemary is known for its strong aroma that can deter pests. The bonus with rosemary is that it's hardy and easy to grow, making it an accessible addition to your herbal toolkit.

Chamomile is another fantastic choice for a dust bath. Known for its calming properties in humans, it can have the same soothing effect on chickens. Adding dried chamomile to the dust bath can create a tranquil environment for your flock. This is especially beneficial during the summer months when heat stress might be a concern.

Marigold petals, with their bright colors and aromatic scent, can be another addition to your dust bath herb blend. They contain potent compounds that may discourage pests and can lend a lovely golden hue to your chickens' dust bath.

Lemongrass is another herb that you might consider. Its refreshing citrusy aroma can make the dust bath even more inviting. Additionally, it contains substances that may have anti-bacterial and anti-parasitic properties.

Creating an herbal dust bath for your chickens can be a simple process. Start by ensuring your dust bath area is clean and dry. Then, mix in your chosen dried herbs with the dust or sand. Remember, the herbs should be dried to prevent them from molding in the bath.

For proportions, a handful of herbs for every few pounds of dust or sand can be a good starting point. However, feel free to experiment with different amounts to see what your flock enjoys best.

These fragrant dust baths not only offer health benefits but also enrich your chickens' environment, providing them with sensory stimulation that can alleviate boredom and promote natural behaviors.

While these herbs have been singled out for their specific benefits in a dust bath context, many other herbs could also work well. It all depends on what you have available and what your chickens seem to enjoy. As the summer heat kicks in, these herbal dust baths can offer a refreshing retreat for your flock, helping them stay cool, clean, and happy. But the fun doesn't stop there. There are other creative ways to incorporate herbs into your flock's summer routine, turning everyday activities into refreshing experiences.

One refreshing trick for your flock is creating herbal ice treats. These are easy and effective ways to keep your chickens cool and hydrated. You can use a variety of herbs that are beneficial for chickens, and they can be a fun treat for your flock on a hot summer day.

To make herbal ice treats, all you need are fresh herbs, water, and a freezer. You can use a silicone mold or even an ice cube tray. For the herbs, consider cooling options such as mint or lemon balm, along with others like parsley and oregano for added nutritional benefits. Simply chop the herbs, distribute them into the molds, fill them with water, and freeze them.

When frozen, these herbal ice treats can be added to the chickens' water or served separately. As they peck at the ice, they'll also consume the herbs, leading to a fun, cooling, and nutritious treat.

Another way to make use of herbs during the hot summer months is by creating an herbal spray for the coop. These sprays can help keep the coop smelling fresh, deter pests, and create a calming environment for your chickens.

An example of an herbal spray can be made using lavender, rosemary, and mint. You'd need to steep these herbs in boiling water, much like making tea and then strain the mixture. Once cooled, this herbal infusion can be poured into a spray bottle and used to mist the coop.

Remember, when using an herbal spray, it's important not to spray directly onto your chickens or their food and water sources. Instead, lightly mist the walls and bedding of the coop.

Yet another fun idea for summer is creating herbal shade stations. Plant tall herbs like sunflowers, which chickens won't typically eat, around the run or free-range area. Then, plant your chickens' favorite herbs under these. The taller plants provide shade, while the lower-growing herbs give your chickens a cool spot to rest and snack.

These are just a few ideas to make the most out of the summer season with your chickens. The herbs not only provide nutritional and health benefits but also introduce variety and enrichment into your chickens' daily lives.

Remember, each flock is unique, and so are the chickens that constitute it. As you try out these herbal additions, keep an eye on your flock's response. What works wonderfully for one flock might not be as well-received by another, and that's okay. The goal is to find what best suits your unique group of feathered friends.

The beauty of herbs lies in their versatility and the simplicity with which they can be integrated into various aspects of chicken care. So, experiment with confidence, knowing that you're making your flock's summer healthier, happier, and undoubtedly more exciting.

But amidst all this excitement, we must not overlook one crucial fact — summer, with its searing heat and high humidity levels, can cause heat stress in chickens. Recognizing and mitigating the effects of heat stress should be a priority for every chicken keeper during these warm months.

Heat stress occurs when chickens are unable to cool their bodies effectively, resulting in increased body temperature. This can cause several issues ranging from decreased egg production and slow growth to severe health issues and even death.

One of the best ways to prevent heat stress is by providing ample shade for your chickens. While trees and shrubs offer natural shade, if they are not present in the coop, consider using tarps, cloth, or even pallets to create shaded areas. Incorporate tall herbs like sunflowers in your chicken run to offer not just shade but also a distraction as they make for good 'chicken TV.'

Hydration is another crucial factor. Chickens need a consistent supply of clean, cool water. On extremely hot days, ensure there are multiple water sources available. Adding some herbs to their water can be beneficial. For instance, lemon balm and mint are known for their cooling properties and can make the water more enticing to drink.

Diet plays a significant role in helping chickens cope with summer heat. Light, easily digestible food can make a difference. Incorporating herbs in their feed not only adds nutritional benefits but also can help in cooling. Herbs like dill, fennel, and cilantro are known to have a cooling effect and can be mixed with the regular chicken feed.

Ventilation is crucial, especially within the coop. Good airflow allows heat to escape and cooler air to circulate. Consider the coop's design and make any necessary modifications to improve ventilation.

Dust baths are not just a fun activity for your chickens; they also help them keep cool. A dust bath area in a shaded part of the coop or run can provide much-needed relief from the heat. Adding herbs like lavender, rosemary, and chamomile to the dust bath mixture can enhance the cooling effect, keep parasites at bay, and offer a calming experience for your chickens.

Monitoring your flock's behavior closely can provide valuable insights. Lethargy, panting, loss of appetite, decreased egg production, and pale combs are some signs of heat stress. By observing your chickens and understanding their normal behavior, you can quickly recognize any changes and act promptly.

Finally, remember that every chicken breed has different heat tolerances. Breeds with smaller body size, large combs and wattles, and lighter color are typically more heat tolerant. So, understanding the specific needs and characteristics of your chicken breed can help in better managing heat stress.

While summer brings along challenges like heat stress, it also provides an opportunity to explore the world of herbs in new and exciting ways. A well-planned, proactive approach can ensure your flock not only survives the summer heat but thrives in it.

Keep this in mind as you navigate the summer months with your flock. Your proactive approach to heat stress prevention, combined with your creative use of herbs, can truly make the difference between a harsh, stressful summer and a season of growth, vitality, and joy for your chickens. So, here's to a summer filled with clucking, pecking, and lots of herbal fun!

Part III: Fall Forage: Autumn Abundance

After the sizzle and bustle of summer, comes the calming embrace of fall. The autumn season ushers in a cooler climate, a changing landscape, and new challenges and opportunities for your flock. One of the significant tasks at hand during this time is preparing your chickens for the upcoming winter.

As the days get shorter and temperatures drop, you'll notice some changes in your chickens. Laying may decrease or even halt completely, especially for the breeds sensitive to light changes. This period is a natural rest phase for hens after the heavy laying cycle of spring and summer. Rather than fretting over fewer eggs, see this time as a well-deserved break for your hardworking girls.

Molting, or the process of shedding and renewing feathers, typically occurs during fall. You might find the coop and run littered with feathers and some bare-looking birds strutting around. As jarring as it may seem, it's a natural and necessary process for chickens to refresh their plumage before the cold winter months.

Molting requires energy, and this can take a toll on your chickens. The nutritional needs of your flock increase, especially the need for high-quality protein, which is vital for feather growth. Regular layer feed might not meet this increased requirement. Consider supplementing their diet with additional protein sources.

Herbs can play a significant role in helping your flock through this transition period. A blend of alfalfa, nettle, and parsley can be a great dietary supplement during molting. Alfalfa is a protein powerhouse and a source of vitamins A, C, E, and K. Nettle provides calcium, magnesium, and iron. Parsley is packed with vitamins A, C, and K and also provides calcium and iron. This herbal blend not only supports feather growth but also enhances overall health.

Ensuring a well-balanced diet, high in energy and protein, can go a long way in preparing your flock for winter. Foods like corn and sunflower seeds are excellent sources of energy. Introduce these gradually into your chickens' diet as the weather starts to cool.

Hydration remains crucial, even though the temperatures are dropping. Chickens will eat snow, but it's not a substitute for clean, unfrozen water. Continue to ensure they have access to fresh water at all times.

Boosting the immune system of your chickens in preparation for the colder months is also a good strategy. Incorporate immunity-boosting herbs like echinacea, thyme, and oregano in their feed.

Fall is a great time to prep the coop for winter. Start by doing a thorough cleaning. Remember those herbal disinfectants we discussed earlier? They are perfect for fall cleaning, too. Add plenty of clean, dry bedding for insulation. Herbs like mint and lavender can be mixed in with the bedding to deter pests and keep the coop smelling fresh.

Just as you adapt your own diet with the changing seasons, incorporating seasonal herbs into your chickens' regimen can have a significantly beneficial impact on their health and well-being. Autumn brings with it a bounty of beneficial herbs that can provide essential nutrients and support for your flock as they navigate through molting and the cooler weather.

Thyme is a fantastic herb to start incorporating into your flock's diet during the fall. It's not just a staple in our kitchen; it's an excellent addition to the chicken diet too. Thyme's secret power lies in its antimicrobial properties, which can help in maintaining respiratory health, something quite crucial as the air gets colder and potential respiratory issues might arise.

Rosehips, the fruit of the rose plant that ripens in early fall, are another splendid addition. High in Vitamin C, they are an antioxidant powerhouse. They help boost the immune system, a needful attribute as your flock prepares to face the harsher winter conditions. You can scatter them around the coop or run, and watch as your chickens enjoy their little game of seek and snack.

Another herb that deserves a special mention is Echinacea. Known commonly as coneflower, Echinacea is a powerhouse of immune-boosting properties. It has been used traditionally to combat colds and flus, making it a fitting herb for your chickens as they enter the colder months. The plant's leaves, flowers, and roots can all be safely consumed by your flock.

Garlic might not be an herb in the traditional sense, but its medicinal properties cannot be ignored. As the days get shorter, adding fresh minced garlic to your chickens' water can help in maintaining their general health. Garlic is known for its anti-fungal, antibacterial, and antiviral properties, which makes it a perfect all-rounder for boosting chicken health.

And let's not forget the sage, another fall-friendly herb. Known for its antioxidant and anti-parasitic properties, sage can be a useful addition to your chickens' diet during fall. The flavorful herb can be mixed in feed or scattered around the run for a fun foraging activity.

During fall, consider making a nutritional herbal blend for your flock. You could mix chopped thyme, rosehips, echinacea, garlic, and sage and add it to their feed. It's a fantastic way of ensuring that your chickens are receiving a range of nutrients and health benefits.

As you clean and prep the coop for winter, remember to take advantage of the unique herbs that autumn provides. Whether you're using them for their nutritional benefits, medicinal properties, or pest-repelling abilities, the right herbs can go a long way in ensuring a healthy, happy flock ready to face the winter.

Autumn brings a lot more than just herbs to your flock. It's also a season of abundant leaves, those beautiful, falling natural elements that we often consider more decorative than utilitarian. But when it comes to chicken keeping, fall leaves can provide a plethora of benefits for your coop and your flock.

First and foremost, fall leaves make an excellent natural bedding for your chicken coop. Dry leaves provide a fluffy, comfortable surface for your chickens to rest and sleep. They act as a wonderful insulator, helping to keep the coop warm as the temperatures start to drop. Additionally, leaves mimic the natural foraging environment of chickens, leading to a more enriching environment for them.

Composting is another fantastic use of autumn leaves in your chicken care routine. If you're not already composting, fall is an ideal time to start, as you'll have plenty of leaves at your disposal. Consider creating a compost pile or bin in or near the chicken run. Add in your leaves, chicken droppings, and other organic matter like kitchen scraps. With time, this pile will decompose into a nutrient-rich compost that can be used in your garden.

Adding autumn leaves to the compost pile has another benefit; it attracts bugs and worms. As the leaves start to break down, they become a hotspot for these little creatures, which your chickens will love to snack on. This gives them a fun and enriching foraging experience while also providing them with a protein-rich diet.

Dried leaves can also be used to create a simple and natural dust bath for your chickens. Chickens use dust baths to keep their feathers clean and free from parasites. Fill a shallow tub or a corner of the coop with dried leaves and you've got yourself a no-cost dust bath that your chickens will love.

Lastly, autumn leaves can be used as a natural and eco-friendly way of managing odors in the chicken coop. They absorb moisture and trap odors, making the coop a more pleasant place for both you and your chickens.

While the falling leaves of autumn may seem like just another task on the clean-up list, these leaves are a resource that should not be overlooked. They can be used to improve the health of your chickens and the fertility of your soil while also reducing waste. It's a win-win for everyone!

It's important to remember that all leaves are not created equal. Some trees, such as walnut, can have harmful effects on chickens. Always be sure to identify the types of trees in your area and avoid using leaves from potentially harmful species.

So, as the trees begin to shed their leaves, instead of sighing at the thought of raking them up, celebrate the fact that your chickens' coop is about to get a whole lot cozier. Add those leaves to their run for some interesting foraging, or perhaps start a compost heap that will eventually feed back into the circle of life by enriching your garden. The chickens will appreciate the addition of this season's bounty to their environment. With the autumn leaves falling and the air turning crisper, it's time to think about adding some herbal blends to your chicken's diet to help them build their immunity and be prepared for winter.

The first step in creating fall herbal blend remedies is to understand the specific herbs that are most beneficial for chickens in the fall. Thyme, for instance, is not only a culinary delight but also a powerful medicinal herb. It is packed with thymol, a natural antibiotic that boosts the chicken's immunity and keeps them healthy.

Rosehips, another autumn herb, are high in vitamin C, which is a crucial antioxidant for your flock, enhancing their immune system and keeping their skin, feathers, and beaks healthy. Besides, they are a tasty treat that your chickens will love.

Echinacea, often associated with boosting human immunity, serves the same purpose for chickens. It can help prevent and fight off diseases in your flock. In addition, the plant is hardy and easy to grow, making it a great addition to your garden.

So, how can you incorporate these herbs into your flock's diet? One simple way is to create an autumn forage mix. Combine dried thyme, rosehips, and echinacea along with other dried leaves, seeds, and grains. Scatter this mix in the run for a natural and enriching foraging experience for your chickens.

You could also create an herbal feed blend. Grind up dried herbs and mix them with your chicken feed. This not only gives your chickens a nutrition boost but also keeps their feed interesting and varied.

A "winter-ready" herbal tea could be another great addition to your chicken care regime. Brew a strong tea using thyme, rosehips, and echinacea. Allow it to cool and then serve it to your chickens in place of their regular water. This will not only hydrate them but also provide them with essential nutrients that help boost their immunity.

Fall is also a great time to introduce herbs into your chicken's dust bath. Adding thyme and echinacea to the dust bath can provide health benefits, while rosehips can add an interesting element for your chickens to peck at while they bathe.

As the seasons change and the leaves begin to fall, encouraging your chickens to forage becomes a natural part of their daily activities. Free-range chickens love to scratch and peck at the ground, seeking out bugs, seeds, and fresh greenery. They will naturally supplement their diets with what they find, but you can enhance this process by preserving late-blooming herbs and creating a plentiful fall foraging area.

Consider the value of herbs like sage, parsley, and calendula, which are hardy late bloomers that can provide ongoing nutrition and health benefits. Sage is not only a flavorful herb that chickens love but also packed with antioxidants and known to improve overall chicken health. Parsley, a cold-tolerant herb, is high in vitamins and can support chicken's respiratory health. Calendula, with its bright orange flowers, can add color to egg yolks and offer antifungal and anti-inflammatory properties.

Preserving these herbs for later use can be as simple as drying them. Cut the herbs at their peak, tie them in small bundles, and hang them upside down in a dry, well-ventilated area. Once they are thoroughly dried, store them in a cool, dark place, and they'll be ready to use when needed.

To create an enticing forage area for your flock, scatter some of the preserved herbs in a designated area of the chicken run. You could also plant a fall garden with some hardy, chicken-friendly plants like kale, spinach, and collard greens.

Chickens are natural foragers and providing them with a designated area where they can scratch and peck to their heart's content not only keeps them busy but also helps reduce their feed costs, keep them healthy, and contributes to higher quality eggs.

Another brilliant fall foraging strategy is using the fall leaves as a natural form of bedding in the coop and the run. The leaves not only serve as insulation but also attract a variety of insects that chickens love to snack on. Plus, once they're done with the leaves, you have a rich compost ready for your spring planting.

Setting up a compost pile within the chicken run can be a win-win situation. Your flock gets to enjoy the insects and worms that are attracted to the compost, and you get a high-quality fertilizer for your garden. Plus, the composting process generates heat, which can be particularly beneficial as the temperatures begin to dip in fall.

One more fall activity that you can encourage is pumpkin pecking. Pumpkins are a fall favorite and a great source of vitamins and fiber. The seeds can act as a natural dewormer. Simply cut a pumpkin in half and let your chickens enjoy it at their leisure. Not only will they relish the treat, but they'll also be getting a ton of nutritional benefits.

Every change in season brings about new opportunities to improve your flock's health and happiness. It's about understanding the unique attributes of each season and using them to your advantage. Fall, with its abundance of late-blooming herbs, fallen leaves, and harvest produce, offers plenty of resources that you can use to create a nutrient-rich, exciting environment for your chickens.

Fall is a special time in the world of chicken keeping. The changing colors and crisp air make it a pleasure to be outside tending to the coop. It's a season of harvest, gathering, and preparation. As you and your flock move through these tasks together, remember to enjoy the beauty of the season and the plentiful gifts it provides for our chickens and us. It truly is a season of abundance, an abundance that we can all be grateful for. The goal is to use these herbal blends to build your chickens' immunity, making them healthier and more resistant to disease. But beyond that, these herbs add a variety of flavors to their diet, making their daily meals more exciting.

Each flock is unique, and what works best for one may not necessarily be the same for another. Don't hesitate to try new things and experiment with different herbs and fall produce. What matters most is that you're making an effort to provide your chickens with a varied diet and stimulating environment, which will not only help them physically but also mentally, keeping them content and stress-free. Just make sure to introduce new herbs gradually and monitor your flock for any adverse reactions. Providing your flock with an enriched, diverse environment and diet will lead to happy, healthy chickens. Enjoy the autumn season, and remember, your flock will appreciate all your efforts to keep them thriving throughout the year.

As you enjoy the beauty of the autumn leaves and the crisp fall air, remember that this season is a time of preparation. Every step you take to ensure the well-being of your chickens during this period is an investment in their health and happiness during the winter months. Let this spirit of preparation guide you as you use the abundance of fall to create a safe, nourishing, and enriching environment for your flock. Embrace the season's changes, and enjoy the journey of getting your flock ready for winter. It's all part of the unique, rewarding experience that is chicken keeping. After all, as we've discovered, a well-prepared chicken is a happy chicken!

Part IV: Winter Warmers: Herbs for Cold Weather Comfort

Winter has a beauty of its own, but it brings its share of challenges for backyard chickens. Decreased daylight hours can affect egg production, the chilly winds can cause cold stress, and the snow might limit the outdoor foraging opportunities for your flock. However, just like the other seasons, winter too offers unique ways to utilize herbs to make this time more comfortable for your chickens.

A decrease in daylight hours is one of the first signs of winter's arrival. Chickens, like many animals, are highly influenced by natural light patterns, and as days shorten, it affects their laying cycles. Many backyard chickens will slow down or stop laying eggs completely during the winter months. While this is a normal process and gives the hens a much-needed break, you can still support their health during this time by providing a balanced diet and an enriched environment. Certain herbs like fenugreek can be beneficial in supporting egg production and overall health. It's an excellent source of protein and can also aid digestion.

Cold stress is another significant challenge that chickens face during winter. It can result in weight loss, decreased egg production, and, if not managed properly, can even lead to frostbite. But you can help your chickens combat cold stress by incorporating herbs into their diet and environment. Herbs like oregano, thyme, and rosemary are not only packed with vitamins and antioxidants, but they also have powerful natural warming properties. Adding these herbs to your chickens' diet can help them generate heat and maintain their body temperature.

Let's not forget about garlic. While not an herb, it is an excellent dietary supplement for chickens during the winter. Garlic has natural antibiotic properties that can help boost the immune system and combat potential diseases. It also helps in blood circulation, which is vital in cold weather to keep all parts of the chicken's body warm.

In the coop, herbs can also serve another essential function: insulation. A thick layer of dried herbs like straw, pine, and fir not only provide physical warmth to your chickens but also carry aromatic compounds that can deter pests and keep the coop smelling fresh. Herbs like lavender and mint are particularly effective in this regard.

Incorporating herbs into your chickens' water supply can also be a game-changer. Adding herbs like sage, thyme, or oregano to their water can boost their immune system and help keep them hydrated. Hydration is crucial in winter as chickens often forget to drink water when it's cold, leading to dehydration. Having aromatic herbs in their water can encourage drinking.

One of the most significant winter challenges is the lack of foraging opportunities. With snow covering the ground, your chickens might not be able to scratch and peck as much as they would like to. This can lead to boredom and potential behavioral issues. However, you can create an indoor foraging environment for your chickens by providing a mixture of dried herbs, grains, and seeds. Herbs like parsley and calendula, dried fruits like cranberries, and a variety of seeds can keep your chickens busy and entertained.

Moreover, there's a whole arsenal of herbs that serve dual purposes in the coop during winter, providing not only dietary benefits but also natural heat. Chief among these are garlic, ginger, and cayenne. These herbs, when used strategically, can turn the coop into a winter fortress that keeps your chickens warm, healthy, and content.

Let's start with garlic. We have discussed garlic in previous chapters however it is a very useful herb for your flock! More than just a kitchen staple, garlic is a powerhouse of nutrition and medicinal properties that are beneficial for your flock, especially during winter. Regular consumption of garlic boosts the immune system, helping your chickens fight off potential illnesses. What's more, garlic is known to improve circulation, a crucial function that ensures all parts of your chicken's body stay warm in cold weather.

A tip to incorporate garlic into your flock's diet is to mince or crush the cloves and mix them in with their regular feed. Doing so can be a game-changer, particularly in winter. Moreover, adding minced garlic to their water can work wonders as well, as the aroma can encourage your chickens to hydrate more often.

Moving on to ginger, another herb that's a real winter warmer. Just like garlic, ginger is also packed with vitamins, minerals, and antioxidants. Most importantly, it has natural warming properties, which make it an excellent choice for your flock in winter. Ginger aids digestion, increases circulation, and boosts the immune system. You can mix ginger powder into your chickens' feed or provide fresh, finely chopped ginger for them to peck at.

Lastly, cayenne, the fiery spice that can literally heat up your coop. Capsaicin, the compound that gives cayenne its heat, is beneficial in maintaining body temperature. When chickens consume cayenne, it boosts their metabolism and body heat. However, use cayenne with caution and always in moderation as too much can be too hot for your chickens to handle. Mixing a small amount into their feed is the best way to incorporate it into their diet.

In addition to garlic, ginger, and cayenne, there are many other herbs like thyme, oregano, and rosemary that can contribute to maintaining a warm coop environment. Thyme and oregano have excellent immune-boosting properties, while rosemary is known for its calming effects, making it a great stress reliever for chickens during the cold, dark winter months.

As we explore the subject of winter diets,, it's crucial to remember that a chicken's dietary needs change with the seasons. During winter, their energy demands increase as they work to keep their body temperature up in the face of plummeting temperatures. This calls for an adjustment in their diet, boosting calories and nutrient intake to match their heightened metabolic needs.

Let's start with herbs like fenugreek and fennel seeds. Fenugreek is a legume that is packed with protein, a vital macronutrient for your flock, particularly in winter. Protein is needed not only for egg production but also for maintaining feather health, which is crucial for insulation against the cold. You can sprout fenugreek seeds and add them to your chickens' feed or scatter them in the coop for foraging.

Fennel seeds, too, are a nutritional powerhouse. They contain high amounts of antioxidants, which are beneficial for your chickens' overall health. Fennel seeds also stimulate appetite and aid digestion, ensuring your flock eats well and extracts the maximum nutrition from their feed. You can mix these seeds into your chicken feed or offer them separately in a treat dish.

Flaxseed is another herb to consider during winter. It's an excellent source of omega-3 fatty acids, which are known to improve egg quality. The nutrient-dense seeds can help maintain your chickens' energy levels during the cold days. Ground flaxseed can be mixed into chicken feed, or you can sprinkle whole flaxseed in the coop for your chickens to scratch and peck at.

Herbs like alfalfa and nettles should also feature in your winter herb strategy. Alfalfa is rich in protein and calcium, the latter being especially crucial for hens laying eggs during winter. You can provide dried alfalfa leaves for your chickens to nibble on. Nettles, on the other hand, offer a range of minerals and vitamins, making them a highly nutritious winter supplement. Dried nettles can be added directly to your chicken feed.

When it comes to boosting calories, herbs alone might not be enough. It's a good idea to supplement your flock's diet with grains like corn, oats, and barley. These grains are high in calories and can provide the energy your chickens need to stay warm. You can offer them separately as a treat or mix them into your chicken feed.

It's equally important to ensure your flock has constant access to fresh, unfrozen water. Chickens need to stay hydrated to maintain their metabolic functions, and this is equally important in winter as it is in summer. Therefore, you might want to consider investing in a heated waterer to prevent the water from freezing.

Now let's shift gears a bit and talk about how to create a cozy environment in your coop with winter herbal remedies. Using herbs to create warm broths and other comfort measures can help make the coop a welcoming place for your chickens during the cold months.

A great starting point is a warm herbal broth. This is essentially a strong herbal tea that your chickens can drink to keep warm and receive an extra dose of nutrients. A blend of echinacea, oregano, and garlic makes a potent immune-boosting broth that can help fend off cold-weather illnesses. Add a tablespoon of each herb to a quart of boiling water, let it steep for about 20 minutes, then cool before offering it to your chickens in place of their usual water. Be sure to provide fresh water alongside the broth.

Another remedy involves creating a "winter warmer" grain mix. This mix incorporates warming herbs like ginger and cayenne into a base of calorie-dense grains like corn, oats, and barley. Adding a couple of tablespoons of ground ginger and a teaspoon of cayenne to a pound of mixed grains can provide a subtle warmth that's beneficial for your chickens in winter. The grains can be soaked in the herbal broth mentioned earlier for an added nutrient boost before feeding it to your flock.

Heated perches are another interesting concept to explore. Though not directly involving herbs, they can significantly contribute to a cozy coop. Essentially, these are perches that have a heating element inside, providing a warm spot for your chickens to roost on cold winter nights.

Herbal bedding can also help to keep your coop warm and cozy. A mixture of straw bedding with dried herbs like lavender, mint, and rosemary can create a fragrant and comfortable environment for your chickens. These herbs not only have pest-repelling properties but also have a calming effect that can be beneficial during the stressful winter period.

If you're looking for a way to provide your chickens with a warm treat, consider making a herbal suet cake. Suet is essentially fat, and it's a fantastic source of energy and heat for chickens in winter. You can melt suet or lard, mix in a variety of seeds, grains, and finely chopped herbs like parsley, thyme, and calendula, then pour the mixture into a mold and let it harden. Hang these suet cakes in your coop for your chickens to peck at.

While herbs and proper nutrition are key to ensuring a healthy and comfortable flock during winter, there are more aspects to consider when it comes to managing the coop. Let's discuss some crucial factors like ventilation, insulation, and lighting that contribute to maintaining a comfortable coop during winter.

Firstly, ventilation is crucial, regardless of the season. Chickens generate a significant amount of moisture through their breath, droppings, and even perspiration. In a poorly ventilated coop, this moisture accumulates and can condense on colder surfaces, potentially leading to health problems like frostbite and respiratory diseases. Make sure that your coop has adequate ventilation, but avoid creating drafts, which can chill your birds. The aim is to enable moist air to escape without allowing cold wind to blow directly on your chickens.

Insulation is equally essential. Your coop's walls, ceiling, and floor should ideally have insulation to keep the cold out and warmth in. A variety of materials can serve as insulation, ranging from commercial insulation materials to more natural ones like straw. Besides using materials, you can also strategically place the roosting bars away from doors and windows to avoid drafts.

Heating the coop might be something to consider if you're in a particularly cold region. However, it's generally not recommended due to fire hazards and because chickens are quite good at keeping themselves warm. Instead, focus on providing them with a dry and draft-free environment, and let their feathers do their job. If you're still concerned about the cold, consider breeds that are well-suited for colder climates when starting or adding to your flock.

While I do not recommend substituting their lighting it is another element that may require attention for some. As the days get shorter in winter, the reduction in daylight can affect egg production. Supplemental lighting can help maintain production levels. A light source set on a timer to provide 14-16 hours of light overall can be beneficial. However, sudden changes in light exposure can be stressful for your birds, so it's better to increase the light duration gradually. Winter is a time for hens to get a well-deserved break from the demand spring and summer put on their bodies. This is the season that they get a well-deserved break from constantly laying eggs which in turn also ensures their health. As a natural chicken keeper, I do not support creating unnatural lighting in your coop.

Herbs can also play a part in keeping your coop comfortable in winter. Certain herbs like mint and lavender have insect-repelling properties and can be used in the coop bedding to deter parasites that could stress your chickens. Others like rosemary, thyme, and oregano can be hung in bunches around the coop. They'll release their essential oils, creating a soothing environment that also helps keep the air fresh.

Maintaining clean, dry bedding is vital, especially in winter. Bedding helps to insulate the coop floor, and it also absorbs droppings and other moisture, helping to keep the coop dry. Good choices for winter bedding are straw and wood shavings. Adding a layer of dried herbs to the bedding not only infuses the coop with a pleasant aroma but also helps deter pests and parasites.

Winter can be a challenging season for chickens, but with a well-managed coop and the strategic use of herbs, you can help your flock stay healthy and comfortable. While herbs are valuable, they are a part of the bigger picture of coop management that includes considerations like ventilation, insulation, and lighting. The objective is to keep your chickens comfortable and healthy during the cold months. Creative use of herbs can help you achieve that, and your chickens will thank you for it with their continued good health and productivity. With these strategic additions to your chickens' winter diet, you can help ensure they stay healthy and productive despite the cold. The aim is not just survival but thriving, and a well-thought-out diet can go a long way in achieving that.

While these herbs and grains can bolster your chickens' diet, it's important to remember that they are supplements and not substitutes for a balanced chicken feed. Your flock still needs a good quality poultry feed that meets all their dietary requirements. However, these herbs and grains can definitely enhance the nutritional value of their diet and help them navigate the harsh winter months.

The aim isn't just to get through winter but to have a thriving, healthy flock when spring arrives. Armed with this knowledge of winter herbs and their benefits, you can ensure that your flock gets the very best care, no matter how harsh the winter is. These are natural, effective strategies that you can employ to maintain the health, productivity, and happiness of your chickens, even during the coldest months of the year. The power of herbs is immense, and winter is the perfect time to harness this power for the well-being of your flock. By understanding their needs and challenges, you can use herbs to create a warm, enriched environment throughout the cold months. I will say it again, the happier and healthier your chickens are, the better their egg production and overall performance will be. So, don't let the cold weather deter you. Embrace the winter season and use it as an opportunity to explore new ways to enhance your flock's health and happiness with herbs. So, get your dried herbs ready, keep your garlic handy, and get ready to face the winter months head-on. With a little planning and a lot of love, you can ensure your chickens stay warm, happy, and healthy, no matter how low the temperature drops.

Raising chickens is much more than an engaging hobby; it's a journey filled with learning and discovery. The process of understanding your flock's needs, knowing the value of various herbs, and learning to incorporate them effectively can seem like a lot. Yet, it's a fulfilling process that leads to a healthy and content flock. And, in the end, that's what truly matters. Your journey through each season with your chickens is filled with opportunity and growth - for them and for you, too. Remember, every step you take is an integral part of creating a natural, thriving, and vibrant environment for your chickens. And in doing so, you create the same for yourself. Enjoy the journey, and embrace the change each season brings.

Chapter 4: Herbal Treats for Happy Clucks

Part I: Herby Snacks: Delicious Herbal Treat Remedies

Before we jump into the herby goodness we are going to kick things off with an essential discussion about the place of treats in a balanced chicken diet. Understanding the limits and benefits of these little indulgences can make a world of difference to the health and happiness of your chickens.

Chickens, like people, enjoy variety in their diets. The joy of scratching and pecking, exploring new flavors, and the sheer excitement that comes from finding something different in their usual feed - it all adds up to happier, more contented chickens. And that's precisely where treats come in.

However, before we dive into the world of homemade herbal treats, let's clarify one essential point: treats are just that - treats. They're not meant to replace a balanced chicken diet but to complement it. A chicken's daily intake should predominantly consist of complete chicken feed, which is specifically formulated to provide all the nutrients they need. Consider treats as the icing on the cake, an occasional delight rather than the norm.

So, what benefits can herbal treats provide apart from brightening up your chickens' day? For starters, many herbs have nutritional benefits. Take dandelion leaves, for example. They're a fantastic source of vitamins A, C, and K, not to mention calcium and potassium. Or consider parsley, which is rich in vitamins A and C and iron. These nutrients contribute to your chickens' overall health, enhancing their immune systems and aiding in the production of high-quality eggs.

The advantages of herbal treats go beyond nutrition, though. Many herbs have properties that can support the well-being of your flock in other ways. From aiding digestion to deterring pests, the benefits can be surprisingly diverse. For instance, adding a touch of oregano to your treat mix can help boost your chickens' immune systems. Incorporating some garlic can enhance respiratory health and deter pests. Sprinkling in a bit of mint could help keep the coop smelling fresh, and as a bonus, it's believed to be a natural insecticide. However, moderation is key. Overloading on treats can lead to dietary imbalances and potential health problems down the line. Obesity can be a serious issue in chickens, just as it is in humans, leading to a host of associated health problems, not least of which is a decline in egg production. An excellent guideline to follow is the '90/10' rule: 90% of your chickens' diet should come from complete feed and fresh water, while treats make up the remaining 10%.

Consider also the size of your treats. Larger pieces can encourage natural behaviors like pecking and scratching, which contributes to a more stimulated and thus happier flock. However, ensure any large pieces are safe to consume, not posing choking hazards. For instance, if you're treating your chickens to a sizable pumpkin chunk, it would be a good idea to remove the stringy innards to prevent any potential blockages.

Let's take a walk through the veritable herb garden of options you can utilize in creating herbal treats for your chickens. There's a world of flavors and benefits to explore, from the robust flavors of parsley and basil to the potent wellness-enhancing properties of oregano.

Parsley sits high on the list of chicken-friendly herbs. Renowned for its vitamins A, C, and E, as well as iron and antioxidant properties, parsley provides a myriad of benefits. It aids in blood vessel development, supports immune function, and enhances overall health. To chickens, parsley is a gourmet treat they'll likely flock to, pecking and scratching eagerly. Try mixing chopped parsley with grains or scattering it among their regular feed for a vitamin-packed surprise.

Another flavorful herb your chickens are likely to enjoy is basil. This herb isn't just about great taste; it's packed with vitamins A and K, and it also possesses anti-inflammatory properties. Basil helps improve skin and feather health, boosts the immune system, and even repels flies. Offering fresh basil leaves will not only encourage natural foraging behaviors but also keep your coop smelling wonderful.

As for oregano, it's much more than a favorite pizza topping. For chickens, it serves as a potent health booster. Oregano has antibacterial and anti-parasitic effects, making it an excellent addition to your poultry wellness toolkit. Adding it to your herbal treats can provide your chickens with essential nutrients while helping keep them disease-free. Moreover, oregano aids in respiratory health, something particularly beneficial in the colder months.

Speaking of potent herbs, let's not forget garlic. This herb is a superfood known for its antimicrobial and immune-boosting qualities. While not every chicken might take to its strong flavor immediately, many will come to enjoy it when mixed with other ingredients. Garlic helps maintain overall health, improves respiratory conditions, and can even help in external parasite control. Imagine that—a treat that also keeps pests at bay!

How about some mint? It's not only a refreshing treat, but mint also helps keep the coop cooler in the summer months due to its natural cooling properties. Additionally, mint can aid in respiratory health, deter rodents, and keep your coop smelling fresh. Offering your chickens a peck at a hanging bunch of mint can entertain them, promoting pecking and scratching behavior.

Rosemary is another herb worth mentioning. Not only does it smell divine, but it's also packed with benefits for your flock. It's known for its calming properties and is also rich in antioxidants and anti-inflammatory compounds. It's a fantastic herb for overall wellness and can be used in many forms – dried, fresh, or even as a sprig for them to peck at.

Thyme, rich in antioxidants, is an excellent herb to enhance your flock's health. It promotes respiratory health, acts against certain harmful organisms, and even helps chickens cope with stress. It can be given fresh or dried, mixed in with their feed, or in a treat block.

Marjoram is an excellent laying stimulant, making it beneficial for egg production. Moreover, it's believed to have anti-inflammatory, antibacterial, and antioxidant properties. If your flock is in a laying slump, a marjoram-infused treat might be just what they need.

The herbal world offers a bounty of flavors and health benefits to explore. Each herb has something unique to offer, be it nutritional value or health-boosting properties. Treat time can be more than just a fun interlude; it can be an opportunity to enhance your chickens' health and happiness in a way they're bound to love.

Enhancing your chickens' health and happiness is a goal that's easily achievable through the power of herbs. We've touched on the benefits of numerous herbs, and now, we're going to explore the art of crafting simple, delicious herbal treats for your chickens.

1. Now, let's start with a simple but highly nutritious treat: Parsley Pea Pods. These are not only easy to make but also pack a nutritional punch with the combined benefits of peas and parsley. Here's how to make them:

- Hollow out a few large pea pods, removing the peas.
- Finely chop fresh parsley and mix with the removed peas.
- Spoon the mixture back into the pea pods.
- Serve these to your chickens and watch them have a pecking good time!

2. Another herbal delight your chickens will love is Basil and Berry Surprise. This treat is a combination of antioxidant-rich berries and vitamin-packed basil. Here's how it's done:

- Take a handful of fresh or frozen berries - strawberries, blueberries, raspberries, whatever you have on hand.
- Roughly chop a handful of fresh basil leaves.
- Mix the berries and basil together and serve it up. Watch your hens flock to this fruity and herby surprise!

3. Let's not forget about garlic. Despite its strong flavor, it's a superfood for chickens, offering many health benefits. So, here's a simple remedy: Garlic and Grains Medley.

- Cook a cup of grains (like quinoa or brown rice) as per instructions.
- While the grains are still warm, mix in a couple of finely minced garlic cloves.
- Let the mix cool down before serving it to your hens. This treat is a fantastic way to introduce garlic to your flock.

4. A refreshing summer treat could be Minty Watermelon Cooler. It's as simple as it sounds:

- Cut watermelon into cubes or scoops.
- Sprinkle with finely chopped fresh mint leaves.
- Serve it chilled. It's a fantastic way to keep your chickens cool and hydrated during the hot months.

5. Thyme is an excellent herb to help your chickens cope with stress, and here's a simple treat remedy: Thyme and Corn Mingle.

- Cook some fresh corn on the cob and let it cool.
- Lightly brush the corn cob with olive oil and then sprinkle dried thyme over it.
- Give the cob to your chickens. They'll love pecking at it, and it'll serve as an enriching activity.

6. Lastly, let's consider a treat that could stimulate egg-laying: Marjoram Oat Clusters.

- Mix two cups of oats with a handful of finely chopped fresh marjoram.
- Add in a couple of whisked eggs and mix well to combine.
- Shape the mixture into small clusters and bake at 350°F (175°C) for about 15 minutes or until golden.
- Once cooled, these clusters are ready for your hens to enjoy.

The world of homemade chicken treats is not only exciting but also filled with opportunities for nutrition and delight for your hens. But how exactly do you offer these treats? When is the best time? What methods should you use, and what are the appropriate portion sizes? Let's explore these queries together to get the most out of our herby treats.

First off, timing is crucial. Generally, it's best to offer treats to your chickens in the afternoon. This strategy ensures your hens have had plenty of time to fill their crops with their regular feed, which should always be the main part of their diet. If treats are offered too early, chickens might overindulge, potentially leading to an unbalanced diet. A late afternoon treat not only works well with their eating schedule but also gives your hens something to look forward to during the day.

In terms of methods, the way you present treats can affect both the enjoyment of your chickens and their health. One way to offer treats is by scattering them in the coop or run. This method encourages natural foraging behavior and provides physical and mental stimulation. It helps to mimic the way chickens would naturally find their food in the wild, pecking and scratching around to find delicious morsels.

On the other hand, if you're introducing a new treat, it might be best to offer it in a controlled way, perhaps in a separate dish or feeding trough. This way, you can observe how your hens react to the new food item. It's also a great method if you're offering treats that can be messy, like the Parsley Pea Pods or Minty Watermelon Cooler we mentioned earlier.

Now, onto portion sizes. A good rule of thumb is the 90/10 rule. This means that treats, including your homemade herby treats, should make up no more than 10% of your chickens' daily intake, with the remaining 90% being a balanced chicken feed. This rule helps ensure that treats remain treats and don't overshadow the essential nutrients your hens need from their primary food source.

The size of the treat can significantly influence how your hens interact with it. Larger treats like the Marjoram Oat Clusters might be a fun challenge for your hens, encouraging them to peck and nibble, promoting natural behaviors. On the other hand, smaller, easier-to-peck foods like the Basil and Berry Surprise may be quickly gobbled up by eager beaks, making them perfect for a quick and enjoyable snack. However, determining the right treat isn't just about the size or the remedy; it also involves observing your chickens, understanding their preferences, and figuring out why they prefer certain treats over others.

To begin, observation is a significant aspect of chicken keeping that often goes unnoticed. Spending time with your chickens, watching their behaviors, their interaction with their environment, and each other can tell you a lot about their preferences. It's a delightful exercise, a time to bond with your flock and gain insight into their little chicken lives.

For instance, you might observe that your chickens enjoy pecking at the Basil and Berry Surprise more when it's scattered around the coop rather than served in a dish. This observation could be because chickens are natural foragers and scattering treats taps into this instinct, making the treat not just a food source but also an entertaining activity.

In contrast, you might notice that your chickens prefer the Marjoram Oat Clusters when they're hung from a string in the coop. This method could simulate the challenge of pecking at something that moves, much like pecking at insects in the wild. The added challenge might make the treat more appealing, not just filling their bellies but also providing mental stimulation.

Another factor in treat preference can be the individual personalities of your chickens. Yes, chickens do have personalities! Some may be more adventurous and willing to try new treats, while others may be more cautious, sticking to tried-and-true favorites. Observing these personality traits can help you cater to each chicken's preferences, ensuring all members of your flock are happy and satisfied.

Of course, the health benefits of the herbs you use can also factor into your chickens' preferences. For example, you might notice your chickens are particularly fond of treats containing garlic or oregano. These herbs are known for their immune-boosting properties, and it's possible that your chickens, in their own way, recognize these benefits.

Finally, the freshness and quality of your ingredients can play a substantial role in your flock's preferences. Fresh, high-quality ingredients are more likely to be a hit with your chickens, packed with flavors and nutrients that might be missing in less fresh or lower-quality ingredients. Remember, the quality of the treats you offer can directly impact the health and productivity of your flock.

An essential aspect to remember when offering treats is to watch your flock's reaction. Chickens can have preferences, just like us, and might enjoy some treats more than others. Some might gobble up certain herbs, while others turn up their beaks. It may take some trial and error to figure out which herbs your flock likes best, so feel free to experiment and monitor their reactions. If you notice a particular treat isn't a hit, don't be disheartened. It's all part of the learning process. You're getting to know your flock better, understanding their likes and dislikes.

Observing your chickens' preferences and understanding the factors that influence them can enhance your chicken-keeping experience. It's not just about providing treats but about understanding your flock, their behaviors, and their preferences. It's an ongoing process, a continual learning experience filled with surprises and delightful discoveries. So, the next time you whip up a batch of herbal treats, take a moment to watch your chickens enjoy them. You might be surprised at what you discover!

In essence, while herbal treats are a delightful addition to your chickens' diet, they should be given thoughtfully and in moderation. They're an excellent way to diversify your flock's diet and encourage natural behaviors, all while providing additional nutritional benefits. And remember, treat time is also an opportunity for interaction and bonding - a moment to relish in the simple pleasure of making your chickens cluck with happiness.

In conclusion, the key to offering treats lies in balancing enjoyment with health considerations. With the right timing, methods, and portion sizes, treat time can be a source of happiness and health for your chickens, enriching their lives and diet in a flavorful way..

Part II: Scratch and Peck: Fun Foraging Mixes

Foraging is more than just an activity for your chickens; it's an essential part of their daily routine that greatly contributes to their overall health and well-being. The action of scratching and pecking at the ground isn't simply a way for chickens to find food; it's a form of physical exercise, mental stimulation, and a way for them to engage in their natural behaviors.

Think about it: chickens in the wild spend a significant part of their day foraging for food, and they've developed a range of behaviors and skills around this activity. They scratch the ground to uncover hidden treats, peck at different objects to figure out if they're edible, and explore their surroundings to find the best foraging spots. This activity keeps them physically fit and mentally stimulated, ensuring their health and well-being.

In a backyard setting, where chickens might not have as much space to roam and explore, foraging can still play a crucial role in maintaining your flock's health. As a chicken keeper, it's important to encourage this natural behavior as much as possible. This can be done by providing a variety of foraging materials and opportunities for your flock.

Creating your own foraging mixes can be a fun and rewarding way to encourage this natural behavior. These mixes can contain a variety of ingredients like grains, seeds, dried herbs, and even dried insects. The diversity of ingredients not only provides a range of flavors and textures for your chickens to enjoy but also ensures they get a balanced diet.

For instance, grains like wheat, oats, and barley can be the base of your foraging mix. These grains are high in energy and easy for chickens to digest. Seeds like sunflower seeds, flax seeds, and pumpkin seeds are packed with essential nutrients like protein and healthy fats. Dried herbs can add a flavorful kick to your mix while also providing health benefits. For example, lavender is known for its calming properties, and adding it to your foraging mix can help create a more peaceful coop environment.

Dried insects like mealworms or crickets can also be a big hit with chickens. In the wild, insects form a significant part of a chicken's diet, providing them with protein and other essential nutrients. Adding dried insects to your foraging mix can help replicate this aspect of a chicken's natural diet.

In addition to providing nutrition, these foraging mixes also serve another important purpose: they stimulate your chickens mentally and physically. Scratching and pecking through the mix to find their favorite treats can keep your chickens entertained for hours, reducing boredom and associated behaviors like feather pecking.

The very act of foraging requires chickens to be active, keeping them physically fit. Their innate curiosity drives them to explore and sample a variety of ingredients in the mix, from seeds and grains to a colorful array of herbs. It's this wonderful world of herbs that we will dive into next.

Incorporating herbs into the foraging mix isn't just about adding variety. Each herb has unique qualities that contribute to a hen's health. From boosting immune function to calming stress, herbs work wonders in promoting poultry health. Let's look at some herbs that your flock might find irresistible.

First on our list is the dandelion. You might see it as a pesky weed, but to chickens, it's a nutrient-packed treat. Dandelions are rich in calcium and vitamins A, C, and K. These nutrients are critical to eggshell formation and overall health.

Next, we have plantain. Not to be confused with the banana-like fruit, plantain is a common weed with ribbed leaves and tall flower spikes. Chickens adore plantain for its tender leaves, but they also get the bonus of plantain's anti-inflammatory and wound-healing properties.

Clover is another favorite in the poultry world. This hardy plant is not only easy to grow but also packed with protein, making it a healthy addition to your foraging mix. Chickens usually love both red and white clover, and as a bonus, these plants are excellent soil improvers.

Adding mint to your foraging mix can also bring about benefits. Mint is a known insect repellent, so it might help keep pesky bugs away from your coop. Plus, its cooling flavor could be a hit during the summer months.

Thyme is an aromatic herb known for its antibacterial properties, and chickens generally love its flavor. It's a great choice if you want to boost your flock's immunity.

Lastly, consider adding some sage to your mix. This herb is not only a flavorful treat but is also known for its antioxidant and anti-parasitic properties.

But these are just a few examples. The world of herbs is vast, and your foraging mix can include any combination of herbs based on what's locally available and what your chickens prefer. Whether you grow these herbs in your garden or source them locally, be sure to use only untreated, safe-to-consume plants.

Now, let's dive into the fun part: creating engaging foraging mixes. The key here is variety, presentation, and portion sizes. Foraging mixes are at their most engaging when they incorporate a wide array of ingredients. A diverse mix keeps chickens intrigued and motivates them to peck and scratch to discover the different textures and flavors. As we have already mentioned, include herbs like dandelion, plantain, clover, mint, thyme, and sage. But don't stop there! You can also add grains, seeds, and even dried fruits and vegetables to add even more depth to your mix.

In terms of grains, options like corn, wheat, and oats are a hit with most flocks. For seeds, consider pumpkin seeds, sunflower seeds, and sesame seeds. Dried fruits like raisins or apples and dried vegetables like carrots or peas can add a sweet or savory surprise to the mix.

While creating a foraging mix, pay attention to the size and texture of the ingredients. Different sizes and textures not only keep your chickens mentally stimulated but also ensure they exercise different parts of their beak and neck muscles.

Also, consider the presentation. Instead of simply throwing the mix onto the ground, consider creating engaging 'foraging spots.' For instance, you can hang a head of lettuce or a bunch of herbs from a rope in the coop or bury treats in a sandbox. Encourage your flock to work a bit to get their treats, imitating the challenge of foraging in the wild.

Another fun idea is to use treat balls or similar feeding devices that require some manipulation. Stuff the foraging mix into these devices and watch your hens have a blast pecking and kicking to get their treats. Not only does this add an element of play, but it also slows down the eating process, helping prevent issues like crop impaction.

In terms of portion sizes, it's essential to remember that foraging mixes, while nutritious, should not replace a balanced chicken feed. Aim for the foraging mix to make up no more than 10% to 20% of your chickens' daily diet. This way, they get the enjoyment and benefits of foraging without risking nutritional imbalances.

Remember to scatter the foraging mix over a wide area to encourage more movement and prevent crowding. Doing so also reduces competition among your flock and ensures that even the lower-ranking chickens get their fair share of the treats. Creating a harmonious and stress-free environment is a significant part of ensuring a happy, healthy flock.

Adjusting the foraging mixes in response to your flock's preferences and nutritional needs is an integral part of flock management. You can't just set a standard mix and forget it. It's a dynamic process that needs regular attention and tweaking. After all, chickens, like us, have their own individual preferences, and their nutritional needs can vary based on factors such as age, breed, and health status.

To start, spend some time observing your flock during their foraging sessions. Which ingredients do they peck at first? Which do they seem to ignore or leave till the end? Do they have a particular liking for certain herbs or grains over others? This kind of chicken-watching might seem time-consuming, but it's actually a delightful way to spend a sunny afternoon and will provide invaluable insights into your flock's tastes.

As previously mentioned, it's not just about preferences but also about their nutritional needs. For instance, if your flock is molting, they may benefit from a foraging mix rich in protein. This could mean adding more seeds and legumes into the mix during this time. If your hens are laying, consider incorporating more calcium-rich ingredients, such as crushed eggshells or oyster shell.

Suppose you notice your chickens looking a bit dull or showing signs of low energy. In that case, they might benefit from herbs known for their health-boosting properties, such as thyme and oregano. On the other hand, if it's the height of summer and the heat is intense, consider herbs like mint or lemon balm, known for their cooling effects.

Also, remember to take seasons into account. The availability of herbs and other fresh ingredients will vary throughout the year, and so too should your foraging mix. An autumn mix might feature more root vegetables and hearty grains, while a spring mix might lean heavily on fresh, leafy greens and seeds.

And let's not forget that variety is the spice of life, especially for your chickens! Continuously offering the same foraging mix could lead to boredom, and a bored chicken is often an unhappy or disruptive chicken. So, even if you've found a mix that your chickens seem to love, don't be afraid to switch things up and introduce new ingredients from time to time.

Finally, keep in mind the balance of the entire diet. While the foraging mix is a delightful and beneficial part of your chickens' food intake, it is not the entirety. The foraging mix must be balanced with the other components of their diet, including their main feed, grit for digestion, and other treats or supplements they may receive.

So, armed with this knowledge, feel free to experiment with your foraging mixes. Your goal is not just to feed your chickens but to nurture them. By paying attention to their preferences, adjusting for their nutritional needs, and continually offering variety, you're doing more than just providing food. You're creating an environment where your chickens can thrive. Keep an eye on your flock as they explore the mix, noting which ingredients they seem to prefer and whether they enjoy certain presentations over others. With time, you'll become an expert in crafting foraging mixes that keep your flock healthy, entertained, and happily clucking all day long! The goal is to mimic your flock's natural foraging environment as closely as possible while also providing them with nutritional boosts. This means you can get creative with your mix – there's no one-size-fits-all remedy. So, have fun crafting your unique blend of foraging mix, and watch as your chickens delight in the scratch-and-peck adventure that awaits them! This can help keep your chickens healthy and happy, ensuring they live fulfilling lives. There's nothing more satisfying than watching a flock of healthy, happy chickens enthusiastically exploring a foraging mix you've lovingly prepared just for them. It's one of the many joys of chicken keeping! So, the next time you feed your chickens, don't just give them food - give them a foraging adventure!

Part III: Fresh is Best: Sprouting Your Own Herbs

Sprouting your own herbs is a delightful activity that pays off in multiple ways. Not only does it provide you with a ready supply of fresh, flavorful herbs for your kitchen, but it also offers a bounty of health benefits for your chickens. The process of sprouting enhances the nutritional value of the herbs, making them a supercharged treat for your flock.

Let's delve into the specifics. The magic of sprouting lies in the transformation that the seeds undergo during the process. Seeds are nature's powerhouses, crammed with nutrients needed for a plant's initial growth. However, these nutrients are typically locked away and are not easily accessed by our chickens.

When a seed is sprouted, however, this changes. The process of germination begins to break down the seed's outer protective layers, which means that those hard-to-digest nutrients suddenly become more accessible. At the same time, the sprouting process also triggers the seed to begin converting its stored nutrients into a form that can be used to fuel growth. This includes breaking down complex carbohydrates into simple sugars, proteins into amino acids, and fats into simpler fatty acids.

What does this mean for your chickens? In a nutshell, it means that sprouted herbs offer a nutritional boost compared to their unsprouted counterparts. They are richer in a range of essential nutrients, including vitamins, minerals, and enzymes. Plus, they also have higher protein content, a critical component for egg production, feather growth, and overall health of your hens.

Take, for instance, sprouted alfalfa. This humble herb, when sprouted, turns into a high-protein, high-energy food source that's loaded with essential amino acids, the building blocks of protein. Similarly, sprouted fenugreek can offer a powerful nutrient boost, including iron, magnesium, and a host of other vital minerals.

In addition to their enhanced nutritional profile, sprouted herbs are also easier for chickens to digest compared to whole seeds. This is again thanks to the sprouting process, which begins to break down the seed's outer layers. When your chickens consume sprouted herbs, they're able to extract more nutrients compared to consuming the seed in its unsprouted form. This can lead to improved digestion, more efficient nutrient absorption, and overall better health for your flock.

Let's not forget that sprouted herbs can also provide enrichment for your flock. Chickens love the process of pecking and scratching at the sprouts, which offers both mental and physical stimulation. Plus, the vibrant green of the sprouts can be a welcome sight in the coop, particularly during the colder months when fresh greens can be scarce.

Chickens enjoy variety, and sprouting different herbs for your flock can create a rainbow of flavors and nutrition that keeps them interested and promotes good health. The selection of herbs to sprout is vast, and each one brings its own unique qualities to the table.

Alfalfa is a top choice when it comes to sprouting. It's a rich source of protein, making it ideal for chickens in their prime laying years. The increased protein can help boost egg production and contribute to healthy feather growth. Additionally, alfalfa is packed with vital vitamins and minerals, including calcium for strong eggshells, magnesium for heart health, and potassium for overall cellular function.

Fenugreek is another herb worth considering for your sprouting adventures. This herb is known for its slightly sweet, nutty flavor that chickens seem to adore. Sprouted fenugreek is packed with iron and other minerals, contributing to the overall health of your flock. It's also high in fiber, promoting good digestion and absorption of nutrients.

Next on the list is mustard. Now, this may seem like an odd choice given its pungent flavor, but chickens are often more adventurous eaters than we give them credit for. Mustard sprouts bring a zing of flavor and a host of health benefits, from high levels of Vitamin A for eye health to selenium for healthy feather growth and egg production.

Clover sprouts are another excellent option. These sprouts are high in protein, similar to alfalfa, and contain an abundance of vitamins and minerals. Furthermore, their sweet and mild flavor makes them a favorite among many chickens. Clover sprouts also have the added benefit of being a rich source of isoflavones, compounds known to have anti-inflammatory and antioxidant benefits.

For a sprout with a mild, sweet flavor and a crispy texture that chickens enjoy, consider sprouting lentils. Sprouted lentils are a powerhouse of nutrition, boasting high levels of protein, fiber, and a multitude of essential vitamins and minerals. These include iron, potassium, and B vitamins, which are crucial for a chicken's overall well-being.

Beyond these, there are plenty more options to explore. Broccoli sprouts, sunflower sprouts, flax sprouts - the list goes on. Each brings a unique set of nutrients and flavors, making your sprouting journey a never-ending adventure.

Sprouting herbs at home is an engaging and rewarding process. It's as much a joy for you, the sprouter, as it is for your chickens who will relish the results. To ensure the process is successful, there are some important steps to follow.

The first task on your to-do list is assembling the necessary equipment. You'll need a container for sprouting, a strainer or cheesecloth, and of course, your chosen herb seeds. Mason jars are commonly used containers due to their wide opening, but any glass or food-safe plastic container will work. If using a jar, consider getting a sprouting lid - they make rinsing and draining the sprouts a breeze.

With your container in hand, you're ready to start. Rinse your seeds under cool, running water. Then place them in the container, filling only about one-eighth of it as sprouts need room to grow. Afterward, fill the container with cool water. The seeds should be covered by about two inches of water as they'll swell up during soaking.

Now comes the waiting game - let the seeds soak. Smaller seeds like alfalfa might only need four to six hours, while larger seeds like fenugreek might require up to twelve. This soaking phase is crucial as it activates the seeds, waking them up from dormancy and kickstarting the sprouting process.

After soaking, it's time to drain. If you're using a sprouting lid or a jar with cheesecloth secured with a rubber band, it's as simple as turning the jar upside down and giving it a good shake. Make sure to drain all the water - any remaining can lead to mold growth, which is a big no-no in the sprouting world.

Then begins the rinse and drain cycle, which will continue until your sprouts are ready. At least twice a day - morning and evening would be ideal - rinse your seeds with cool water and drain thoroughly. This rinse and drain cycle is important to provide the sprouts with moisture without letting them sit in water, which could cause rot.

In just a few days, you should start to see some action. Tiny white roots - these are the actual sprouts - will begin to emerge from the seeds. This is a good sign. It means your seeds are sprouting and growing.

As your sprouts continue to grow, remember to keep them out of direct sunlight and at room temperature. Sunlight can cause your sprouts to green, which might seem like a good thing, but it can actually make the sprouts tough and bitter. Room temperature is ideal as warmer temperatures can encourage mold growth.

Once your sprouts have grown to an ideal size - typically when the sprouted root is about the same length as the original seed - they're ready for your chickens. Do one final rinse and drain, and then it's treat time. Your chickens will appreciate the effort you've put into growing these nutritious and delicious sprouts.

With your sprouts ready and rinsed, the anticipation builds. You've put effort into sprouting these herbs, and now it's time for the real judges - your chickens - to have their say. Introducing sprouted herbs to your flock isn't complicated, but there are a few things to keep in mind to make the process smooth and beneficial for everyone involved.
But hold on, not so fast. Remember to introduce these new sprouts gradually, adding a small amount to their diet at first and then increasing it over time. This will give their digestive systems time to adjust to the new food.

Let's start with the 'when.' Sprouts are typically introduced to chickens in the morning. This ensures your flock has the entire day to explore, peck, and scratch at these new additions to their diet. It also means the sprouts won't sit uneaten overnight, which can attract unwanted pests to your chicken run or coop.

Now, onto the 'how.' Resist the temptation to simply toss the sprouts into the run or coop. Remember, these sprouts are new to your chickens, and we want to make their introduction as enticing as possible. Instead, consider presenting the sprouts in a shallow dish or scatter them on a clean surface where the chickens are sure to find them.

Observation is key here. Watch how your flock reacts to the sprouts. Are they intrigued, pecking at them immediately? Or are they hesitant, maintaining a safe distance from the unfamiliar greenery? Both reactions are normal. Chickens, like people, have their individual preferences and habits. Some might dive right in, while others may take their time. The goal here is not to rush the process.

Portion sizes are another factor to consider. A good rule of thumb is to offer sprouts as no more than 15% of your chickens' total daily intake. So, if you're feeding your chickens about two pounds of feed per day for a small flock, that's roughly five ounces of sprouts. Remember, sprouts are a treat, not a complete diet. Your chickens still need their regular feed for a balanced diet.

Introducing a new type of sprout? Consider mixing it with a variety your chickens are already familiar with. This approach helps ease the transition to the new sprout and encourages your chickens to try something new.

Additionally, keep a keen eye on the sprouts' condition. They should be consumed within a day of being offered to the chickens. Sprouts left uneaten for longer than that can start to degrade or mold, posing a health risk to your flock. Remove any uneaten sprouts at the end of the day.

What about young chicks? Can they enjoy the sprouted goodies as well? Absolutely! Sprouts are an excellent addition to chicks' diets. They offer a bounty of nutrients, are easy to digest, and provide a fun foraging experience. For chicks, make sure the sprouts are tender and easy for them to peck at and digest.

Ultimately, introducing sprouted herbs to your chickens should be an enjoyable experience for you and them. This is a time of discovery and enrichment for your flock, allowing them to explore new flavors, textures, and foraging opportunities. But as with anything new, there might be bumps along the way. It's all part of the journey. Sometimes, you might face sprouting issues like mold, poor germination, or even sprouts that just won't grow. Don't worry, though, these problems are usually easy to fix once you know what to look for and how to adjust your sprouting process.

First, let's tackle the issue of mold. Mold on your sprouts is a sign of too much moisture and insufficient airflow. To prevent this, ensure your sprouting containers have ample drainage. After rinsing the sprouts, make sure they're well-drained before you leave them to grow. A good practice is to rinse and drain the sprouts at least twice a day, morning and evening, to keep them clean and hydrated without being waterlogged. Keep your sprouting container in a well-ventilated area with indirect sunlight.

On to the next common issue - poor germination. When seeds don't sprout, or only a few do, it can be disappointing. The culprit here is often the quality of the seeds. Always use seeds meant for sprouting, as they're tested for germination and are untreated. Expired seeds or those stored improperly might not sprout well. Also, remember that each type of herb seed has a different sprouting time, so don't lose hope if you don't see sprouts right away.

There are times when your seeds may sprout, but the sprouts just won't grow. This usually points to an issue with the sprouting environment. Like all plants, sprouts need the right balance of water, air, and warmth. Too cold, and they won't grow; too hot, and they might wilt. Aim for a room temperature between 65-75°F for optimal sprouting conditions. If your sprouts are still not growing, they might not be getting enough air. Make sure your sprouting container is not overcrowded and has plenty of ventilation.

Now, let's say your sprouts are growing, but they look weak or spindly. This issue often comes down to insufficient light. While sprouts don't need direct sunlight, they do require bright, indirect light to grow strong and healthy. If you're sprouting indoors, consider placing your sprouting container near a north-facing window or under fluorescent lighting.

Lastly, if your sprouts have a strange smell, it's often a sign that they're fermenting, usually due to too much warmth or inadequate rinsing. Make sure you're rinsing your sprouts thoroughly at least twice a day, and store them in a cooler location.

While these are the most common sprouting issues, remember that every sprouting journey is unique. You might face different challenges, and that's okay. Consider them opportunities to learn more about the sprouting process and your unique growing environment.

If a batch of sprouts doesn't work out, don't be disheartened. Even experienced sprouters encounter failed batches from time to time. The key is not to give up. Try to identify what went wrong, make the necessary adjustments, and start again.

Sprouting is as much an art as it is a science. It requires patience, observation, and a willingness to learn. Each batch of sprouts brings with it a new opportunity to better understand the process and refine your skills. And remember, the goal is not perfection but progress.

So, carry on sprouting. Be mindful of these common issues, make adjustments as needed, and keep nurturing those nutritious sprouts for your chickens. Introducing sprouted herbs to your chickens is more than just a feeding process; it's a testament to the symbiotic relationship between you and your flock. You provide them with nutrient-rich sprouts, and in return, they reward you with healthy egg production, natural pest control, and their quirky, entertaining behaviors.

And that, in a nutshell, is the home sprouting process. It might seem daunting at first, but once you get the hang of it, it becomes second nature. The joy of watching tiny seeds transform into vibrant sprouts ready for your flock to enjoy is truly rewarding. Plus, you can rest easy knowing you're providing your flock with fresh, nutrient-packed food. Always choose seeds that are organic and untreated. This ensures that they are safe for your chickens to consume and will germinate properly. Incorporating sprouted herbs into your chicken's diet can be a delightful experience. Not only will your chickens benefit from the enhanced nutritional content of the sprouted herbs, but they'll also enjoy the variety of flavors and textures. It's a win-win for both you and your feathered friends!

It's important to note that sprouting is as much an art as it is a science. You might find that your sprouts aren't quite right the first time around, and that's okay. Just like any new skill, it takes practice. You might need to adjust the soaking time or the frequency of your rinse and drain cycles or even try different types of seeds. That's the beauty of sprouting - you can always experiment and find what works best for you and your flock. With a bit of patience and perseverance, you'll be a sprouting pro in no time.

Don't worry if you're new to this sprouting business. Like any new skill, it might take a bit of practice to get the hang of it, but once you do, there's no going back. Your chickens will love you for it, and their health will show it. So, gather those seeds and start sprouting today! It's easier than you think, and the benefits for your flock are immeasurable. Sprouting your own herbs can be a fun, satisfying project that benefits both you and your chickens. With a little bit of time and patience, you can provide your flock with these power-packed treats, reaping the rewards in terms of their health, vitality, and egg production. While the process might seem a bit daunting at first, it's actually quite straightforward and becomes easier with practice. Plus, the joy of watching a tiny seed transform into a sprout and then offering it to your excited flock makes it all worthwhile.

Have fun with it! Sprouting can be a fun and engaging project that not only enriches your flock's diet but also brings a bit of nature into your home. So go ahead, take the leap, and embark on your sprouting journey. The cluck of approval from your hens will be all the thanks you need.

Remember, sprouting is a journey. It may take a bit of trial and error to find which sprouts your chickens love most, and that's part of the fun. So keep on sprouting and savor the process as much as the end result - happy, healthy chickens enjoying the fruits (or in this case, sprouts) of your labor. Enjoy the journey!

In the world of chicken treats, sprouted herbs stand out for their nutritional boost, digestibility, and the sheer joy they bring to your flock. Whether you're a seasoned chicken keeper or just starting your journey, sprouting herbs could be a delightful addition to your chicken-keeping routine. So why not give it a try? Your flock will certainly thank you for it! Happy sprouting!

Part IV: High Flyers: Herbal Additions to Homemade Feed

Step into the world of homemade chicken feed, and it's hard not to feel like an artisan, crafting a unique, wholesome blend that's tailor-made for your flock. There's a sense of empowerment in taking control of your chickens' nutrition. You get to handpick the ingredients, ensuring every seed, grain, and herb contributes to a balanced, healthy diet that meets your flock's specific needs.

Why go the homemade route? Well, that's where we delve into the realm of customization. Every flock is unique, and what works for one might not work for another. Chickens of different breeds, ages, and life stages have varying nutritional requirements. Layer hens need more calcium for eggshell production, while roosters don't. Young chicks need a higher protein content for growth, while mature hens need less. When you make your own feed, you're the master blender, adjusting the ingredients and proportions to create a feed that's just right for your flock.

Freshness is another compelling reason to consider homemade feed. Fresh ingredients are packed with flavor and nutrients. When you make your feed, you know it's fresh. There's no wondering about the production date or how long the feed has been sitting on a store shelf. And let's face it, chickens, like us, appreciate a fresh, tasty meal.

Hand in hand with freshness comes quality. When you're the one sourcing the ingredients, you can prioritize quality. You might opt for organic grains, high-quality protein sources, and herbs from your own garden. You can avoid feeds with questionable additives or fillers. This control over the ingredient quality can lead to better overall health and productivity for your flock.

Making your own feed can also be cost-effective. Purchasing ingredients in bulk and mixing them at home can be cheaper than buying commercial feed, especially if you're feeding a large flock. Plus, by growing some ingredients yourself, like herbs and sprouts, you can further reduce the cost while adding a boost of freshness and nutrition.

Now, let's consider the benefits of adding herbs to homemade feed. Herbs are not just flavor enhancers; they are a powerhouse of nutrients and health benefits. Different herbs have different properties. Some are known for their calming effects, others for boosting immunity, and others for improving respiratory health. Including a variety of herbs in your homemade feed can boost its nutritional profile and add a touch of flavor that your chickens will love.

When it comes to choosing herbs for your homemade chicken feed you have a plethora of options! As we have discussed each herb has its own unique benefits, flavor profiles, and nutrient contents, all of which can add depth and richness to your homemade chicken feed. Let's explore some of these wonderful herbal additions.

First on our list is calendula. This brightly colored herb is a favorite among chicken enthusiasts for good reason. Calendula petals, known for their vibrant orange hue, can actually enhance the color of your chickens' egg yolks. But that's not all; they also possess anti-inflammatory properties and can support skin health. Moreover, calendula is relatively easy to grow, making it a sustainable and economical choice.

Next, we have mint. Mint is a powerhouse herb that's known for its potent smell and cooling properties. It can help to naturally repel pests in the coop, thanks to its strong aroma. On the nutritional front, mint is rich in vitamins A and C, which can support your chickens' overall health. Moreover, its cooling properties can be especially beneficial during the hot summer months, providing some much-needed relief to your chickens.

Garlic is another herb worth considering. While not an herb in the traditional sense, its health benefits are too significant to ignore. Garlic is known for its immune-boosting properties, and adding it to your chicken feed can help your flock ward off disease. Moreover, it's been suggested that garlic can help with internal parasites, acting as a natural dewormer. But remember, moderation is key with garlic. Too much can affect the taste of the eggs.

Let's not forget oregano, often termed the "super herb". Oregano is packed with antioxidants and has strong antimicrobial properties. It's been suggested that it can help prevent common poultry diseases, making it a valuable addition to your homemade feed. Plus, chickens seem to enjoy the taste!

Thyme, another herb from the Mediterranean, is worth mentioning. Thyme is known for its respiratory benefits, and it's been used in poultry farming to help with respiratory issues. This herb is rich in vitamin A, which supports eye health, and vitamin C, which aids in immunity.

Finally, consider adding basil to your homemade feed. Basil is more than just a staple in your kitchen; it's a great source of protein, vitamin E, and iron. Chickens love the taste, and it can provide a nice variety to their diet.

In essence, herbs can offer a unique blend of health benefits, flavor, and visual appeal to your homemade feed. Whether it's the vibrant colors of calendula, the cooling properties of mint, the strong aroma of garlic, or the powerful nutrients of oregano, thyme, and basil, each herb adds its own touch. But the beauty of homemade feed is that you can experiment. Try different combinations, see what your chickens prefer, and adjust accordingly.

Creating a balanced, herbal homemade feed is an exercise in creativity and attention to nutritional detail. This activity allows you to cater to your chickens' specific tastes, needs, and even moods while also taking full control over the quality of their diet. Let's embark on this culinary journey for our feathered friends together.

Firstly, it's crucial to remember that while herbs can be a delightful addition, the bulk of your chickens' diet should still comprise grains, protein, and other essential nutrients. A well-balanced chicken feed generally contains around 60-70% grains. This category includes foods like corn, wheat, barley, oats, and rice, which provide a hearty supply of energy.

Next, protein. Chickens need a good amount of protein for feather growth, egg production, and overall vitality. Around 20-30% of the feed should consist of protein-rich ingredients like soybean meal, fish meal, or other poultry-approved protein sources. In this respect, herbs like alfalfa can be useful. Known as a "protein herb," alfalfa can add to the protein content of the feed.

Now, let's talk about the fun part: herbs. As we've discussed earlier, herbs like calendula, mint, garlic, oregano, thyme, and basil can offer fantastic health benefits and flavors. Ideally, herbs should make up around 5-10% of the feed mix. You can adjust this percentage based on your chickens' preferences and the specific herbs you're using.

Don't forget about the additional ingredients, which can enhance the nutritional value of the feed. These can include items like shell grit for calcium, sunflower seeds for healthy fats, or sea kelp for trace minerals.

So, let's dive into a basic remedy for herbal chicken feed.

Ingredients:
- - 60% Grain mix (You can use a mix of corn, barley, wheat, and oats)
- - 25% Protein source (Soybean meal or fish meal are good options)
- - 10% Herbal mix (Use any combination of calendula, mint, garlic, oregano, thyme, and basil)
- - 5% Additional ingredients (Oyster shell, grit, sunflower seeds, and sea kelp are all great choices)

Directions:
- Start by gathering your grains. These should be ground but not too finely; a mixture of textures will encourage natural pecking behavior.
- Mix in your chosen protein source. Ensure it's well-distributed to prevent the chickens from picking out only the grains.
- Now add your finely chopped or crushed herbs. Don't worry about making the pieces too small; chickens love a good peck.
- Lastly, incorporate your additional ingredients. Give everything a good mix to evenly distribute the components.
- Store your feed in a cool, dry place to keep it fresh. Remember to make it in batches that can be used within a couple of weeks to ensure optimal freshness.

And there you have it! A homemade, herbal chicken feed that's balanced, nutritious, and absolutely cluck-worthy. Remember, this remedy is merely a guide. Feel free to adjust proportions, substitute ingredients, or experiment with other herbs based on what's available and what your chickens enjoy.

Switching to a homemade feed is a transition that should be handled with care. A sudden change in diet can stress your chickens and may even lead to digestive issues. Here's a guide to smoothly introducing homemade, herbal feed to your flock.

Firstly, you need to remember that any transition should be slow and steady. Chickens are creatures of habit and prefer stability, especially when it comes to their food. You want to start by mixing a small amount of the homemade feed into their regular feed. A good rule of thumb is to start with 10% homemade feed and 90% commercial feed.

Over the next week or so, you can gradually increase the proportion of homemade feed and decrease the commercial feed. Watch your chickens carefully during this period. Healthy chickens should be active, have bright eyes, and have a good appetite. Their feathers should be shiny and full, and they should be regularly laying eggs if they are of laying age.

Another key aspect to monitor is their droppings. Normal chicken droppings should be firm and brown with a white part, which is the urine. Any change in color, consistency, or frequency might indicate a problem.

If you notice any negative changes in your chickens' behavior or droppings, this could be a sign that the transition is happening too fast or there's something in the new feed that doesn't agree with them. In this case, you might need to slow down the transition, adjust the remedy, or consult with a poultry expert.

Once you have fully transitioned to the homemade feed, it's essential to keep a close eye on your chickens. Each chicken is different, and while one might thrive on the new feed, another might not. Adjustments might be necessary, and that's perfectly okay. Remember, the goal is a healthy, happy, and productive flock.

Also, don't forget about the water. Chickens should always have access to fresh, clean water. This becomes even more important when changing their diet, as ample hydration can help prevent digestive issues.

It's crucial to ensure that your homemade feed is stored correctly to maintain its freshness and nutritional value. A cool, dry place is ideal. Using your feed within a couple of weeks of making it will also help ensure it's consumed when at its best.

Even after successfully transitioning your chickens to a homemade feed, the journey isn't over. In fact, you could say it's just beginning. This is because one of the key benefits of homemade feed is the ability to adjust and tweak the remedy based on the needs of your flock.

The adjustment period of your flock to the homemade feed may bring about some insights. For instance, you might find that your chickens have a particular love for the marjoram you added, pecking enthusiastically whenever it's feeding time. Or you might notice that they're not quite as fond of the mustard seeds, often leaving them behind. These observations are valuable. They give you a sense of your chickens' preferences, which you can then use to tailor your homemade feed.

But taste isn't the only factor to consider. Nutritional needs are also important. Chickens at different stages of life require different nutrients. Layers need plenty of calcium for egg production, while chicks need more protein for growth. If you notice that your layers' eggshells are becoming thin, for example, it might be time to increase the amount of calcium-rich ingredients, like oyster shell or dandelion, in your feed. Similarly, if your growing chicks seem less active than usual, a boost in protein might be necessary.

Health is another key consideration. If your flock is going through a stressful period, perhaps due to a move or a change in weather, you might want to add more stress-busting herbs like lavender and chamomile. Or if a respiratory issue is going around, herbs known for their respiratory benefits like thyme and peppermint could be beneficial.

One of the joys of creating a homemade feed is that it's a dynamic process. It's not about finding one perfect remedy and sticking to it. It's about constantly learning, observing, and adjusting based on the needs and preferences of your flock. Making your own chicken feed offers a wonderful blend of benefits: customization, freshness, cost-effectiveness, and quality control. You're in the driver's seat, able to steer the nutrition of your flock based on their specific needs and preferences. Plus, the addition of herbs can take your homemade feed to a new level of nutrition and taste. As you embark on this journey of homemade feed, remember that the goal is not just to feed your chickens but to nourish them.

I know I keep saying it but remember that each flock is unique, and what works for one might not work for another. It's all about finding what works best for you and your chickens. It may take a little time and a few iterations, but the end result - a feed that's tailored specifically to your flock, boosting their health, productivity, and happiness - is well worth it. Transitioning your chickens to a homemade feed is not something to be rushed. It requires patience, careful observation, and potentially some trial and error. But the reward - having complete control over your chickens' diet and providing them with fresh, nutrient-rich, herbal feed - is certainly worth the effort. And remember, this is a journey. So, take it one step at a time and enjoy the process.

"Tend to your flock, and your heart will grow with them."
— Mary Butler

Chapter 5: Nests That Pass the Peck Test

Part I: The Nest Is Best: Herbal Bedding Blends

The humble nest bedding. It's something many chicken keepers may not give much thought to, but it plays an important role in the lives of your chickens. It's not just about providing a place for your chickens to lay their eggs. It's also about comfort, cleanliness, and even egg production.

To understand why nest bedding is important, let's first look at what happens when a chicken decides it's time to lay an egg. This process is not as simple as it may seem. A chicken will often spend a fair amount of time preparing for this. She will inspect various nesting spots, turning around, fluffing up the bedding, and maybe even removing pieces that don't meet her standards. Only when she's satisfied will she finally settle down to lay her egg.

From this behavior, it's clear that chickens are quite particular about their nests. And with good reason - a good nest makes the process of laying eggs more comfortable and stress-free. Nest bedding provides a soft, cozy spot for the chicken to rest on. It cushions the egg, reducing the risk of breakage. It also insulates the nest, helping to maintain a comfortable temperature.

But comfort is not the only benefit. Cleanliness is another key factor. Nest bedding helps to absorb droppings and other fluids, keeping the nest clean. This is important not only for the health and hygiene of your chickens but also for the quality of your eggs. Eggs laid in a dirty nest can get soiled, which may make them unsuitable for consumption or sale. Fresh, clean bedding reduces this risk.

Egg production is another aspect that can be influenced by nest bedding. Comfortable, attractive nests encourage chickens to lay their eggs in the nest rather than elsewhere. This not only makes it easier for you to collect the eggs, but it also reduces the risk of egg loss due to breakage or predation.

Given these benefits, it's clear that nest bedding is a crucial part of chicken keeping. But don't just settle for any bedding. Why not make your chickens' nests even better with herbal bedding blends?

Herbs bring a lot to the table. Not only do they add a pleasant aroma, which can make the coop a more enjoyable place for both you and your chickens, but they also offer a variety of health benefits. Some herbs, for example, have insect-repelling properties. Adding these to your nest bedding can help to keep pests at bay. Others have calming effects, which can make the nest an even more appealing place for your chickens to lay their eggs.

In other words, incorporating herbs into your nest bedding can take it from good to great. And the best part? It's easy to do. Just imagine walking into a chicken coop and being greeted not by the usual barnyard aroma but by the gentle scent of lavender, mint, and pine wafting from the nests. It's a delightful experience, and it's one you can easily create by incorporating herbs into your nest bedding.

First on our list of herbs for bedding is lavender. Renowned for its calming and relaxing properties, it's a great choice for nesting boxes. Chickens, like humans, can benefit from a relaxed atmosphere when it comes time to lay eggs. Plus, the sweet, floral scent of lavender can help mask any unwanted odors in the coop, making it a more pleasant place for both you and your flock.

Next, we have mint. Mint is a powerful aroma that many pests, including mice and insects, find off-putting. Including this herb in your nest bedding can, therefore, help to deter these unwelcome visitors. Additionally, mint has a cooling effect, which can be particularly beneficial during the warmer months.

Pine is another excellent choice for nest bedding. Pine needles are soft, making them comfortable for your chickens to sit on. They also have a fresh, clean scent that can help keep the coop smelling good. Moreover, pine has natural antibacterial properties that can help keep your nests clean and healthy.

There are many other herbs you can consider, too. Rosemary, for example, is another herb with insect-repelling properties. Chamomile can help to calm nervous chickens, making it a good choice for flocks that are a little on the skittish side. Marigold flowers can be used to add a pop of color to your nests, making them more visually appealing.

When choosing herbs for your nest bedding, consider not only their potential benefits but also their availability and cost. While it's great to add a variety of herbs, there's no need to break the bank. Even just one or two herbs can make a difference.

Using herbs in your nest bedding is not just about adding a nice scent. It's about creating a more pleasant and healthy environment for your chickens. It's about taking a simple, everyday aspect of chicken keeping and turning it into an opportunity to improve the well-being of your flock.

Creating herbal bedding blends can be as simple or as complex as you want it to be. You can use a single herb, or you can experiment with different combinations to create your own unique blend. Feel free to get creative! The goal is to create a nest that not just passes the peck test but excels at it! Crafting herbal bedding blends for your chickens can be a fun and rewarding process. It's a chance to get creative, play with different combinations, and create a unique blend that suits your flock's needs.

The base of your herbal bedding blend will be your usual nesting material. This could be straw, wood shavings, or any other bedding material you typically use. This will provide a comfortable and absorbent layer for your chickens to lay their eggs on.

The next step is to choose your herbs. As we discussed earlier, different herbs offer different benefits. Lavender, for instance, can create a calming environment and mask unpleasant odors. Mint can deter pests and has a cooling effect, which can be useful in warm weather. Pine needles add a fresh scent and have natural antibacterial properties. Consider what benefits you want to provide to your chickens and choose your herbs accordingly.

When it comes to proportions, a general guideline is to aim for about one part of herbs to four parts of bedding material. However, these proportions are not set in stone. Feel free to adjust them based on your preferences and your chickens' reactions. If you notice that your chickens seem to enjoy the herbs, you might want to add a little more. If they seem put off by the strong scents, you might want to use less.

Once you have your materials, the process of creating the blend is simple. Just mix your chosen herbs into your bedding material until they're evenly distributed. Then, replace the old bedding in your nesting boxes with your new herbal blend.

There are a few best practices to keep in mind when creating and using your herbal bedding blends. First, make sure the herbs you're using are safe for chickens. While most common culinary herbs are safe, there are some plants that are toxic to chickens, so it's always a good idea to double-check.

Second, remember to replace the bedding regularly. While the herbs can help mask odors and deter pests, they're not a substitute for good coop hygiene. Regularly removing soiled bedding and replacing it with a fresh blend can help keep your coop clean and your chickens healthy.

Lastly, pay attention to your chickens' reactions. Not all chickens will react the same way to all herbs. Some might love the scent of lavender, while others might prefer mint or pine. Experiment with different blends and see what your chickens seem to enjoy the most.

So, why not give it a go? Creating your own herbal bedding blends can be a fun way to enhance your chickens' nesting environment. Whether you're aiming for a pest-free coop, a calming atmosphere, or simply a nicer smell, the right blend of herbs can help you achieve your goals. And, of course, it's another great way to ensure your nests pass the peck test with flying colors!

However, before we get too excited we have to remember that just like with any change in your chicken's environment, introducing herbal bedding should be done gradually. It's crucial to give your hens time to adjust and observe their reactions carefully.

First off, you'll want to introduce your chickens to the new bedding material. This can be done by adding a small amount of the herbal blend to the existing bedding. This helps to familiarize your chickens with the new scents without overwhelming them.

Next, watch your chickens closely. Pay attention to how they interact with the new bedding. Do they seem interested? Are they pecking at it curiously, or are they shying away? Remember, your goal is to create a nest that your hens feel comfortable in. If they seem to be avoiding the nest or showing signs of stress, you might need to adjust your blend.

Not all hens will respond the same way to all herbs. Just like people, chickens have their own individual preferences. Some might love the strong aroma of rosemary, while others might prefer the subtler scent of chamomile. That's why it's important to try different herbs and combinations to see what works best for your flock. You might even find that different hens in your flock prefer different herbs, in which case, you can create custom blends for each nest.

Remember, this is a process of trial and error. It's unlikely that you'll find the perfect blend on your first try, and that's okay. Don't be discouraged if your first blend isn't a hit. It's all part of the process. And when you do find a blend that your chickens love, the satisfaction will be worth it.

After you've introduced the herbal bedding and made any necessary adjustments, you'll need to maintain it. This includes regularly replacing the bedding to ensure it's fresh and clean. Remember, while the herbs can help mask odors and deter pests, they're not a substitute for regular cleaning. A clean nest is crucial for the health of your chickens and the quality of their eggs.

A vital aspect to keep in mind is that chickens are creatures of habit. Any change, no matter how beneficial, can initially cause some confusion or discomfort. But don't worry. With time, your chickens will get used to the new bedding and start to enjoy the benefits of the herbs. The key is to be patient, observant, and ready to make adjustments as necessary.

In the chicken rearing world, one aspect cannot be stressed enough – cleanliness is crucial. This golden rule applies as much to the nest boxes as it does to the coop at large. But how can you keep that beautifully scented herbal bedding blend in tip-top shape? Let's discuss the steps you can take to maintain freshness, hygiene, and comfort in your nest boxes.

First off, we have the changing schedule. Nest bedding should be replaced regularly to keep the boxes clean and reduce the risk of disease. The frequency of replacement can depend on various factors like the size of your flock, the weather, and your hens' laying patterns. However, a good rule of thumb is to change the bedding every one to two weeks, or when it becomes soiled or wet.

But there's no need to wait until change day to maintain cleanliness. Spot cleaning is a vital everyday practice. This simply means removing any soiled or wet bedding as soon as you notice it, and replacing it with fresh herbal bedding. Spot cleaning helps to keep the nest boxes clean and inviting and can extend the life of your bedding between full changes.

Another factor that can impact the freshness of your bedding is pests. Let's face it, chickens aren't the only ones who find a cozy nest box appealing. Mites, lice, and other critters can make themselves at home in your hens' nests. This is where your herbal bedding blends come into their own. Certain herbs like mint, lavender, and wormwood are known for their pest-repelling properties. Incorporating these herbs into your blend can act as a natural deterrent, helping to keep those pesky intruders at bay.

On top of these pest-repelling herbs, good coop hygiene practices can help prevent infestations. These include regularly cleaning and disinfecting the coop, checking your hens for signs of pests, and treating any infestations promptly.

Another pro tip? Rotate your herbs. Changing the blend of herbs in your bedding can help maintain the effectiveness of their pest-repelling properties. Different pests are repelled by different herbs, so a rotating selection can help keep a wider range of critters at bay. Plus, it gives your hens a bit of variety, which is always a good thing!

To conclude, keeping your herbal bedding fresh is a combination of a regular changing schedule, daily spot cleaning, and using pest-repelling herbs. These practices help create a clean, comfortable, and healthy environment for your hens. Not to mention, they make your nest boxes smell downright delightful.

Remember, creating a nest that passes the peck test doesn't stop at choosing the right bedding. It's also about keeping that bedding fresh, clean, and inviting. So roll up your sleeves, prepare your herbal blends, and get ready to provide your hens with the luxury nests they deserve.

Part II: Egg-citing Herbal Mists: Calm and Quiet Nests

Let's imagine for a moment. You're a hen; it's time to lay an egg, and you're looking for the perfect spot. Would you prefer a dark, dull, stressful corner? Or a bright, calming, fragrant nest box? The answer is clear, isn't it? Ambiance plays a key role in a hen's decision about where to lay her egg. And one of the ways we can enhance the ambiance of nest boxes is through the use of herbal mists.

Now you might be wondering, what does ambiance have to do with egg laying? Well, quite a lot. Just like us, hens need to feel safe and relaxed to carry out certain activities. Laying an egg is a vulnerable time for a hen, and a quiet, calm environment can help reduce stress and make the process easier.

Reducing stress in chickens isn't just about making them feel better, though that is a crucial aspect. Lower stress levels can also improve overall health, leading to a stronger immune system and increased longevity. And let's not forget about egg production. Happy, relaxed hens tend to be more productive layers. They're also more likely to lay their eggs in the nest boxes rather than hiding them in random spots around the yard.

So, how do you create this serene nest box atmosphere? One way is through the use of herbal mists. Herbal mists, also known as hydrosols or flower waters, are a byproduct of the process of distilling essential oils. They contain many of the same beneficial properties as essential oils but are milder and safer for chickens.

Misting your nest boxes with herbal mists can help create a calming, aromatic environment. Some herbs that are excellent for this purpose include lavender, chamomile, and lemon balm. These herbs are known for their soothing properties and can help create a tranquil nest box ambiance.

Let's dive into the benefits of these herbs a bit more. Lavender is widely known for its calming properties. It's often used in aromatherapy to reduce anxiety and promote sleep. In the context of a nest box, lavender can help create a peaceful environment that encourages laying.

Chamomile is another herb that's a powerhouse of calming properties. It's commonly used in teas to promote relaxation and ease stress. Spraying a chamomile mist in your nest boxes can help soothe your hens and make them feel safe and relaxed.

Lemon balm, a member of the mint family, is another great option. This herb has a fresh, uplifting scent that can help reduce stress and promote a sense of well-being. It can create an inviting, pleasant ambiance in your nest boxes.

To create an herbal mist, you simply need to steep your chosen herbs in boiling water, strain the mixture, and then let it cool. Once cool, you can pour it into a spray bottle, and it's ready to use. Spritz your nest boxes with the mist regularly to maintain a calming atmosphere.

Creating a calming ambiance in your nest boxes isn't a one-size-fits-all endeavor. It's about observing your flock and finding what works best for them. Try different herbs, observe your chickens' reactions, and adjust as needed. The goal is to create a nest box environment that your hens love and feel comfortable in.

In essence, the ambiance in your nest boxes can significantly impact your hens' laying habits and overall well-being. So why not give herbal mists a try? With their calming properties and delightful scents, they're a wonderful tool to help ensure your nests pass the peck test.

Plants and herbs have been used for thousands of years for their therapeutic properties, not just for humans but also for animals. For our feathered friends, certain herbs can contribute significantly to a calming, soothing ambiance that makes their nest boxes a preferred location for laying eggs. Among the vast variety of herbs out there, a select few stand out for their calming effects: chamomile, rosemary, and lemon balm. And they're just the start!

Let's delve deeper into the calming world of chamomile. This daisy-like plant, famed for its comforting aroma, is often found in bedtime teas intended to promote a good night's sleep. In avian terms, it's equally beneficial. A chamomile mist in the nesting box can soothe your hens, easing any restlessness or stress. Imagine them, then, walking into a nest box that exudes the gentle aroma of chamomile. The calming scent could be just the touch needed to ensure they lay their eggs in comfort.

Next up, rosemary. You might recognize this herb from the kitchen, as it's a popular addition to many dishes. But rosemary is more than just a flavor enhancer. The herb also has stress-relieving properties, which can work wonders in creating a serene environment for your hens. An added bonus is its pest-repelling abilities, helping to keep your nest boxes free of unwanted insects.

Lemon balm, with its delightfully fresh aroma, is another fantastic herb for your nest box mists. This member of the mint family is known for its stress-reducing effects, and the scent alone can create an inviting ambiance that your chickens will love. It's a particularly good choice for those hot summer months, with its light, refreshing scent.

While chamomile, rosemary, and lemon balm are fantastic choices, the world of calming herbs doesn't stop there. Other herbs that can be used in your mists include lavender, with its well-known relaxing properties, and marjoram, which can be particularly comforting for hens laying their first eggs. And let's not forget about mint, which not only adds a fresh aroma but can also help deter pests.

The herbal mist you choose to use will depend on what works best for your flock. Start with small amounts of mist, observe your chickens' reactions, and adjust accordingly. Some hens might prefer the sweet aroma of lavender, while others might be more inclined towards the refreshing scent of mint. It's all about finding what helps your hens feel calm, safe, and ready to lay.

The key to using herbal mists effectively lies in their regular application. A one-time spritz won't sustain the calming ambiance you're aiming for. Instead, make misting a part of your regular chicken care routine, spritzing the nest boxes every few days to maintain a relaxing environment.

Creating your own herbal mists is a rewarding journey that lets you cater to the specific needs of your chickens while indulging your creative side. It's a way to provide a soothing, tranquil atmosphere that will be appreciated by your feathered friends. So, how do you get started? With a few basic materials and a pinch of patience, you'll be spritzing your homemade mists in no time.

First things first, gather your materials. You'll need some fresh or dried herbs of your choice, distilled water, a pot for boiling, a strainer, a spray bottle, and a cool, dark place for storage. Sounds easy enough, right? Let's delve into the process.

Select your herbs. We've already discussed some excellent options: chamomile, rosemary, and lemon balm are stellar choices. But don't let that limit you! Consider the preferences of your chickens, the availability of herbs, and the specific effects you're aiming for. Maybe you'd like to try a lavender and mint blend for a calming, refreshing mist. Or perhaps marjoram and chamomile for a comforting, stress-relieving mist. The choices are numerous, and the experimentation is part of the fun!

Once you've chosen your herbs, it's time to prepare the infusion. For this, you'll want to add about a cup of herbs to around two cups of distilled water. Bring this to a boil, then let it simmer on low heat for around 15 to 20 minutes. Afterward, turn off the heat and let the mixture cool. This process allows the herbs' essential oils—the components carrying the scent and beneficial properties—to be released into the water.

Once your infusion has cooled, strain it into a clean, glass spray bottle, taking care to remove all the plant matter. There you have it: your homemade herbal mist, ready to create an enchanting, calming environment for your hens.

Now, let's talk about storage and usage. When it comes to storage, it's crucial to keep the mist in a cool, dark place. The reason for this is simple: heat and light can cause the essential oils in your mist to degrade, reducing their efficacy and aroma. A cupboard or a drawer can serve as excellent storage spots.

When it comes to using your mists, a light spritz every few days is all it takes to maintain a soothing ambiance in your nest boxes. Be mindful not to overdo it; you don't want your bedding to get damp. The goal is to lightly disperse the scent into the environment, inviting your hens to a stress-free, relaxing nest box.

Also, consider the time of day when using your mists. Early morning, before your hens start their egg-laying routine, can be an ideal time. This way, your hens will enter the nest boxes just as the calming scent of the herbs begins to fill the air.

Creating your own herbal mists can seem like a daunting task, but in reality, it's a simple, rewarding process that offers an array of benefits for your chickens. With a little creativity and patience, you'll be well on your way to providing an environment that's not just comfortable for your hens but also an olfactory delight.

Let's begin with a simple calming mist, perfect for chickens who seem a bit stressed or anxious. For this remedy, we'll focus on chamomile and lavender, two herbs renowned for their calming properties.

A. Calming Chamomile-Lavender Mist

Ingredients
- 1 cup of water
- 2 tablespoons dried chamomile flowers
- 2 tablespoons dried lavender buds
- Spray bottle

Directions:
- Bring the water to a boil in a pot.
- Once boiling, remove the pot from the heat and add the chamomile flowers and lavender buds.
- Cover the pot and let the herbs steep for about 20 minutes or until the water has cooled.
- Strain the mixture, pressing the herbs to extract as much of the beneficial oils as possible.
- Pour the strained liquid into your spray bottle.

Your Calming Chamomile-Lavender Mist is now ready to use! Remember, this is not a cleaning spray, so it's intended to be used in addition to, not in place of, regular nest box cleaning.

Let's proceed to another remedy. This time, we'll craft a Refreshing Mint-Rosemary Mist that's perfect for hot summer days. Both mint and rosemary are known for their fresh and invigorating scents. This spray not only creates a pleasant environment for your hens but also helps deter pests.

B. Refreshing Mint-Rosemary Mist

Ingredients
- 1 cup of water
- 2 tablespoons dried mint leaves
- 2 tablespoons dried rosemary leaves
- Spray bottle

Directions:
Follow the same steps as in the previous remedy. The resulting mist will have a fresh, invigorating aroma that's sure to make your nest boxes an inviting place for your hens.

Lastly, let's whip up an Herbal Pest-Deterrent Mist. While the previous two mists are focused on creating a calming and refreshing environment, this one is all about keeping pests at bay.

A.   Herbal Pest-Deterrent Mist

Ingredients
- 1 cup of water
- 1 tablespoon dried rosemary leaves
- 1 tablespoon dried mint leaves
- 1 tablespoon dried lavender buds
- 1 tablespoon dried wormwood leaves
- Spray bottle

Directions:
Again, follow the same steps. The resulting mist will not only provide a pleasant scent but also help deter a range of pests thanks to the properties of these specific herbs.

Using herbal mists effectively isn't just about creating a delightful concoction of herbs. A key component of its successful implementation lies in understanding how and when to apply these fragrant sprays. Creating a rhythm that aligns with your hens' natural behaviors, timing, and close observation are essential to ensure your efforts yield the best results.

Firstly, let's talk about frequency. Your hens are hardworking ladies, and their coop sees quite a bit of activity. To maintain a calming and fresh-smelling ambiance, regular application of your herbal mist is crucial. How regular, you ask? A good rule of thumb is to aim for a light spritz every two to three days. This frequency ensures that the calming effects and pleasant aroma of the mist are consistently present in the nest boxes, encouraging relaxation and contentment amongst your hens.

But it's not just about frequency. The timing of application can be a game-changer in maximizing the benefits of your herbal mists. A great time to spritz the herbal mists is in the early morning hours, right before your hens start their daily egg-laying ritual. The soothing scents wafting through the nest boxes, as they settle down to lay, can create an incredibly calming and inviting atmosphere, promoting successful egg-laying and reducing stress levels.

Another good time to apply the mist is during cleaning routines. A fresh, clean coop coupled with the invigorating aroma of herbs can make the space feel welcoming and relaxing for your hens. It's about creating an environment that not just looks clean but also smells fresh and feels comforting.

Just as the sun sets and your chickens are winding down for the day, another light misting can help encourage a peaceful and restful night for your flock. The goal here is to create an environment that promotes not just physical but also emotional well-being, contributing to overall health and happiness.

While we've established a basic guideline for frequency and timing, remember that each flock is unique. What works wonderfully for one may not be as effective for another. This is where close observation becomes key. Keep an eye on your hens, observing how they react to the herbal mists.

Do they seem calmer and more content? Are they laying more consistently? On the flip side, if you notice any signs of distress or discomfort, don't hesitate to make changes. Perhaps a certain herb is not to their liking, or maybe the scent is too strong. Observation and adjustment are an essential part of the process, allowing you to create an environment tailored to your hens' preferences and needs.

When applying the mist, aim for a light spray around the nest boxes, avoiding any direct application on your hens. Keep the spray bottle at a reasonable distance to ensure a light mist rather than a heavy spray. It's about creating a subtly scented atmosphere, not overwhelming the space (or your hens) with a strong aroma. Using herbal mists is a multifaceted process involving more than just selecting calming herbs and preparing a fragrant mix. It's about understanding the rhythm of your flock, timing your applications appropriately, and constantly observing and adjusting based on your hens' reactions. Above all, it's about creating a peaceful, stress-free space where your hens can thrive.

One of the fundamental aspects of chicken keeping, particularly when utilizing holistic practices such as herbal mists, is that it's not a one-size-fits-all approach. It's a journey of exploration and adjustment, guided by your flock's unique characteristics, preferences, and needs. It's about creating a synergy between your actions and your flock's reactions.

Think of your flock as a community. Each hen is an individual with her own set of preferences and behavior patterns. What one hen finds calming, another may find irritating. It's crucial to observe your flock and note their reaction to the herbal mist you're using. Observation can tell you whether your hens are comfortable with the current blend or if they're showing signs of discomfort or distress.

Signs of distress can be subtle. A change in egg-laying patterns, increased agitation, or avoidance of certain areas in the coop could all be indicators that something isn't quite right. If your hens are suddenly laying fewer eggs or seem more nervous, it might be time to take a closer look at the mist blend you're using. Could a specific herb be the culprit? Or perhaps it's the strength of the aroma?

Adjusting your herbal mist blend in response to your hens' reactions can sometimes feel like a guessing game, but it's a critical part of the process. Start by considering the potential irritants. If you suspect a particular herb might be causing discomfort, try eliminating it from your blend and observe any changes in your flock's behavior.

Remember, the strength of the aroma can be just as impactful as the choice of herbs. While we might enjoy the strong scent of certain herbs, your hens might find it overpowering. If you suspect that the aroma might be too strong, try reducing the quantity of herbs in your blend or diluting it further with water. Again, it's all about observation and adjustment.

Another crucial aspect of adjusting your herbal mist blend is to consider the seasonal needs of your flock. What works well during the warm summer months might not be as effective during the cooler seasons. For instance, in summer, you might want to focus on herbs with insect-repelling properties like basil or lemongrass. In contrast, during the cooler months, warmer, soothing herbs like sage or rosemary might be more beneficial.

And of course, don't forget about the specific needs of your flock. Do you have hens who are particularly anxious? Incorporating more calming herbs like chamomile or lavender might be helpful. Or maybe you have older hens that could benefit from herbs with anti-inflammatory properties, like yarrow or marjoram.

In essence, adjusting your herbal mist blend is a dynamic process, one that requires patience, observation, and a willingness to experiment. It's about listening to your flock, interpreting their signals, and responding in a way that best supports their well-being. It's a journey of mutual understanding and respect, culminating in a peaceful, nurturing environment that meets the needs of every member of your flock. In the grand scheme of things, the well-being of your flock is at the heart of every decision you make and every action you take.

Part III: Feather Soft Liners: DIY Herbal Nesting Pads

There's something quite magical about nest pads, especially when they're infused with the right mix of herbs. They serve a variety of purposes, adding an extra layer of functionality to your nest boxes. They're a bit like a cozy, feather-soft bed for your hens, providing comfort while serving practical roles related to insulation, cleanliness, and egg protection.

Let's delve a little deeper into these benefits and how they contribute to a nest that passes the peck test.

In terms of insulation, nest pads work wonders in maintaining a steady temperature within the nest boxes. This aspect is crucial as chickens are sensitive to drastic temperature shifts. During cold winter months, these pads can help keep your hens warm, providing an extra layer of comfort as they settle down to lay their eggs. On the flip side, in the warmer months, the pads can help keep the nest boxes cool by preventing the transfer of heat from the surrounding environment. So, not only do the pads offer a soft, comfortable laying spot, but they also help create a more stable and hospitable environment for your hens.

Cleanliness is another major benefit of using nest pads. We all know how messy a chicken coop can get. Between the feathers, dirt, and inevitable chicken droppings, maintaining a clean coop can be a challenge. But that's where the nest pads step in. They serve as a barrier between the hen and the nest box floor, catching droppings and other messes. This not only helps keep your hens clean and comfortable but also makes your coop cleaning duties a whole lot easier.

Next up, let's talk about egg protection. When a hen lays an egg, there's always a risk of the egg cracking, especially if the nest box floor is hard or uneven. Nest pads offer a soft landing spot for freshly laid eggs, significantly reducing the risk of cracks or breaks. This is particularly beneficial for those of us who raise chickens for their eggs. After all, there's nothing quite as disappointing as finding a nest box full of cracked eggs.

But the benefits of nest pads don't stop at insulation, cleanliness, and egg protection. When you infuse your nest pads with herbs, you add a whole new layer of benefits to the mix. Herbal-infused nest pads can help deter pests, promote relaxation, and even enhance the overall health of your flock. Just imagine a nest pad filled with lavender and chamomile, promoting a calming environment for your hens. Or one with basil and lemongrass, helping to keep those pesky insects at bay.

In essence, nest pads serve as a versatile tool in your chicken-keeping toolkit. They go beyond providing a comfortable spot for your hens to lay their eggs. They actively contribute to the creation of a healthier, happier, and more efficient coop. So, whether you're battling cold winters, aiming for a cleaner coop, or striving to protect those precious eggs, nest pads can be a game changer.

As we venture deeper into the art of creating nests that pass the peck test, keep these benefits in mind. Nest pads, especially when thoughtfully crafted and herbal-infused, can transform your nest boxes into a haven for your hens, a place where they feel safe, comfortable, and relaxed. And that, dear friends, is what the peck test is all about.

So, you've got your nest pads ready, and now comes the fun part - deciding which herbs to incorporate. It's like having a spice rack but for your chicken coop! And just like spices in a remedy, different herbs have different properties and can create diverse sensory experiences for your hens.

One classic material for nest pads is straw. Straw might not be a herb, but it forms the basis for a sturdy, breathable nest pad. Its structure allows for good airflow, reducing the risk of mold and providing a comfortable base for your hens. Remember, straw is the canvas; herbs are the paint. It's on this base of straw that you can begin to add your selected herbs, enhancing the nest pad's benefits.

Calendula, for example, is a popular herb in the world of chicken keeping. Known for its vibrant orange flowers, calendula not only makes your nest boxes look pretty, but it also has numerous health benefits. It's packed with antioxidants and has antibacterial properties that can help keep your coop clean. It's also known to stimulate egg-laying, which is always a bonus.

Eucalyptus is another great choice for nest pads. This potent plant has a distinct scent that's known to deter pests, acting as a natural insect repellent. It also has antimicrobial properties, contributing to a cleaner, healthier coop. Not to mention, its fresh, crisp scent can help combat coop odors, keeping your nest boxes smelling fresh.

Mint is another herb that's great for deterring pests. In fact, rodents particularly dislike the strong scent of mint. Including this herb in your nest pads can help keep mice and rats at bay. On top of that, mint has a cooling effect that can be particularly beneficial during the warmer months, helping to keep your hens comfortable.

For a calming effect, consider herbs like lavender and chamomile. These herbs are known for their relaxation properties and can help create a peaceful environment for your hens. Lavender has the added benefit of being a natural antiseptic, promoting a clean and healthy coop.

And let's not forget about rosemary. This herb has a number of benefits for chickens. It's thought to boost respiratory health, a vital factor especially in colder months when coops are closed up more tightly. Rosemary's strong aroma also makes it a good choice for masking any unpleasant coop smells.

Lastly, herbs like marjoram and parsley can be beneficial for their egg-laying stimulation. Marjoram is known to stimulate the hormone systems responsible for egg production, while parsley is packed with vitamins and minerals that support overall hen health.

Incorporating herbs into your nest pads is not just about picking one and sticking to it. You can create blends based on the specific needs and preferences of your flock. You might have a summer blend that focuses on cooling herbs like mint, or a winter blend that includes more warming herbs.

Remember, the key is to observe your flock and see how they react to different herbs. You're an artist creating a masterpiece, and your flock's behavior and well-being are the best indicators of whether your blend is a hit or a miss.

This is by no means an exhaustive list of herbs you can use. There's a wide world of herbs out there, each with its own unique properties and benefits. In the appendix you'll find more detailed information on a wide variety of herbs you might consider for your nest pads.

Creating herbal-infused nest pads is a creative, dynamic process. It involves understanding the benefits of different herbs, experimenting with blends, and watching your flock's reaction. It's yet another tool you can use to craft a nest that truly passes the peck test.

Once your homemade, herbal-infused nest pads are ready, it's time to introduce them to your hens. This might sound straightforward, but remember, chickens are creatures of habit, so any change in their environment needs to be introduced carefully and gradually. There's a finesse to it, a strategy that involves empathy, patience, and careful observation.

The first step to introducing nest pads to your flock is the process of placement. The change should occur during a time of day when the chickens are least likely to be laying eggs. Early morning or late evening is best, as your hens are less likely to be disturbed at these times. Quietly replace the old bedding with your new, aromatic nest pads. Remember, the goal is to minimize disruption.

Once the nest pads are in place, observe your hens. At first, they might seem perplexed by the changes in their nest boxes. The unfamiliar sight and smell may take them by surprise, causing them to peck at the pads out of curiosity. They may even avoid the nest boxes completely for a time. This is natural and to be expected. With time and familiarity, your hens will get used to their new bedding.

If you find your hens are hesitant to use the nest boxes after the introduction of the pads, don't panic. A gentle nudge might be all they need. Place a few dummy eggs or golf balls in the nest boxes to encourage them. Chickens have a strong instinct to lay their eggs in a communal spot. Seeing 'eggs' in the new bedding can signal to them that it's a safe place for laying.

As your hens adjust to the new bedding, pay close attention to their behavior. Are they relaxed and comfortable when they're in the nest boxes? Are they laying regularly? Is egg production steady or even improved? Keep an eye out for signs of distress as well, such as loud, repetitive clucking, or avoiding the nest boxes altogether.

Maintain this period of observation for at least a week or two. This gives your hens enough time to adjust to the change and allows you to gather enough data on their reaction.

Another key aspect of introducing nest pads is the maintenance of cleanliness. Ensure that you're changing or refreshing the nest pads regularly. The frequency of change depends on the size of your flock and how quickly the pads get dirty. A good rule of thumb is to replace or refresh the pads every 2-3 weeks or as soon as they appear soiled. Remember, a clean nest box is paramount for the health of your flock and the quality of their eggs.

If your hens are not taking to the herbal nest pads, don't be disheartened. It may take some tweaking and experimenting. Perhaps a different herb blend will be more appealing, or maybe your hens prefer a lighter or heavier herbal infusion. Don't be afraid to go back to the drawing board.

This whole process may require a bit of trial and error. But that's okay. The primary goal is to create a comfortable, soothing environment that encourages your hens to lay and keeps them healthy and happy. If that requires some adjustment and fine-tuning, then it's all part of passing the peck test.

The magic of this whole endeavor lies not in immediate success but in the journey itself. It's about understanding your hens, responding to their needs, and being willing to learn and adjust. That's the key to creating a nest box environment that doesn't just pass the peck test but excels at it. After all, a contented hen is a productive hen. Part of ensuring that your hens stay contented lies in maintaining and replacing the nest pads regularly. Just like any bedding, herbal nest pads need to be kept clean and fresh to continue providing benefits to your hens.

Cleaning and refreshing your nest pads is an essential part of your routine chicken care. It helps keep the nest boxes hygienic, ensures the comfort of your hens, and contributes to the overall success of your eggs. As for how often to refresh or replace the pads, this will depend on a few factors, such as the size of your flock and how quickly the pads get soiled. As a rule of thumb, you should aim to refresh or replace the pads every two to three weeks or as soon as they appear dirty.

The process of cleaning your nest pads involves removing them from the nest boxes and shaking out any dirt or droppings. If the pads are still in good condition but the herbal infusion has lost its potency, you can simply refresh them. This involves sprinkling them with a fresh batch of your chosen herb blend, ensuring an even distribution. Once refreshed, the pads can be placed back in the nest boxes, ready to provide a soothing and clean environment for your hens.

In some cases, the nest pads might be too dirty or worn out to be refreshed. In these instances, it's best to replace them entirely. Creating a new set of herbal nest pads offers an opportunity to experiment with different herb blends, and it ensures that your hens always have fresh, comfortable bedding.

The lifespan of your nest pads will depend on several factors. These include the quality of the materials you used, the size of your flock, and the cleanliness of the nest boxes. With good care, nest pads can last for several months. However, it's essential to keep an eye on them and replace them as needed. If the pads begin to fall apart or if the herbs lose their scent, it's time for a new batch.

Apart from the regular cleaning and refreshing routine, it's a good practice to do a deeper cleaning of your nest boxes every few months. This involves thoroughly scrubbing the boxes, letting them dry, and then adding fresh bedding. It's an opportunity to keep your coop in the best condition and ensure the health and happiness of your hens.

Remember, maintaining and replacing nest pads is not just about hygiene and aesthetics. It plays a significant role in the comfort and well-being of your hens. The cleanliness of the nest boxes directly affects the health of your hens and the quality of their eggs. Furthermore, a clean, fresh-smelling nest box can encourage regular laying and help prevent issues like egg eating or laying outside of the boxes.

On a final note, keep in mind that every flock is different. What works for one may not work for another. As a chicken keeper, you know your hens best. You are in the best position to observe their behavior, understand their preferences, and make the best decisions regarding their care.

Keeping your hens happy and healthy is a journey. There might be some trial and error involved, and that's perfectly okay. Each step you take, every decision you make, and every change you introduce brings you closer to creating the ideal environment for your flock—an environment that doesn't just pass the peck test but goes above and beyond to ensure the health, happiness, and productivity of your hens. Keep up the good work, and remember, the journey is just as important as the destination.

Part IV: The Art of Egg-Laying: Herbal Nurturing Nests

Let's step back a little and examine the intriguing world of chicken egg-laying. The process is a symphony of biology, playing out in an intricate cycle that's influenced by a plethora of factors. To truly understand the value of our nest-enhancing efforts, it's vital to have a grasp of what exactly happens when our hens are hard at work.

When talking about egg-laying in chickens, we're looking at a process that's as much about internal physiology as it is about external influences. So, let's break down the cycle and shed some light on how we can help optimize conditions for our hens.

The egg-laying process in hens begins in the hen's ovary. Unlike mammals, hens are born with all the potential eggs they can lay in their lifetime in the form of tiny yolks in their ovaries. When a hen reaches maturity, usually around 5 to 6 months old, these yolks start to develop one by one. Each mature yolk is then released into the oviduct, a long tube leading from the ovary to the outside of the hen. This is called ovulation, and it usually occurs early in the morning.

Once in the oviduct, the yolk travels down this passage, and the egg white, or albumen, is added. The egg then receives its shell in the shell gland, usually taking about 20 hours in total.

This delicate yet robust shell not only protects the potential chick inside but also allows for gas exchange, which is crucial for chick development.

Once the egg is fully formed, the hen lays the egg, and the cycle starts all over again. Depending on the breed, a healthy hen can lay an egg approximately every 24 to 27 hours, meaning that with a dawn ovulation, the next egg is typically laid a little later each day.

However, this is where it gets interesting. You see, chickens, unlike some animals, don't have a strictly regulated reproductive cycle. They're heavily influenced by external conditions—light exposure being one of the key factors. The pineal gland in the chicken's brain is sensitive to changes in daylight, influencing the release of hormones that stimulate egg production. This is why hens usually lay more eggs during long summer days and fewer during shorter winter days. Providing a consistent light source can help maintain regular egg production during the darker months.

But light isn t the only influencer. Nutrition plays a significant role in a hen's ability to lay eggs consistently. Essential nutrients, particularly protein, and calcium, are vital for egg production. Without adequate nutrition, hens may lay fewer eggs, or the eggs they do lay might have thin shells or other abnormalities.

Stress also plays a significant role in egg-laying. Stressed hens often decrease their egg production or stop laying altogether. This can be caused by changes in their environment, predator threats, illness, or even a disruption in the pecking order. This is where our nest-enhancing efforts come in. By providing a safe, comfortable, and calming nest box environment, we can help reduce stress levels and promote consistent egg-laying.

Temperature, too, can impact a hen's egg-laying abilities. Both extreme cold and extreme heat can cause a drop in egg production. Chickens are hardy creatures, but they do best in moderate, stable conditions. In hot weather, ensure they have access to shade and fresh water. In cold weather, providing adequate coop insulation can help keep your hens comfortable and laying.

Aage has a say in egg-laying. Hens typically start laying at around 5 to 6 months of age and reach peak egg production at about 1 to 2 years of age. After that, egg production gradually decreases. By understanding these influencing factors, we can provide targeted care and create an environment that supports our hens in their egg-laying mission.

Egg laying is an intricate ballet of hormones, biological processes, and environmental influences. As chicken keepers, the more we understand about it, the better equipped we are to support our hens. With this knowledge in mind, we can appreciate the value of creating nurturing nests and why every effort we make towards this is a step in the right direction.

With our understanding of the egg-laying process, we can take a step further into the world of herbal support for our hardworking hens. Mother Nature has gifted us with an array of herbs that can assist our flock in their egg-laying endeavors. With the right blend of herbs, we can create an enriched environment that supports their health and productivity.

Raspberry leaf, for instance, is a powerhouse of nutrients. It's packed with magnesium, potassium, iron, and B vitamins, which are all essential for a hen's overall health and egg production. Raspberry leaf has been used by farmers for generations due to its potential to strengthen the reproductive system, making it a fantastic addition to our nesting boxes.

Another potent herb is nettle. It's chock-full of essential nutrients including iron, calcium, magnesium, and vitamins A, D, and K. The high calcium content is particularly beneficial for egg-laying hens, as calcium is a critical component of eggshell production. Nettle also boasts general health benefits and can help strengthen the immune system, promoting overall well-being.

Dandelion, often dismissed as a common weed, is another excellent herb for supporting egg-laying. It's a powerhouse of vitamins and minerals, including calcium, iron, magnesium, and vitamins A, C, and K. The leaves and flowers can provide an excellent nutrient boost for your hens, and the bright yellow flowers can also add a pop of color to your nesting boxes, making them more attractive to your hens.

These are just a few examples of herbs that can aid in egg-laying support. There are many others, including mint for its calming properties, alfalfa for its high protein content, and fennel, believed to stimulate egg-laying. Including a variety of these herbs in your nest boxes can offer numerous health benefits for your hens and potentially improve their egg-laying prowess.

But the fun doesn't stop there! In addition to adding these herbs directly to the nesting boxes, they can also be used to create herbal blends, tinctures, and treats to further support egg-laying.

Always remember, though, that while herbs can provide many beneficial nutrients and support egg-laying, they should not replace a balanced diet. High-quality feed, fresh water, and grit for digestion are fundamental necessities for your hens. The herbs are supplements, there to offer extra support and enrich the environment for your flock.

Think of these herbs as another tool in your chicken-keeping toolkit. By understanding their benefits and learning how to use them, you can provide the best possible environment for your hens to lay their eggs. In doing so, you create a nurturing nest promoting not only the quantity but also the quality of the eggs produced.

Creating an egg-supporting nest doesn't end with just understanding the herbs and their benefits, however. The real magic lies in the application, in seeing how your hens react and adjust, in continually learning, and in creating an environment that truly supports your hens. It's about taking steps, however small, towards better understanding and caring for your flock.

Establishing a nurturing nest environment takes a holistic approach that extends beyond the introduction of beneficial herbs into the nest. It encompasses everything from the physical layout of the nest to the social structure of the flock to the dietary considerations and general health of your hens.

From a physical perspective, remember that hens seek comfort and privacy when laying their eggs. Design your nest boxes to be cozy and inviting, shielding them from the hustle and bustle of the coop. A good nest box provides ample space for your hen to move around comfortably. Too small, and the hen may feel cramped; too large, and it may feel exposed. As a general guideline, a nest box should be at least 12 inches by 12 inches, with a height of about 18 inches to prevent eggs from being kicked out.

Next, consider the placement of your nest boxes. Hens prefer low light when laying, so position your nest boxes in a spot that avoids direct sunlight. Also, ensure they are easily accessible but off the ground to provide a sense of security. Raising the nests off the floor also deters predators and reduces the likelihood of egg breakage.

Social dynamics within the flock also play a significant role in egg-laying. Hens can be surprisingly particular about where they lay their eggs, and many will often prefer to lay in the same nest as others. This behavior is known as nest fidelity and is a remnant of their wild ancestors' behavior where shared nests were safer from predators. However, this can lead to nest box congestion and stress among hens. Mitigate this by providing one nest box for every four to five hens.

On the dietary front, remember that egg-laying is a physically demanding process, and hens require a balanced diet to stay healthy and produce eggs consistently. High-quality layer feed should be the primary source of nutrition, providing essential proteins, vitamins, and minerals. Calcium is particularly important as it directly contributes to eggshell strength. Providing a separate dish of oyster shell or crushed eggshell can help fulfill this need.

Hydration is equally important. Chickens need a constant supply of fresh water for digestion and overall body function, including egg production. Not only does it aid in food digestion, but it also plays a crucial part in maintaining body temperature and nutrient transportation.

Of course, we can't overlook the benefits of integrating herbs into the hens' environment. As mentioned earlier, herbs like raspberry leaf, nettle, and dandelion can provide additional nutritional support and promote calmness among the flock. Consistently refreshing these herbs in the nesting boxes will ensure their effectiveness and enhance the overall nesting experience for your hens.

Health checks are an essential part of maintaining a nurturing environment for your flock. Regular observation and interaction will help you notice any changes in behavior or appearance that may indicate health issues. If a hen is unwell, her egg production can be affected. Therefore, proactive health management is critical for egg-laying support.

Finally, remember that each flock is unique. What works for one may not work for another. It's crucial to pay attention to your hens, observe their habits, and respond to their needs accordingly. Patience and flexibility are key in creating an environment that supports your hens throughout the egg-laying process.

By incorporating these strategies, you're not just aiming for more or better eggs. You're supporting the overall well-being of your hens, providing an environment where they can thrive. And when your hens are healthy, comfortable, and happy, they'll reward you with a bountiful supply of fresh, delicious eggs.

No onto a situation that all of us chicken keepers inevitably face: issues with egg-laying. It can be concerning to find soft-shelled eggs, irregular egg-laying patterns, or even a hen who seems to have stopped laying altogether. But don't fret. Armed with your observation skills, a bit of knowledge, and the magic of herbs, you can respond effectively to these situations.

Soft-shelled or shell-less eggs can be a common occurrence, particularly with new layers whose systems are still fine-tuning the art of egg production. However, in older hens, it can indicate a calcium deficiency. Calcium is critical in the formation of strong eggshells. Providing a separate dish with oyster shell or crushed eggshell can help supplement their calcium intake.

You might also consider incorporating herbs known for their high calcium content. One such herb is nettle. Besides being a good source of calcium, it's also rich in iron and other vital minerals. Make nettle available in their diet, or try adding it to the nesting boxes.

Another herb to consider is dandelion. Often seen as a pesky weed, it's a powerhouse of nutrition. Its leaves are rich in calcium and beneficial vitamins. Chickens usually love dandelions, and it's safe for them to eat in abundance. Dandelion can be provided fresh or dried in their feed or nesting areas.

Irregular egg-laying patterns or a decrease in egg production can stem from several factors. Stress, whether from changes in the environment, flock dynamics, or health issues, can impact egg-laying. Providing a stable, calm, and safe environment can help mitigate this. Herbs known for their calming properties, like lavender and chamomile, can be added to nesting boxes to create a more tranquil environment. These herbs release their essential oils when crushed by the hens, providing a calming atmosphere.

A sudden stop in egg-laying can be quite concerning. However, it's crucial to remember that hens naturally have laying cycles influenced by daylight hours and their age. They typically slow down or cease laying during winter months or as they get older. However, if you notice a sudden stop in egg-laying outside of these reasons, it might be a sign of health issues, and a vet check may be necessary if you are unsure how to diagnose the reason.

While you explore potential health issues, try supporting your hen's health with raspberry leaf. Known as the "woman's herb" for its use in human female reproductive health, it's equally beneficial for hens. It's rich in vitamins and minerals, including calcium, and is believed to support the reproductive system.

Another egg-laying issue is egg-binding, where the hen has difficulty passing an egg. It's a potentially life-threatening condition that requires immediate veterinary attention if you are unsure how to help your girl. However, prevention is always better than cure. Keeping your hens healthy with a balanced diet, sufficient calcium, and regular exercise can help prevent this condition.

Observation is key in responding to egg-laying issues. Take time to watch your hens. Note their behavior, interactions, eating habits, and, of course, their egg-laying patterns. Unusual behavior or changes in egg-laying can be the first sign that something's amiss.

Remember, though, that not all egg-laying issues are cause for alarm. Some irregularities are normal, particularly in new layers or older hens. What's important is to know your hens and support them with a good diet, a comfortable environment, and a bit of herbal magic.

After spending considerable effort understanding the egg-laying process recognizing and responding to potential issues, it's now time to appreciate and celebrate the miracle of fresh eggs. The moment when you reach into the nest box and feel the warmth of a newly laid egg, the delightful heft of it in your hand, the smoothness of the shell under your fingers - that is a magical moment that never gets old.

Your hens, these wonderful, feathered creatures you've nurtured and cared for, are giving you the gift of sustenance. Each egg is a testament to the cycle of life and a tangible reminder of the bond between you and your hens. It's a connection that goes beyond pet and keeper - it's a shared dance with nature itself.

And what a dance it is! Each egg that your hen lays involves a symphony of biological processes. From the development of the yolk in the ovary, its release into the oviduct, the formation of the egg white or albumen around it, the creation of the shell, and finally, the egg's journey out into the world, it's an astounding marvel of nature.

The eggs themselves are tiny packets of nourishment. Packed with high-quality protein, essential vitamins, and minerals, eggs are truly a "superfood". Each egg yolk is a golden storehouse of Vitamin A, D, E, and B12, along with iron, phosphorus, and folate. The egg white is a clean source of protein, with little to no fat. Your hens aren't just giving you a gift; they're providing you with a versatile and nutritious food source.

The beauty of the egg isn't just in its nutritional profile but in its versatility in the kitchen. Fried, scrambled, poached, baked, or boiled eggs are a staple in cuisines around the world. Each fresh egg from your hens opens up a world of culinary possibilities. From breakfast scrambles to baking, sauces to desserts, the humble egg is a key ingredient in countless dishes.

Beyond the kitchen, eggs have cultural and symbolic significance, too. They symbolize fertility, rebirth, and the cycle of life and death. In many cultures, eggs are used in rituals, celebrations, and as offerings. The egg isn't just a source of food, it's a symbol steeped in cultural and spiritual meaning.

It's easy to take for granted the regular gift of eggs from your hens. But remember to take a moment every now and then to appreciate this everyday miracle. Look at each egg with wonder, acknowledging the complex biological processes that went into its creation, the care you've given your hens, the herbs that you've incorporated into their lives, and the time and attention that you've invested.

The next time you collect eggs, pause. Feel the warmth of the egg and the smoothness of the shell. Look at the color, shape, and size. Each egg is unique, just like each hen in your flock. It's a direct reflection of all the love and care you've put into creating a nurturing environment for your hens.

Celebrating the miracle of fresh eggs is about acknowledging the cycle of life, the bond between you and your hens, and the care and attention you've put into creating an environment where your hens can thrive. So, here's to you, the dedicated chicken keeper, and to your hens, the extraordinary egg layers. Here's to the humble egg, a symbol of life, a source of sustenance, and a testament to the wonderful dance of nature. Here's to the journey you've undertaken with your hens, the lessons learned, the small victories, and the joy of finding that perfect egg in the nest box. Let's celebrate the miracle of fresh eggs every day.

"The art of healing comes from nature, not from the physician."
— Paracelsus

Chapter 6: Flock First Aid with Herbs

Part I: Don't Wing It: Herbal First Aid Basics

Let's discuss the specifics of recognizing the need for first aid in your flock. Despite our best efforts to keep our flock healthy and safe, chickens can be prone to a variety of injuries and ailments. Knowing how to identify and react to these can be the difference between a quick recovery and a tragic loss.

Let's start with physical injuries. Chickens can suffer from a wide array of injuries - from minor scratches and pecks to more serious conditions like sprains, broken bones, and deep wounds. In many cases, injuries occur due to their social behaviors, environmental hazards, or predators.

Cuts and scratches, often from interactions with coop fixtures or during friendly squabbles, are among the most common. A bit of blood can cause a frenzy among flock members, as chickens are instinctively attracted to the color red. Therefore, treating even minor injuries promptly is crucial to prevent pecking and subsequent harm.

Injury from predators is a more serious matter. If a predator has managed to access your chickens, they might suffer from deep cuts, missing feathers, or worse. Immediate attention and treatment can be lifesaving. The careful use of herbs in these instances can aid in the healing process and fight potential infection.

Respiratory issues are also common among chickens. Symptoms such as sneezing, coughing, nasal discharge, and wheezing could indicate a respiratory infection. In such cases, you'll need to act quickly to prevent the disease from spreading to the rest of the flock. Certain herbs can assist with boosting immune response and alleviating symptoms.

Parasites, both internal and external, are a common occurrence in chickens. External parasites include mites, lice, and fleas, which can cause itching, irritation, feather loss, and restlessness. Internal parasites like worms can result in weight loss, diarrhea, and decreased egg production. A variety of herbs have been used for centuries in parasite management, providing a natural and gentler alternative to chemical treatments.

Common internal ailments include egg binding, where a hen is unable to pass an egg, and sour crop, a yeast infection in a chicken's crop often due to an imbalanced diet. These issues can quickly become life-threatening and demand immediate attention. Some herbs may aid in alleviating symptoms and support recovery.

Chickens, like any animal, can suffer from a variety of other health issues such as eye problems, foot issues like bumblefoot, and reproductive complications. These conditions can be hard to diagnose without the help of a vet, but there are still steps you can take at home to provide comfort and care.

Observation is key in all these situations. Daily interaction with your flock allows you to notice any changes in behavior, appetite, or physical appearance. By getting to know your flock, you'll be able to detect when something isn't quite right. Look for signs of discomfort, changes in demeanor or energy level, or any physical signs like limping or changes in their droppings.

A well-prepared chicken keeper is equipped with not just the right tools and treatments but also the knowledge to handle common chicken injuries and ailments. The ability to recognize these conditions is the first step in providing effective care.

Bear in mind, though, that the use of herbs is a complement, not a substitute, for veterinary advice. It's always best to consult with a vet for severe injuries, unknown ailments, or when you're unsure. The information you gain from your vet combined with a well-prepared herbal first aid kit can help ensure your hens receive the care they need when they need it.

Understanding common chicken injuries and ailments is critical for any chicken keeper. From minor pecking injuries to more severe conditions, knowing what to look for and how to respond can greatly affect the outcome. It's the difference between a quick recovery and a slow deterioration. Never underestimate the importance of keen observation, swift action, and, when needed, professional advice.

Recognizing the role that herbs play in first aid allows us to better understand how these natural remedies can work alongside more traditional methods to support the health of our flock. The healing properties and benefits of herbs extend far beyond their culinary uses. They serve as an essential part of a chicken keeper's first aid toolkit.

Let's delve into the role of herbs in first aid, exploring the healing properties and benefits they offer. It's fascinating how these plants, which we might casually use in cooking or see in our garden, harbor powerful medicinal benefits.

Consider comfrey, for instance. This plant is recognized for its remarkable wound-healing properties. Comfrey leaves contain allantoin, a substance that stimulates cell growth, speeding up the healing process. Therefore, applying a comfrey poultice to a chicken's wound can aid in faster healing.

Yarrow, another remarkable herb, is known for its ability to stop bleeding. In fact, it's been used for this purpose since ancient times. When applied to a wound, yarrow can help slow down or even stop bleeding, making it a great addition to your herbal first aid kit.

Then there's the versatile plantain – not the banana-like fruit, but the common plant found in yards and fields worldwide. Plantain has anti-inflammatory and antimicrobial properties, making it effective for treating minor skin irritations and wounds. It can also soothe the digestive tract, offering relief for conditions such as sour crop.

Garlic, a kitchen staple, is beneficial in warding off both internal and external parasites. Given regularly, it can serve as a natural preventive measure against worm infestations. Garlic also possesses antibacterial and antiviral properties that support the general health of your flock.

Echinacea, often associated with immune support in humans, holds similar benefits for chickens. It can help strengthen their immune system, making them more capable of fending off diseases.

Calendula is another herb that deserves a spot in your chicken first aid kit. It is known for its skin-healing properties, promoting the healing of wounds and burns. Moreover, its vibrant flowers can add a golden hue to egg yolks when added to your chickens' diet.

Aloe Vera, known for its soothing and healing properties, can be used to treat minor skin irritations and burns. The gel from the Aloe Vera plant is rich in compounds that reduce inflammation and promote healing.

Lavender, apart from its delightful aroma, is known for its calming effect. Its antiseptic properties make it a good choice for minor cuts and wounds. Moreover, when added to nesting boxes, it can promote a relaxing environment that encourages laying.

Thyme, loaded with antiseptic properties, is excellent for respiratory issues. Infused in a hot water vapor, it can help alleviate symptoms of respiratory infections, providing a natural way to help your chickens breathe easier.

While herbs offer numerous health benefits, they should be used judiciously. It's crucial to educate ourselves on the correct uses, potential side effects, and correct preparation methods of these herbs. Overuse or incorrect use can lead to problems, and not all herbs are safe for all animals or in all situations.

That being said, the judicious use of herbs can enhance the health and well-being of your flock. Integrating them into your chickens' environment and diet allows for a proactive approach to health care – a way to fortify their defenses before problems arise.

The prudent application of herbs certainly strengthens your flock's health and well-being. By weaving them into your chickens' habitat and diet, you're establishing a preemptive healthcare strategy, bolstering their defenses before any issues surface.

Let's have some fun and construct a chicken herbal first aid kit. What are the must-have herbs, necessary tools, and supplies you need to address common poultry problems? Equipping yourself with the right set of resources gives you the ability to act swiftly when an issue arises, offering instant relief and increasing the chances of a quicker recovery.

Starting with herbs, you might wonder, 'Which ones should I include?' Well, previously we've explored numerous beneficial herbs and their various properties, and these certainly make a good starting point. Comfrey, Yarrow, Plantain, Garlic, Echinacea, Calendula, Aloe Vera, Lavender, and Thyme should be staples in your chicken herbal first aid kit. Each herb possesses unique medicinal properties that can cater to different ailments.

While these herbs form the basis of your kit, a broader selection might include herbs like chamomile, known for its calming properties, and elderberry, which can help boost immunity during those tough winter months. Parsley is another herb that aids in egg-laying while offering a nutritional boost. Oregano acts as a natural antibiotic, and sage offers anti-parasitic properties, making them worthwhile additions as well.

Moving on to tools and supplies, it's all about keeping it practical and versatile. A pair of sharp, clean scissors is indispensable for cutting herbs or bandages. Tweezers come in handy when you need to remove splinters or debris from wounds. A magnifying glass can be useful in providing a closer look at injuries or identifying tiny parasites.

Having a good selection of bandages is a no-brainer. These include gauze, self-adhesive bandages, and regular adhesive strips for minor cuts and scrapes. You might also want to keep on hand some wound spray, preferably an herbal one, for disinfecting wounds before dressing.

Consider having a set of droppers or syringes (without needles) for administering herbal tinctures or oils. Speaking of oils, having a basic selection of carrier oils such as olive or coconut oil is beneficial. Many herbs are most effective when infused in oil, and these oils can also serve to soothe dry or irritated skin.

Natural, unscented soap is necessary for cleaning wounds, as is saline solution. Saline is gentle on injuries and is excellent for washing out dust or debris before applying any herbal remedies.

A quick digital thermometer is another must-have. Detecting a rise in body temperature can be the first sign of an illness brewing, so it's an essential part of your kit.

If you're planning to prepare herbal remedies in advance, small containers or jars are also a necessity. Whether it's a salve, a poultice, or an infused oil, having somewhere clean and airtight to store your concoctions is essential. Just remember to label everything clearly, including the date it was made.

On that note, a small notepad and pen might not seem like typical first-aid kit items, but trust me, they're invaluable. Jotting down symptoms, temperatures, or changes in behavior can provide useful information in diagnosing and tracking an illness.

An herbal guide or handbook is always a good idea to include in your kit. Even with a solid base of knowledge, in times of stress, having a guide to quickly reference can be a real lifesaver.

Even with a sturdy foundation of knowledge in your grasp, during stressful times, having a quick reference guide can indeed prove to be a lifesaver. It's not just about having a well-stocked first aid kit but also about knowing how to use it effectively. To that end, let's explore some basic first-aid procedures that you can carry out using herbs. We'll be focusing on cleaning wounds, applying dressings, and some additional strategies to ensure your feathery friends are on the path to recovery in no time.

Before diving in, remember one crucial fact – every situation, every chicken, is unique. What works in one situation may not be as effective in another. Therefore, flexibility, coupled with observation and intuition, forms the foundation of successful chicken care.

Cleaning wounds is an integral first step in any first-aid situation involving injury. It helps prevent infection and promotes healing. In our herbal kit, we have natural, unscented soap and saline solution, both of which are gentle on wounds. Now, here's where we can add some herbal magic: Calendula, known for its antimicrobial properties, can be infused into the saline solution. Alternatively, you can create a tea using the flowers and use it to gently clean the wound area. Aloe Vera, widely recognized for its soothing and healing properties, can also be applied to cleaned wounds to promote healing.

Applying dressings comes next in the line of action. As per the severity and nature of the wound, different types of bandages can be used. However, before the dressing comes the application of a suitable herbal remedy. Comfrey, with its powerful wound-healing properties, can be made into a salve and applied to cleaned wounds before dressing. Infusing some lavender into your salve can add the benefits of this calming, antibacterial herb, promoting both physical and emotional recovery for your chickens. For deeper wounds, a poultice made with Plantain leaves can be applied. Known for its antibacterial and anti-inflammatory properties, Plantain helps in drawing out infection and promoting healing.

Additionally, let's not forget the importance of internal health when it comes to recovery. Echinacea, a well-known immune-boosting herb, can be made into a tincture and added to your chickens' water, providing internal support to complement external wound care. Garlic, too, with its potent antibacterial properties, can be added to their diet, providing an extra layer of defense against potential infections.

Moving beyond wound care, herbs offer a plethora of benefits for various other common chicken ailments. Respiratory issues, for instance, are common among chickens, and herbs like thyme and oregano, with their strong antimicrobial properties, can help in alleviating symptoms. They can be used in a variety of ways – from adding fresh or dried leaves to their feed to making a strong tea and using it in a warm vapor bath for your chickens.

Digestive problems are another area where herbs can lend a helping hand. Herbs like dandelion and nettle can support the digestive system and can easily be incorporated into the diet of your chickens. If you suspect your flock has a parasitic infestation, herbs like wormwood and pumpkin seeds can help in flushing out the unwelcome guests.

Now, while these procedures provide a solid starting point, it's vital to remember that severe cases or conditions showing no signs of improvement should be addressed by a professional veterinarian. The information provided here is intended to empower you as a chicken keeper to better care for your flock, foster a more natural, holistic lifestyle for them, and act swiftly and confidently when minor issues arise. However, it's equally important to know when to seek expert advice.

Armed with these procedures, you've laid the foundation for effective first aid in your flock. However it's essential to recognize that dealing with severe conditions or persistent issues is a job for a professional veterinarian. The advice shared here empowers you to provide better care for your flock, foster a more natural, holistic lifestyle, and act swiftly and confidently in the face of minor challenges. Just as crucial, however, is recognizing when professional help is needed.

Stepping in as a caretaker, it is your responsibility not only to administer first aid but also to monitor your chickens during their recovery. Observing and gauging their progress, looking out for signs of healing or potential complications, and determining when and how to follow up are all integral parts of post-treatment care.

When observing healing signs, keep in mind that chickens, like all living beings, have their own unique healing timeline. Factors like the severity of the condition, the hen's overall health, and her age can all play a part in how quickly or slowly she recovers. An essential marker of healing is a gradual return to normal behavior. Is she eating and drinking properly? Has she rejoined the flock or is she still keeping to herself? Is she preening and keeping her feathers clean? These are all good signs that her health is on the mend.

Physical signs of healing, especially in the case of wounds, include reduced swelling and redness, the formation of new skin, and lessening discomfort. As time goes by, the area should look cleaner, feel less painful, and start returning to its normal color.

At the same time, vigilance is key in spotting potential complications. Excessive swelling, heat, and redness around the wound even after a few days could indicate an infection. Also, watch for pus, which is a clear sign of an ongoing bacterial infection. In such cases, immediate veterinary attention is necessary.

Behaviorally, if your hen seems unusually listless, refuses to eat or drink, or is visibly in pain, these are tell-tale signs that she may not be healing as expected and that something more serious might be afoot. Similarly, a sharp decline in egg production, changes in droppings, or continued isolation from the rest of the flock can also suggest complications.

Follow-up care depends greatly on the initial issue. Cleaning and dressing of wounds should continue until they're completely healed. Herbal support, like Echinacea tincture or garlic in their diet, can continue as these natural additions not only aid in healing but also contribute to overall health.

After the initial treatment of respiratory or digestive issues, a close eye on the chickens' behavior will inform if and when further intervention is necessary. If symptoms persist or worsen, it's time to consult your vet.

Your role in the healing process extends beyond the first aid administered at the onset of an issue. It involves careful observation, the ability to identify potential complications, and the judgement to determine when professional advice is needed. As a chicken keeper, you're not only charged with the health of your flock but also their well-being.

With time and experience, you'll become increasingly adept at reading the subtle signs your chickens give off, developing a deeper understanding of what's normal for your flock, and when to intervene. This ongoing interaction and the deep connection you forge with your flock is, in many ways, the true joy of chicken keeping.

Every flock is unique. What works for one may not work for another. It's about understanding, observing, and responding to the specific needs of your hens. It's about arming yourself with knowledge and then applying it to create the best possible environment for your flock.

There is a certain magic that comes with integrating these natural remedies into our care routines. A sense of being more connected to the land, to the ancient wisdom of the herbalists who came before us. But beyond that, there is a sense of empowerment that comes from knowing that we have the ability to help our feathered friends when they need us most. This is the beauty of embracing the role of herbs in first aid. And as we learn more, we become better stewards, more in tune with the needs of our flock, and more capable of providing the care they need.

Chicken keeping is a journey of discovery, of learning to care for and understand another species. Armed with knowledge, intuition, and a well-stocked herbal first aid kit, you are well-prepared to face the challenges that come your way. And remember, each challenge overcome is an opportunity to learn and grow, both for you and your flock. Together, you'll navigate through the ups and downs of this rewarding endeavor, with each day bringing with it the promise of fresh eggs, happy clucks, and the simple joy of being a part of this amazing journey.

In the end, herbal first aid isn't about replacing professional veterinary care. Instead, it's about understanding how you can bolster your chickens' health with nature's bounty, treating minor issues effectively, and nurturing a resilient flock able to bounce back from life's little hiccups. It's about harnessing the power of nature for the welfare of your chickens and fostering a lifestyle that is as natural and wholesome as it is fulfilling for both you and your feathered friends.

Part II: Peck and Heal: Herbs for Wound Care

The world of chickens is fascinating and lively. Their social interactions, the pecking order, the squabbles over food, and favorite perching spots - it's a flurry of feathers and clucks. However, this active lifestyle can also lead to injuries. As a chicken keeper, it's essential to understand different wound types, how to identify them, and how they can impact your flock's health.

At the top of the list are scratches. Scratches are superficial wounds, usually caused by sharp objects in the environment, rough handling, or other chickens' claws during the usual bustle. They are often shallow, affecting only the skin's surface. While generally not serious, they can become a gateway for bacteria if not cared for promptly.

Pecks, as the name suggests, are injuries inflicted by other chickens using their beaks. Chickens can peck each other due to various reasons - establishing dominance, boredom, or stress, to name a few. It's a natural behavior, but it can lead to significant injuries if it escalates. Pecks can range from mild, hardly noticeable ones to severe ones, leading to open wounds.

Cuts, on the other hand, are deeper wounds that often involve both the skin and the underlying tissues. These could be caused by sharp objects in the chicken's environment, accidents, or predatory attacks. Cuts are usually more severe than scratches or pecks, requiring immediate attention as they have a higher risk of infection and complications.

Puncture wounds are also common in a chicken's life. These happen when a pointed object pierces the skin, creating a small, deep wound. The danger of puncture wounds lies less in their size and more in their depth - they can introduce bacteria deep into the body, leading to serious internal infections.

Bumblefoot, though not a wound in the traditional sense, is a common condition in chickens that deserves mention. It's an infection caused by the bacterium Staphylococcus, entering usually through a scratch or cut on the foot. It's characterized by a hard, swollen, and often painful lump on the footpad.

Each wound type presents unique challenges and requires specific attention. The good news is that, aside from deep, serious wounds, most minor injuries can be effectively managed using herbs and proper wound care.

Herbs come in with their anti-inflammatory, antibacterial, and wound-healing properties. For instance, calendula, known for its skin healing benefits, can be used as a poultice or in a salve for treating scratches and mild pecks. A strong tea made from yarrow, a herb reputed for its ability to stop bleeding, can be used to clean deeper cuts.

For puncture wounds, after a thorough cleaning, a compress of plantain, a common garden weed with powerful drawing properties, can help draw out any residual debris or infection. Bumblefoot, being a more complex issue, often requires an integrated approach of both conventional treatment and herbal support for effective healing.

In a world where chickens scratch in the dirt, dust bathe, and occasionally squabble with each other, injuries are inevitable. Understanding these wound types helps you provide the first line of defense for your flock's health. It enables you to react swiftly, addressing minor injuries before they escalate, keeping your flock happier, healthier, and more productive.

Of course, severe wounds, wounds that don't heal or are associated with other signs of illness should always be evaluated by a veterinarian. But in many cases, being prepared with the knowledge of wounds and having an herbal first aid kit on hand can make all the difference. Armed with herbs and a little know-how, you'll be well-equipped to tackle the majority of minor injuries in your flock.

Now, for minor injuries, herbs are the unsung heroes. They offer healing and antiseptic properties, they can aid in quick recovery, reduce the risk of infection, and, in some cases, even provide pain relief. Understanding which herbs to use and when to use them is key. In this section, we'll be talking about some essential herbs that should be part of your chicken first aid kit - Yarrow, Plantain, Comfrey, and many more.

Let's begin with Yarrow, one of the most versatile herbs in your herbal arsenal. Known scientifically as Achillea millefolium, it's named after the Greek hero Achilles, who used it to treat his soldiers' wounds during the Trojan War. Yarrow's astringent and antiseptic properties make it an excellent choice for cleaning wounds. Moreover, it's reputed to stop bleeding, which makes it a go-to herb for cuts or pecks that result in open wounds.

Next up, Plantain, a common weed found in almost all parts of the world, is a treasure trove of medicinal properties. Also known as Plantago, this humble plant is a powerful anti-inflammatory and antiseptic. It's excellent at drawing out toxins and other foreign materials from wounds, which is particularly useful in the case of puncture wounds. A poultice made from its leaves can help speed up the healing process.

Comfrey, or Symphytum officinale, often referred to as 'knit bone', is a key player when it comes to wound healing. Its leaves are rich in allantoin, a compound that stimulates cell growth, thereby speeding up healing. It's especially effective for healing scratches, as it not only aids in closing the wound but also helps minimize scarring.

Chickweed, a common garden weed, is another useful herb. Not just a tasty treat for your chickens, it also boasts anti-inflammatory properties. Its soothing effect makes it an excellent choice for treating irritated skin and minor pecks.

Lavender, apart from smelling divine, is a natural antibacterial and anti-inflammatory herb. It's particularly useful for calming stressed chickens. A bundle of lavender hung in the chicken coop can work wonders for a stressed flock. Its healing properties can also be utilized in a salve form for treating scratches or mild pecks.

Calendula, with its vibrant orange flowers, is a valuable addition to your chicken first aid kit. Known for its wound-healing and antimicrobial abilities, it's often used in salves or as a poultice. Its petals can also be dried and added to chicken feed, offering internal support for the immune system.

Herbs are potent, and while they offer a natural way to support healing, they should be used with knowledge and respect. Understanding each herb's properties will help you make the right choice depending on the type of injury. Also, quality matters. Whether you're growing your own herbs or sourcing them, ensure they are free from pesticides and other harmful chemicals. Quality is key, and no truer words have been spoken when it comes to herbs. Pure, natural, and pesticide-free - these should be your guiding principles while sourcing herbs. After all, you wouldn't want to risk the health of your flock by using herbs laced with harmful chemicals. Once you have good quality herbs at hand, the next step is to transform these raw ingredients into remedies that can be effectively used for wound care. Poultices, ointments, and infusions are the primary forms of herbal remedies that you would be preparing. Let's dive into each one and understand how you can make these at home.

Starting with poultices, these are a traditional form of remedy that involves applying herbs directly to the wound. The essence of a poultice lies in its simplicity. You take fresh or dried herbs, crush them or heat them up to release their healing oils, place the resulting mixture onto a clean cloth, and then apply this directly to the wound. For instance, plantain leaves can be made into a poultice crushing the leaves and applying them directly to a wound. The enzymes in the plantain help draw out infection and speed up healing. Another example is a comfrey poultice. You could simmer fresh comfrey leaves in a bit of water, mash them into a pulp, and apply this warm paste to the wounded area.

Next in line are ointments. These are a bit more sophisticated than poultices and require some additional ingredients. The basic idea is to infuse oil with the healing properties of herbs and then solidify the oil using beeswax. Let's take an example of yarrow ointment, known for its ability to stop bleeding and disinfect wounds. You would begin by infusing dried yarrow in a carrier oil (like olive oil or almond oil) for several weeks. Once the oil has been thoroughly infused, you would strain out the yarrow, heat the infused oil slightly, and then add beeswax to solidify the mixture. Once cooled, you have a potent yarrow ointment ready to be applied to wounds.

Finally, we have infusions. In the simplest terms, infusions are like herbal teas prepared for external use. They are made by steeping herbs in hot water, allowing the water to draw out the beneficial properties of the herbs. Infusions are excellent for cleaning wounds or as a base for other preparations. For instance, a lavender infusion, known for its antibacterial properties, can be used to gently cleanse wounds before applying a poultice or ointment. Just add a handful of dried lavender to boiling water, let it steep until the water cools, and strain. The resulting infusion can be used directly on the wounds.

Just as we discussed, infusions like a lavender one work wonders in cleansing wounds. They set the stage for the application of other herbal remedies by ensuring the wound area is clean and free from dirt and debris. Remember, an infusion is a base, a starting point. Once we have our wound cleansed with an infusion, the next steps involve applying the more concentrated herbal preparations - poultices and ointments.

The first step in using a poultice is to ensure that you've prepared it properly. If you're using fresh herbs, these should be crushed or heated gently to release the oils and active compounds. If you're using dried herbs, you may need to add a bit of warm water to rehydrate them and help release their beneficial compounds. Once your poultice is prepared, it's simply a matter of applying it to the wound.

It's best to place the herb material onto a clean cloth and then apply this cloth directly onto the wound. If the injury is small, you might apply the poultice directly. Once applied, cover the poultice with a clean bandage to keep it in place and protect it. The poultice should stay in place for several hours or even overnight to allow the healing compounds in the herbs to do their job. After the poultice is removed, cleanse the area again with an herbal infusion or clean water before applying a new poultice if necessary.

Moving on to ointments, their application is relatively straightforward. First, ensure the wound is clean. Remember, an herbal infusion can be used for this purpose. Once you've ensured the wound is clean, simply apply a thin layer of the ointment directly to the wound. Depending on the wound's location and your chicken's behavior, you may need to cover the ointment with a bandage to keep it in place and prevent your chicken from pecking at it.

It's crucial to note here that herbs, while natural, can still cause reactions in some individuals. Just like people, chickens can have allergies or sensitivities. So, always monitor your chicken's response to any herbal treatment. If you notice any signs of discomfort, inflammation, or increased redness around the wound after applying a poultice or ointment, discontinue use and consult with a vet. I, personally, have never had a chicken have an adverse reaction to natural remedies.

You are your flock's first line of defense. With the right knowledge and skills, you can use herbal remedies effectively and safely to care for minor injuries in your flock. With the poultice applied or ointment smeared, and while watching your feathered patient for signs of improvement, you'll stand a bit taller and feel a bit prouder. It's in these moments of healing and care that we truly embody the spirit of a chicken keeper.

As we continue on this journey of learning about chicken health, it's not just about the immediate actions we take at the onset of an injury. One could argue that the real work, critical care, begins after the initial wound has been addressed. This is when we step into the territory of ongoing wound care – the dressing changes, the constant monitoring, and the attentive tracking of healing progression.

When the poultice is in place, or the ointment is on, it's time for the next phase: maintaining the care. Wound dressings should be changed regularly to prevent infection and promote healing. How often? It depends on the severity and type of wound. Generally speaking, dressing changes once or twice a day are a good rule of thumb for most minor wounds.

When it comes to changing the dressing, cleanliness is of the utmost importance. Just as we did when initially addressing the wound, make sure your hands and any tools used are clean to minimize the risk of introducing bacteria to the wound. Remove the old dressing carefully, clean the wound gently with an herbal infusion or clean water, and then apply fresh herbal remedy – a new poultice or another layer of ointment – before covering it with a new, clean dressing.

Constant monitoring is essential. Be sure to examine the wound each time you change the dressing. Look for signs of improvement such as the wound shrinking in size, a decrease in redness, and the growth of new, healthy skin. Also, keep an eye out for any potential signs of infection like increased redness, swelling, or an unpleasant odor.

Monitoring your chicken's behavior is equally important. Chickens, like most animals, are experts at hiding their pain, so it's up to you to pick up on subtle signs. Is the chicken still active? Eating and drinking well? Do they interact with the rest of the flock as usual? A healthy, healing chicken should maintain their daily habits. Any changes in behavior, especially combined with a wound that doesn't seem to be improving, should warrant a call to your vet.

Last but definitely not least, let's talk about healing progression. Healing doesn't happen overnight. It takes time, especially when it comes to the natural healing process bolstered by herbal remedies. But with patience, you'll begin to see the fruits of your efforts and your chicken's resilience. The wound will gradually get smaller, new skin will start to form, and before you know it, you'll have a fully healed chicken on your hands.

On this healing journey, remember that each chicken is an individual and will heal at his or her own pace. You're there to facilitate this process and provide the best care possible during their recovery. You're doing great work, and your chickens appreciate it - even if they can't tell you so directly.

Incorporating herbs into your flock's first aid kit is a holistic step towards better health and well-being. These green allies have been used for centuries to heal and nourish. By understanding their properties and learning how to use them effectively, you're not just addressing injuries but enhancing the overall resilience of your flock.

Remember, your role as a chicken keeper isn't just about providing food and shelter for your feathered charges. It's also about ensuring their well-being, and that includes being prepared for injuries. Every scratch, peck, or cut offers an opportunity to learn and grow in your journey as a chicken keeper. After all, the more you understand your chickens, the better you can provide for them.

There's an undeniable joy in observing the daily antics of your flock, in hearing the excited clucks as you scatter treats, but there's also a profound satisfaction in knowing you've done your part in tending to their health, that you've offered a bit of comfort in a time of discomfort. Using herbs is not just about addressing specific problems, it's about fostering an environment that enhances the overall health of your flock. You're not just a chicken keeper; you're a steward of these wonderful creatures. Part of that responsibility involves learning and utilizing the gifts of nature in caring for your flock. It's important to keep in mind that while these remedies can be powerful aids in healing, they are not a substitute for professional veterinary advice in severe cases. That being said, for minor injuries and wounds, these herbal remedies can be the first line of defense. They are natural, devoid of synthetic chemicals, and when prepared with quality herbs, they can offer a holistic approach to wound care.

Part III: Combs and Wattles: Herbal Care for Chicken Faces

Now, let's take a step back and focus our attention on some of the most prominent features of our beloved chickens: their combs and wattles. These distinctive, fleshy protuberances on their heads and throats are not just for show, they're functional structures that help chickens regulate their body temperature. However, these exposed appendages can be susceptible to a range of issues, from frostbite and fowl pox to pecking injuries and more.

Let's start with one of the more common issues, especially for those chicken keepers in colder climates: frostbite. This is a condition where the tissue freezes due to exposure to cold temperatures. Frostbite tends to affect the tips of the combs and wattles first since these areas are the most exposed and have a higher surface area to volume ratio, causing them to lose heat rapidly. Signs of frostbite include discoloration (the affected areas turn a pale, whitish color), swelling, and, in severe cases, blackened tissue.

Then there's fowl pox, a viral disease that affects chickens worldwide. This disease presents itself in two forms: dry and wet. The dry form is characterized by wart-like nodules on the non-feathered areas such as the combs and wattles. These nodules can vary in size, and they often first appear as white pinhead-sized spots that develop into brownish-black scabs. The wet form affects the respiratory tract and is marked by canker-like lesions in the mouth and throat.

Pecking injuries are another common issue when it comes to combs and wattles. Chickens can be surprisingly brutal to each other, and a brightly colored, bleeding comb or wattle can be an irresistible target to an aggressive flock mate. This can result in wounds that need to be treated promptly to prevent further pecking and potential infection.

Another common condition is comb and wattle lice. These tiny parasites are often overlooked but can cause significant discomfort and stress for chickens. They tend to cluster on the comb and wattle area and can cause the skin to become irritated and inflamed.

Next on our list are injuries and infections. Chickens can get their combs and wattles caught on coop wire, sharp edges, or other hazards in their environment, leading to cuts and scrapes. These injuries can then become infected if not addressed promptly. Signs of infection can include redness, swelling, pus, and an unwell chicken.

Lastly, we must address tumors, cysts, and abscesses. Though not as common, combs and wattles can develop these growths due to various reasons, including viral infections or injuries. These can often be hard to differentiate from other conditions without the help of a vet.

Being able to identify these common issues is the first step in providing effective care for your chickens' combs and wattles. But knowing what to look for is just the start. Now that we've recognized the problems, the logical next step is to address them using the natural healing power of herbs. This journey will take us through the world of Aloe Vera, Echinacea, Thyme, and many other herbal allies ready to lend a helping leaf to our feathered friends.

Let's start our herbal tour with the humble Aloe Vera. A succulent plant by nature, Aloe Vera has a rich history of use in herbal medicine, primarily due to its potent anti-inflammatory and wound-healing properties. The transparent gel found inside Aloe Vera leaves is incredibly soothing and can be applied directly to the combs and wattles to help heal minor wounds, burns, and frostbite. The moisturizing effect of Aloe Vera can also help prevent cracking and drying, which are common issues during cold, harsh winters.

Next up is Echinacea, a plant with beautiful purple flowers that are revered for its immune-boosting properties. Echinacea is known to stimulate the production of white blood cells, the soldiers of the body's immune system. This makes it an excellent ally in combating infections and helping the body heal from injuries. You can create a simple Echinacea infusion by steeping the flowers and leaves in hot water. Once cooled, this infusion can be applied directly to affected areas to boost healing and fight infection.

Then we have Thyme. Not just a fragrant herb for your chicken's nesting box or your kitchen's spice rack, Thyme is packed with antibacterial and antifungal properties. Thyme oil can be diluted and applied to the combs and wattles to help treat bacterial infections or prevent infection in wounds. The herb can also be steeped in hot water to make an infusion that can be used as a wash for the combs and wattles.

Calendula, also known as Pot Marigold, is another remarkable herb for skin health. It's been used for centuries to heal wounds, burns, rashes, and skin infections. The vibrant orange flowers contain high levels of flavonoids, compounds that exhibit anti-inflammatory, antibacterial, and antioxidant properties. Calendula can be used as an infusion or in an ointment form to promote skin health and speed up healing.

Another beneficial herb to mention is Comfrey. Comfrey is renowned for its ability to promote cell growth and repair skin tissue, earning it the nickname "knit bone." When used externally, Comfrey can help heal cuts and abrasions. However, Comfrey should only be used on clean, uninfected wounds as it can cause the skin to heal over an infection.

Finally, there's Lavender. Besides its calming scent, Lavender has potent antibacterial and anti-inflammatory properties. An infusion or diluted oil can be applied to the combs and wattles to combat bacterial infections, reduce inflammation, and soothe irritations.

These are just some of the many herbs available to us for the care of our chickens' combs and wattles. The world of herbal healing is vast and varied. It's always good to have multiple options on hand to address different issues. Are you ready to learn how to harness these herbs and transform them into useful remedies for your flock's facial care? Sprays, salves, and washes are the forms we will be discussing, as these are the most suited for treating comb and wattle ailments.

Herbal sprays are a convenient, no-contact way to apply herbal treatments to your chickens, ideal for birds that might not enjoy hands-on attention. Sprays can be used for a wide variety of purposes, from simple freshening sprays for a quick perk-up to medicated sprays for treating specific issues. For instance, a thyme spray, lauded for its antiseptic properties, can be created by steeping thyme leaves in boiling water. Once cooled, strain the mixture and put it in a clean spray bottle for easy application. This thyme spray can be used on a chicken's comb and wattles to keep them clean and help prevent bacterial infections.

Next, we come to herbal salves. A salve is essentially a blend of oils and waxes that provides a protective layer over the skin, allowing the healing properties of the herbs to work their magic. They are excellent for treating wounds, protecting against harsh weather conditions, and providing relief from skin irritations. A simple calendula salve, known for its anti-inflammatory and healing properties, can be made by infusing calendula flowers in an oil such as olive or almond for several weeks. Once the oil has absorbed the properties of the calendula, it's strained and gently heated with beeswax to create a soothing salve that can be applied to your chickens' combs and wattles.

Finally, herbal washes or infusions, as they're often called, are another way to utilize herbs for chicken care. They can be used to clean wounds, soothe irritations, and offer relief from a variety of skin conditions. A simple lavender wash, for example, can be made by steeping dried lavender in boiling water. The resulting infusion, with its calming and antibacterial properties, can be used to gently clean your chickens' combs and wattles.

Part IV: Poultry Podiatry: Herbal Foot Soaks

Like with our own health, often it's the smallest problems that can cause the most distress for our feathered friends. One area that's frequently overlooked but can cause significant issues for chickens is their feet. We are going to discuss some of the most common foot problems in chickens and how you, as their caretaker, can be on the lookout for these issues.

One of the most common issues we see in chickens is something called Bumblefoot. Bumblefoot is a bacterial infection caused by Staphylococcus aureus, which is essentially the same bacteria responsible for staph infections in humans. The bacteria enter the foot through a cut or scrape and can cause a painful abscess filled with pus. If left untreated, the infection can spread to the bones and joints and can cause significant pain and lameness. Early signs of Bumblefoot include swelling, redness, and a characteristic black or brown scab on the foot's bottom. Chickens with Bumblefoot might also show signs of pain, such as limping or refusing to walk. Please keep in mind when treating Bumblefoot, be sure to wear gloves to protect yourself from catching or spreading the infection!

Scaly leg mites are another common foot problem in chickens. These microscopic parasites burrow under the scales on a chicken's legs and feet, causing them to lift and appear rough or crusted. In severe cases, the chicken's legs and feet might become swollen, and they may experience difficulty walking. Chickens with scaly leg mites might also exhibit signs of discomfort, such as frequent scratching or picking at their legs and feet.

Foot and leg injuries can also be common in backyard flocks, especially those with access to a large range area where they can roam freely. Cuts, scrapes, and abrasions can happen if chickens step on sharp objects or get their feet caught in fencing or other equipment. Sprains and fractures can also occur, particularly if chickens fly down from a height and land awkwardly. Signs of an injury could include limping, swelling, bleeding, or an apparent deformity. Chickens with a foot or leg injury might also spend more time sitting or lying down, or they may avoid putting weight on the affected leg.

Chickens, like other birds, also have a unique problem related to their nails and spurs. If they don't have access to enough abrasive surfaces to naturally file them down, their nails and spurs can overgrow. Overgrown nails can curve and grow back into the foot, causing pain and infection, while overgrown spurs can make walking difficult and potentially lead to injuries. Chickens with overgrown nails or spurs might also show signs of discomfort or difficulty walking.

Lastly, we have footpad dermatitis, also known as "foot burn" or "pododermatitis." This condition is usually seen in commercial poultry operations where birds are kept in close quarters on wet bedding. The damp, unsanitary conditions cause the skin on the chicken's feet to become irritated and inflamed. Over time, this can lead to the development of sores and abscesses on the feet. Chickens with footpad dermatitis may exhibit signs of pain, such as limping or reluctance to walk, and you might also notice inflammation or sores on their feet.

Spotting these common foot issues early can be a game-changer in maintaining the health and happiness of your flock. Regularly checking your chickens' feet for signs of these problems and addressing them promptly can help prevent minor issues from becoming major ones. As always, remember that even with the best care, chickens can and will get sick or injured. Knowing what to look for and how to respond can make all the difference.

What are herbal foot soaks? What are the beneficial effects on chicken feet? Herbal foot soaks can be extremely helpful in treating and preventing foot problems in chickens. They can cleanse wounds, soothe pain, reduce inflammation, promote healing, and provide a relaxing experience for your chickens.

Epsom salt, while not technically an herb, is a key component in many chicken foot soaks. Magnesium sulfate, better known as Epsom salt, has been used for centuries to soothe aching muscles, reduce inflammation, and draw out toxins. For chickens, an Epsom salt soak can help soften scabs and calluses, draw out infection, and reduce pain and swelling.

Lavender is an aromatic herb widely celebrated for its calming, anti-inflammatory, and antiseptic properties. The scent alone has a calming effect, which can be especially beneficial when you're dealing with an anxious or stressed chicken. Lavender can help clean wounds and promote healing, reduce inflammation and swelling, and provide a soothing experience for your chicken.

Rosemary is another herb that can be highly beneficial in a foot soak for chickens. This aromatic herb has natural antibacterial and anti-inflammatory properties. It can help to cleanse and heal wounds, reduce inflammation and pain, and stimulate circulation to promote faster healing. Additionally, its pleasant aroma can help to calm and relax your chickens.

Calendula, sometimes known as pot marigold, is a bright, cheerful herb that's a powerhouse of healing properties. It's packed with antioxidants and has potent anti-inflammatory and antimicrobial properties. In a foot soak, calendula can help to cleanse wounds, reduce inflammation and pain, promote wound healing, and soothe irritated skin.

Yarrow is a bit of a wild card in the world of herbs, but it's a fantastic addition to a chicken foot soak. This potent herb has been used for centuries to treat wounds and stop bleeding, earning it the nickname "soldier's woundwort." Yarrow can cleanse wounds, reduce inflammation and pain, stop bleeding, and promote healing.

Sage, a common herb found in many kitchens, has more to offer than just flavor. Sage has natural antimicrobial and anti-inflammatory properties. In a foot soak, sage can help to cleanse wounds, reduce inflammation, and promote healing.

Chamomile, another calming herb, is often used in foot soaks for its soothing properties. It can help to cleanse wounds, reduce inflammation and pain, promote healing, and relax your chickens.

The goal of a foot soak is to clean the foot, promote healing, and provide comfort to your chicken. The best part about using herbs is that they are gentle, safe, and beneficial in more ways than one. The world of herbal healing offers a myriad of possibilities, so don't be afraid to explore and learn more about these fantastic plants and their uses.

Now that we have an idea of what herbs we can use, let's dive into making our own herbal foot soak solutions.

Our basic remedy is quite simple. You'll need a container large enough for your chicken's foot or feet, warm water, Epsom salt, and your chosen herbs. Here's the general breakdown:

1. Fill the container with warm water, enough to cover the chicken's feet.
2. Add about 1/2 cup of Epsom salt to the water.
3. Choose two or three of the herbs we discussed earlier - like lavender, rosemary, or calendula. Use about 2 tablespoons of each.
4. Stir the water until the Epsom salt is dissolved and the herbs are well distributed.

Now, you've got your herbal foot soak ready to go. Remember, each chicken is different, and you may need to adjust the ingredients and their amounts to suit the needs of your individual bird. For a chicken with a minor foot issue, a 15-20 minute soak once a day may be sufficient. But for more serious issues, longer or more frequent soaks may be necessary.

Always observe your chicken during and after the soak. Look for any signs of discomfort, like excessive squawking or attempts to escape, and adjust your method accordingly. After the soak, gently pat the foot dry, making sure not to rub or cause further irritation.

As you become more familiar with herbal foot soaks and the responses of your chickens, you can start to experiment with different combinations of herbs. Maybe you'll find that sage and chamomile work best for one bird while another responds better to a combination of yarrow and rosemary. That's part of the beauty of herbal remedies - the ability to customize and experiment to find the best solution for each individual bird.

The soothing comfort provided by a warm, herb-infused foot soak can do wonders for a chicken dealing with foot issues. Not only does it cleanse and heal, but it also offers a moment of relaxation and stress relief. Keep in mind, though, that a foot soak is not a cure-all. If your chicken has a serious foot problem, or if the foot doesn't improve with at-home treatment, always seek professional veterinary care.

These foot soaks can also be used as a preventative measure. Regular foot inspections combined with a calming foot soak can help keep your chickens' feet in tip-top shape. It's a small effort that can go a long way in maintaining the overall health of your flock.

Now, let's get down to business and talk about how to administer these foot soaks. Don't worry, it's not as daunting as it might seem. Follow this step-by-step guide, and soon you'll be a pro.

Step 1: Prepare the Foot Soak
As described earlier, gather your ingredients: a suitable container, warm water, Epsom salt, and your selected herbs. Mix everything together until the Epsom salt dissolves and the herbal essences infuse into the water.

Step 2: Secure Your Chicken
Before starting the soak, it's important to make sure your chicken is secure and comfortable. This might mean having another person hold the bird or perhaps wrapping the bird loosely in a towel with only the foot or feet exposed. Make sure the head and wings are secure to prevent flapping and potential injury.

Step 3: Introduce the Foot to the Soak
Gently lower your chicken's foot into the prepared herbal solution. If your bird seems nervous or uncomfortable, talk softly to them and move slowly.

Step 4: Soak Time
Depending on the severity of the foot problem, soaking time can vary. A general guideline is to aim for 15-20 minutes. Keep the bird calm during this time. Maybe this is when you tell your chicken about your day, or maybe you sing to it. Do whatever works to create a soothing environment.

Step 5: Drying Off
Once soaking time is over, gently remove the foot from the water and pat it dry with a clean, soft towel. Don't rub, as this can cause irritation. Once the foot is dry, inspect it for any changes or improvements.

Safety is always a priority when dealing with your flock. Here are a few things to keep in mind:

Temperature: The water should be warm but not hot. Test it on your wrist to ensure it won't scorch your chicken's sensitive skin.

Handling: Always handle your chickens gently to avoid causing stress or injury. Secure them properly before starting the foot soak.

Supervision: Never leave a soaking chicken unattended. Even a docile chicken might try to escape or knock over the soak container, leading to a mess at best and injury at worst.

Herb Choice: Always use herbs that are safe for chickens. Some plants can be toxic to our feathered friends, so do your research and ensure the herbs you're using are chicken-friendly. In the Appendix you will find a list of herbs that are safe and a list of herbs to avoid as they are toxic to your chickens..

In following these steps, you'll provide an effective, soothing treatment for your chickens' foot problems. The best part is seeing their relief and comfort afterwards. Now, let's move on to discussing how to follow up on this care, observe your chickens for signs of recovery, provide ongoing care, and understand what recovery looks like.

As we've discussed, the foot soak is just one part of a larger picture. It's an important step, no doubt about it, but what follows is equally crucial. When you've finished the foot soak, dried off your chicken's foot, and sent them back to their flock, your job isn't over. Now comes observation and ongoing care.

Observation involves closely watching your chicken's behavior and their foot's appearance. Are they limping less? Has the swelling gone down? Is the chicken more active, showing signs of relief? These are all good signs and indicate that the foot soak is helping.

But if the chicken is still in obvious discomfort, limping, or the foot's condition is not improving or even worsening, it might be time to consider a vet visit. A professional can offer advice, diagnosis, or stronger treatments if needed. Remember, the goal is to support your chicken's health, not to replace professional care when it's required.

Meanwhile, ongoing care involves more foot soaks, cleanliness, and possibly applying additional treatments. You may need to continue the foot soaks for several days or even weeks, depending on the issue at hand. Consistency is key here, as intermittent care will not yield the same results as regular, consistent treatment.

Cleanliness, as always, is crucial. Keeping your chicken's living environment clean can help prevent reinfection or worsening of the foot condition. Regularly clean their coop, remove droppings, and ensure their bedding is fresh and dry. This goes a long way in supporting their recovery.

Applying additional treatments might also be needed. Perhaps a natural salve or ointment is in order to further soothe and heal the foot. If you're in doubt about what to use, refer to the appendix at the end of this book, There, you'll find a comprehensive list of poultices, ointments, infusions, sprays, salves, washes, and herbal foot soaks you can prepare and use for your flock.

Finally, what does recovery look like? In general, a recovering chicken will be more active and show fewer signs of discomfort, and the affected foot will look healthier – less swelling, no visible wounds or injuries, and no limping. Every chicken is different, so recovery might not look the same for every bird, but positive changes in behavior and physical health are always a good sign.

These techniques are all part of a greater whole - your overall approach to chicken keeping. Your flock depends on you to keep them healthy and happy, and with these herbal tools in your chicken-keeping kit, you're well-equipped to do so.

"An herb garden is a quiet rebellion against hurried living."
— Unknown

Chapter 7: Beat the Bugs: Natural Pest Control

Part I: Shake a Tail Feather: Herbal Mite Repellents

We're going to focus our attention on some pesky critters - mites. It's a topic that no chicken keeper enjoys, but it's one we all have to deal with at some point. Understanding these pests, their types, signs of their presence, and the potential harm they can cause is the first step in tackling them effectively.

First, let's get a clear picture of what we're dealing with. Mites. They're tiny arachnids - yes, they're part of the same family as spiders - and they're not fun guests to have in your coop. There are several types that can infest your chickens, including red mites, Northern fowl mites, and scaly leg mites. Each one has its own characteristics and ways of making your flock's life miserable.

Red mites, also known as roost mites or chicken mites, are nocturnal pests that live in the cracks and crevices of your coop during the day, coming out at night to feed on your chickens. Their name comes from their reddish-brown color which deepens after they've had a meal.

Northern fowl mites, on the other hand, are more audacious, choosing to live on the chickens themselves. They're a tad larger than red mites and are a dark brown or black color. You'll often find them on the vent area or under the wings of your chickens.

Scaly leg mites are tiny creatures that burrow under the scales of your chickens' legs and feet, causing them to lift and become crusty. Unlike the first two, these mites are not easy to see with the naked eye due to their microscopic size.

Now that we've covered the common types of mites let's discover the signs of an infestation. Unfortunately, mites can be quite secretive, especially in the early stages of an infestation, but your chickens will start to show signs of discomfort.

They may be restless, especially at night when the red mites come out to feed. You might notice decreased egg production or a loss of weight. Some birds will start feather-pecking or over-preening in an attempt to relieve the discomfort. Northern fowl mites can cause a dirty-looking vent area, and a tell-tale sign of scaly leg mites is crusty, raised scales on the legs.

One of the best ways to confirm your suspicions is to do a coop inspection at night with a flashlight. You're likely to see red mites creeping out of their hiding places, and a quick check under your chicken's wings might reveal the Northern fowl mites. As for scaly leg mites, a close look at your chicken's legs should confirm their presence.

So, what's the big deal, you ask? They're just tiny critters, right? Yes, they're small, but their effects can be big. Mites can cause discomfort, stress and lead to decreased egg production in your flock. They can cause anemia if left unchecked, which can be deadly, especially for young, old, or already weak chickens. Scaly leg mites can cause lameness and deformities if not treated.

In short, while mites are a common issue in chicken keeping, they're not something to be taken lightly. They can harm your flock and decrease their quality of life, which is why understanding them and knowing how to deal with them effectively is so important. Remember that old saying? An ounce of prevention is worth a pound of cure. It is always a best practice to prevent mites rather then having to cure them.

In light of the trouble that mites can cause in our flock, it's understandable why many chicken keepers seek out ways to prevent their presence. And wouldn't you know it, there's a whole world of naturally occurring repellents that are safe, efficient, and kind to our feathered friends.

When it comes to selecting herbs that repel mites, we have several choices that are both beneficial to your flock and quite efficient. Let's start with a crowd favorite, lavender. This fragrant herb is well known for its calming properties, but did you know it's also a potent mite deterrent? The strong scent confuses these pesky creatures, keeping them at bay.

Lavender is also a robust plant that can withstand some pecking from your flock, so feel free to plant it around your coop. Just be sure not to use it excessively as too much can be harmful. Stick to hanging bunches in your coop or adding some sprigs to your nesting boxes.

Next on our list is wormwood. This hardy plant has a bitter taste that most pests, mites included, find unpalatable. It's a great plant to have around the perimeter of your chicken run to deter mites from even considering your coop as a place to set up shop. Wormwood has the added benefit of being a natural wormer for your chickens if they decide to have a nibble.

Tansy is another beneficial herb to consider. Its strong aroma makes it a potent mite deterrent. It can be hung in the coop or planted around your run to help keep these pests at a distance. Like lavender, tansy should be used in moderation due to its strong potency. You also need to keep in mind that consumed in large quantities, tansy can be toxic to your chickens. It is best to hang this herb where your chickens cannot reach it or plant it where they cannot forage in it.

We also have peppermint in our arsenal. This versatile herb is a fantastic addition to any chicken run. Not only does it repel mites, but it also keeps other pests like mice and ants away. It's also beneficial to your chickens' respiratory health and, let's be honest, it makes the coop smell delightful.

Another herb that you may want to consider is lemon balm. Its citrusy scent is pleasant to us and our chickens but not so much to mites. It's a gentle herb, so it's safe for your flock to eat in larger quantities. You can also make a simple spray with lemon balm and water to mist your coop and nesting boxes.

And let's not forget about marigold. This bright, cheerful flower is not only beautiful to look at but is also a great bug deterrent. The scent of marigold is disliked by mites, and the petals have anti-inflammatory properties, which can be beneficial if your flock has been dealing with an infestation.

Garlic and rosemary are also useful herbs to have in your mite-fighting toolkit. Garlic boosts the immune system of your chickens, making them less appealing to mites, while rosemary's strong aroma is a natural deterrent.

Choosing the right herbs is a big part of the battle against mites. It's not just about what deters the pests; it's also about what benefits your flock. When you take the time to select herbs that both repel mites and support your chickens' health, you're taking a holistic approach to chicken keeping. It's an approach that recognizes the complex interactions between your chickens, their environment, and the creatures they share it with.

However, it's important to remember that these herbs play a significant role in a multi-faceted approach to mite control. This approach includes good coop management, regular inspections, and prompt treatment of infestations when they occur. With these herbs in your mite-fighting arsenal, you'll be well-equipped to keep these pesky critters at bay and your flock happy and healthy.

Now that you have an idea about which herbs to use let's explore how we can create potent mixtures that are easy to make, effective, and, of course, safe for your feathered friends. We'll go through some basic remedies, discuss preparation methods, and offer tips for storage to make these mixtures last longer.

Our first remedy is for a simple herbal spray that can be misted in the coop, particularly around roosting and nesting areas where mites are likely to congregate. Start with one cup of fresh or half a cup of dried herbs. A blend of lavender, wormwood, and tansy can create a potent mix. Boil these herbs in a quart of water and let it steep until the water cools. Strain the herbs, then pour the liquid into a spray bottle. Add a couple of drops of natural dish soap as a surfactant to help the spray adhere to surfaces. This concoction can be stored in the refrigerator for up to two weeks.

Another great mite-fighting blend is dusting powder. For this remedy, use dried herbs as they need to be ground into a fine powder. A mix of lavender, peppermint, rosemary, and garlic can be especially effective. Grind these herbs in a blender or food processor until they become a fine powder. Sprinkle this aromatic dust in your coop, paying special attention to crevices and hiding spots. This mixture can be stored in an airtight container in a cool, dark place for up to a year.

A potent nesting box blend is another way to deter mites. This blend uses whole dried herbs that release their scent over time. You'll want to use herbs that are safe for your chickens to ingest as they'll be in close contact with them. Lemon balm, lavender, and marigold are great options for this mix. Simply mix these herbs in equal parts and add them to your nesting boxes. The herbs should be replaced every few weeks or when their scent starts to fade. Store any extra in a breathable bag in a cool, dark place.

It's important to remember that these mixtures should be used as part of your regular coop cleaning routine. They are not a cure for mite infestations but rather a preventative measure to create an environment that's unappealing to mites.

The preparation methods we've outlined are relatively straightforward and do not require specialized equipment. A common kitchen blender or food processor, a pot for boiling water, and a strainer are the main tools you need. The goal is to make it easy for you, the chicken keeper, to incorporate these practices into your routine.

When it comes to storage, the key is keeping the herbs as fresh as possible to preserve their aromatic properties. The herbal spray should be stored in the refrigerator to keep it from spoiling. For the dusting powder and nesting box blend, store them in a cool, dark place to maintain their potency. Make sure the containers are airtight to keep out any moisture. These are just remedies to get you started. You will find a larger list of remedies in the appendix. This appendix should be considered a reference for possible ways to use herbs in parasite prevention.

The next question is, how do we apply these herbal mixtures in the context of a chicken coop? Integrating these strategies into your chicken care routine can help create an environment that's not so welcoming for mites.

First off, let's talk about coop treatments. This should be part of your regular cleaning routine, which means removing soiled bedding, sweeping out dust and cobwebs, and inspecting for any signs of mites. Once you have a clean slate, you can start applying your herbal remedies. The herbal spray we discussed earlier is perfect for this task. Spray it around the coop, paying special attention to corners, cracks, and underneath roosting bars. These are favorite hiding spots for mites. Don't forget the nesting boxes too! Refresh your nesting box blend during this clean-up and remember, a little goes a long way. Mites are tiny creatures, and it doesn't take much to make their environment inhospitable.

Next, let's talk about dust baths. Dust bathing is a natural behavior for chickens. It helps them keep their feathers clean and free of parasites. But we can give nature a helping hand by providing a dedicated dust bath area sprinkled with our homemade herbal dusting powder. A simple tub or a shallow pit in the ground can serve as your dust bath. Chickens will fluff, shake, and roll around in the dust, effectively coating their feathers and skin with the herbal dust. This not only helps to physically remove mites, but the aroma of the herbs can also deter them.

Another strategy to consider is treating individual birds. This is especially important if you notice a chicken showing signs of heavy mite infestation, such as excessive pecking at itself, bald patches, or visible mites. In these cases, a more direct application may be necessary. The herbal spray can be gently misted onto the bird, avoiding the eyes and beak. Alternatively, you can also dust the bird directly with the herbal dusting powder.

It's also essential to maintain a healthy environment around your coop. Mites are often brought into the coop by wild birds or rodents, so discouraging these visitors can help prevent mite infestations. This might involve securing feed in rodent-proof containers or removing bird feeders that attract wild birds close to your coop.

These strategies are not meant to be a quick fix for a mite infestation. They are tools to integrate into your regular care routine to help prevent mites from becoming a problem in the first place. Consistent application is the key to success here.

Ensuring the health and well-being of your flock requires a proactive and watchful eye. Mites, as we've noted, are a common adversary, but with regular checks and an understanding of signs of infestation, you can keep these pests in check. So, how does one undertake the task of regular monitoring for mites?

To start, establish a routine. Ideally, this should include daily observations and more thorough weekly checks. During daily observations, look at your flock's behavior. Chickens that are infested with mites are often restless, especially at night when mites are most active. They may have trouble sleeping, which could result in a drop in egg production. Regular egg checks are another excellent opportunity to observe for any changes or signs of mites.

For weekly checks, you'll want to get up close and personal. Inspect each bird individually. Using gloves, gently part the feathers, particularly around the vent area, under the wings, and on the belly where mites like to congregate. Adult mites are tiny, round, and dark, so they can be challenging to spot, especially on darker-feathered breeds. However, mites also leave a telltale sign - clusters of tiny white or grey specs, which are their eggs. Look out for these signs along the base of the feathers.

It's equally crucial to inspect your coop during these weekly checks. Remember, mites will hide in cracks and crevices in the coop during the day, only coming out at night to feed on your birds. Pay attention to roosting bars, nesting boxes, and any other places where your chickens spend a lot of time. If you notice grayish dust (which is actually mite feces) or a crusty buildup (mite eggs and larvae), these are signs of a mite infestation in the coop.

Remember to maintain your mite control measures as part of this routine. Refresh the nesting box blends and the dust bath areas with your homemade mite-repellent mixtures. Continue to spray your coop with the herbal spray during your cleaning routine. Regular application is the key to keeping these herbal remedies effective.

So, what should you do if you notice signs of a re-infestation? First, don't panic. Despite your best efforts, re-infestations can happen. Mites are pervasive and resilient, but they're also manageable. Increase the frequency of your coop cleaning and herbal treatments, and consider treating individual birds if they show signs of heavy infestation. It might take a little time, but consistency is your best weapon.

Ongoing prevention is the best strategy for dealing with mites. By making these checks and treatments a part of your regular chicken care routine, you'll create an environment that's less attractive to mites. You'll also catch any potential infestations early, making them easier to manage.

Monitoring for mites might seem like a daunting task, but it doesn't have to be. It's a way to engage more deeply with your flock, ensure their comfort, and learn more about their behavior and needs. Plus, you get the satisfaction of knowing you're doing your best to keep your chickens healthy and happy using natural, safe methods. As we journey further into this world of natural pest control, you'll find that these principles of observation, prevention, and treatment apply to many other challenges you might encounter in chicken keeping.

Mites are a common problem for chicken keepers, but they don't have to be a big one. By understanding these tiny pests and taking proactive steps to make your coop a mite-unfriendly place, you can protect your flock and ensure their health and happiness. You're also using natural, non-toxic methods that are safe for your chickens, your family, and the environment. It's a win-win all around!

Part II: No Fleas Please: Herbal Flea Treatments

Now that we've tackled the mighty mite, let's turn our attention to another tiny but troublesome parasite: the flea. Yes, chickens can get fleas, too, and while they're less common than mites, they can cause a lot of discomfort for your flock and can be a nuisance in your coop. Understanding how to recognize a flea infestation is the first step in tackling this problem.

There are several species of fleas that can infest chickens. The most common is the sticktight flea, also known as the hen flea. Unlike mites, fleas are larger and easier to spot. Adult sticktight fleas are small, dark, and flat. They get their name from their habit of sticking tight to their hosts. You'll usually find them congregating around the chicken's head and neck, particularly near the eyes and wattles.

So, what signs should you look for to spot a flea infestation in your flock?

Unlike mites, fleas don't usually cause chickens to lose feathers or to peck and scratch excessively. Instead, the most visible sign of a sticktight flea infestation is the presence of the fleas themselves. You might notice small, black specks around the bird's face, which, upon closer inspection, are fleas.

In addition to the physical presence of fleas, another sign to watch for is changes in chicken behavior. Chickens with fleas may seem stressed or agitated. You might notice a decrease in egg production or that your chickens aren't roosting comfortably.

What about the impact on chickens? Well, in small numbers, fleas are mostly an annoyance to chickens. However, in larger numbers, they can cause significant problems. Fleas feed on blood, and a heavy infestation can lead to anemia in chickens. This can cause your chickens to become lethargic and pale, and in severe cases, it can even be fatal.

It's also worth noting that sticktight fleas can carry diseases such as avian pox and tapeworms. These diseases can further compromise the health of your flock, so swift action to control fleas is essential.

When it comes to the coop, fleas behave a bit differently than mites. Sticktight fleas tend to stay on the host, so you're less likely to find them hiding in the coop. However, fleas do lay eggs, and those eggs often fall off the host into the environment.

The eggs are tiny and whitish, and they're often found in places where the chickens like to dust bathe or in the bedding in the coop. A flea infestation in the coop can be challenging to spot, but if you notice your chickens avoiding certain areas they usually enjoy, it might be worth a closer inspection.

Fleas can be tough customers, but the good news is that they're not invincible. With the right knowledge, a keen eye, and a trusty arsenal of herbal treatments, you can keep your flock flea-free. And like with mites, remember that prevention is always better than cure. So, now that you know what to look for, let's delve into some natural ways to prevent and treat flea infestations in your flock.

Equipping yourself with the right set of tools to combat flea infestations is crucial for maintaining a happy and healthy flock. Among these tools, certain herbs have proven to be extraordinarily helpful due to their insect-repelling properties. In particular, rosemary, peppermint, and eucalyptus are standout champions. These aren't the only herbs that can help with flea control, but they're definitely at the top of the list. Let's dig into each of these and understand why they are so effective.

Rosemary is more than just a delightful aromatic herb for your kitchen—it's also a powerful ally in the fight against fleas. Its strong scent is a natural flea deterrent. It's been used for centuries to repel various pests, fleas included. You can use rosemary in multiple forms—dried and sprinkled in the coop, in dust baths, or as a rosemary tea rinse. When applied to the chickens or their environment, it's like a giant "Keep Out" sign for fleas.

Peppermint, on the other hand, has a cooling effect that soothes the irritation caused by flea bites. Just like rosemary, peppermint has a strong smell that fleas find quite offensive. You can use peppermint in a similar manner—either dried or fresh leaves in the coop or dust bath, or as an essential oil diluted in a spray bottle and misted in the coop and on the chickens. A word of caution though, ensure that the peppermint oil is well-diluted, as it can be too strong in concentrated form.

Eucalyptus is yet another powerful herb in our flea-fighting lineup. It's quite potent in repelling a wide range of pests, including fleas. You can use it in the form of dried leaves or essential oil. Eucalyptus oil diluted in water makes a refreshing and effective spray that not only repels fleas but also masks the scent of your chickens, making it harder for new fleas to find them. Again, remember to dilute it properly, and always do a small patch test to ensure your chickens are not sensitive to it.

Beyond these three, there's a whole host of herbs that can aid in your fight against fleas. Lemongrass, cedarwood, lavender, pennyroyal, and fennel are all known to have flea-repelling properties. In fact, they work so well that you might consider planting some around the coop as a natural pest control measure.

One important thing to remember when selecting herbs for flea control is to know your flock. Some chickens may be sensitive to certain herbs. As I keep saying, always introduce new herbs gradually and monitor your flock for any adverse reactions. And as always, while herbs are a great tool, they're most effective when used as part of an integrated pest management strategy. Regular coop cleanings, dust baths, and monitoring for signs of infestations are all crucial for keeping fleas at bay.

Making herbal flea treatments involves three primary methods: infusions, sprays, and bedding additions. Each method provides its own set of benefits and uses, and together, they create a powerful defense against pesky fleas.

First, let's tackle herbal infusions. Infusions are similar to tea, wherein herbs are steeped in hot water and allowed to infuse their beneficial properties into the liquid. For flea control, you can make an infusion using rosemary or peppermint, both of which are known for their flea-repelling properties. To make an infusion, take a handful of either herb, add it to boiling water, and let it steep for about 20-30 minutes. Once it cools down, you can use it to rinse your chickens after a regular bath. Not only will this leave your chickens smelling fresh, but it also creates an environment that's uninviting to fleas.

Next are herbal sprays, which are fantastic for quick and easy application. These can be made using essential oils derived from the herbs we've mentioned earlier. Mix a few drops of your chosen essential oil—like peppermint or eucalyptus—with water in a spray bottle. Remember, these oils are potent, so a little goes a long way. Always dilute them properly to ensure they're safe for your flock. You can spray this mixture in your coop and even lightly mist it on your chickens. It acts as a deterrent for fleas, and the refreshing aroma can help mask the scent of your chickens, making it harder for fleas to target them.

Lastly, let's talk about adding herbs directly to your chickens' bedding. This method is as simple as it sounds. You can sprinkle dried rosemary, peppermint, or any other flea-repelling herbs onto the coop bedding and nesting boxes. As your chickens move around, they'll naturally distribute the herbs, releasing their aromatic oils. These scents make the coop less appealing to fleas. In all of these methods, the key is consistency. Apply these treatments regularly to maintain their effectiveness. Rotate the herbs you use to prevent fleas from becoming accustomed to any one scent.

While prevention is always our first line of defense, knowing how to effectively treat a flea infestation when it arises is equally important. The application methods, frequency, and safety considerations will all depend on the particular herbal treatment you're using.

For the herbal infusions, your chickens will likely see this as a somewhat exotic bath time. To apply the infusion, pour the cooled mixture over your chickens, being sure to reach all the nooks and crannies where fleas might hide. Remember to be gentle and reassuring; your chickens might not be accustomed to this sort of thing. As for frequency, applying the infusion once a week during a flea outbreak should be sufficient. Be sure to keep a close eye on your chickens' skin for any signs of irritation. If irritation occurs, try diluting the infusion more or switch to a different herb.

As for herbal sprays, the application can be a quick and simple process. Spritz the diluted essential oil mixture around the coop, targeting corners, cracks, and crevices where fleas might lurk. You can also lightly mist your chickens, but avoid spraying directly onto their faces. As the essential oils in the spray can be quite potent, it's best to start with a biweekly application and observe your flock's reaction. If no irritation or discomfort is observed, you can increase the frequency to twice a week.

The direct application of herbs onto your chickens' bedding is a straightforward process. Simply sprinkle the dried herbs onto the bedding and nesting boxes and allow your chickens to do the rest. This method can be performed once a week or more frequently if a flea problem is present. Always monitor your flock for any potential allergic reactions. If you notice excessive scratching or signs of discomfort, remove the herbs and try a different type.

A vital point to remember throughout the treatment process is the safety of your flock. Chickens are hardy creatures, but they can still have adverse reactions to certain herbs, especially in concentrated forms like essential oils. Always start with a lower concentration and watch your flock for any signs of distress or discomfort. If you notice anything amiss, stop the treatment immediately and seek advice from a vet or experienced chicken keeper.

Treating your flock for fleas might seem like a daunting task, but remember, you're not alone in this fight. Countless chicken keepers have successfully dealt with flea infestations using these same methods. With consistency, vigilance, and a little patience, you can help your flock shake off these pesky parasites and return to their happy, healthy selves. The battle against fleas doesn't end with treatment. Ongoing monitoring for signs of re-infestation is crucial to keep your flock flea-free in the long term.

Alright, let's dig into how we can keep that flea-free state going. So, you've treated the fleas, your flock is back to their chipper selves, and the coop is free of unwanted guests. That's a big win in the chicken-keeping world. But the work doesn't stop there. Maintaining a flea-free flock is a continuous process that involves prevention strategies and regular checks.

Regular checks are the foundation of preventing flea infestations. The sooner you can identify and respond to a flea problem, the better. Set a schedule and stick to it, checking your chickens and their coop for signs of fleas. A good starting point could be once a week, but this might need to be adjusted based on your circumstances, such as the time of year, local flea populations, and the health of your flock. Make this a part of your normal chicken care routine, perhaps when you're collecting eggs or refreshing their food and water.

During these checks, you're looking for any changes in your chickens' behavior or appearance that could signal a flea problem. As we discussed earlier, things like excessive scratching, restlessness, and feather loss are all signs to watch out for. Be thorough, as fleas are excellent at hiding. Check under the wings and around the vent area, as fleas often congregate there. If you do spot fleas, act quickly. The sooner you respond, the less established the fleas will become, and the easier they'll be to remove.

Now, for the prevention strategies. These will likely be a combination of methods we've already discussed and some additional ones to bolster your defenses. The first step in prevention is to continue with the herbal treatments, even when there are no visible signs of fleas. These treatments aren't just for eliminating fleas; they're also excellent at discouraging them from setting up shop in the first place. Maintain your routine of applying herbal infusions, sprays, or bedding additions, changing the herbs periodically to keep the fleas guessing.

Maintaining a clean and dry coop is another key prevention strategy. Fleas thrive in damp, dirty environments, so regular coop cleanings can go a long way in keeping them at bay. Depending on the size of your flock and the coop conditions, this could mean a full clean-out every few weeks or more frequent smaller cleanings. Whatever the schedule, consistency is crucial.

Another prevention method is to encourage your chickens' natural dust-bathing behavior. Dust bathing is a chicken's first line of defense against parasites, fleas included. Providing a dedicated dust bath area filled with a mix of sand, soil, and diatomaceous earth can be a great way to promote this behavior. You can also sprinkle in some of your flea-repelling herbs for an extra layer of protection.

Finally, keep an eye on the areas around your coop. If you have a run, ensure it is kept clean and dry, and check for any signs of fleas. It might be necessary to apply your herbal treatments to these areas as well. Similarly, if your chickens free-range, be aware of where they're ranging. If there are areas where fleas are common, it might be worth restricting access to those areas.

There's a lot to consider in maintaining a flea-free flock, but don't be daunted. With each step you take, you're making your flock less attractive to fleas. Over time, these strategies will become second nature, woven into the fabric of your chicken-keeping routine. With vigilance, consistency, and a good understanding of your flock, you'll be well-equipped to keep your chickens flea-free, allowing them to live their best chicken lives. And remember, each chicken keeper's journey is unique, and so is each flock. You'll likely need to tweak and adapt these methods to suit your situation, and that's okay. It's all part of the adventure of chicken keeping.

Part III: Fly Away: Natural Fly Control with Herbs

Flies might seem like an inevitable part of chicken keeping. After all, where there are animals and animal waste, flies seem to follow. While it's true that completely eliminating flies is likely an impossible task, that doesn't mean we should ignore them. Flies can cause significant disturbances to your flock and pose health risks if their population is not managed.

Firstly, let's talk about health risks. Flies are known vectors for disease, capable of transmitting a host of pathogens that can impact the health of your flock. They do this in a couple of ways. One is through their feeding habits. Flies aren't exactly the most sanitary eaters. They regurgitate digestive juices onto their food to dissolve it before consuming it, leaving behind a trail of potential pathogens. Another is through their life cycle. Fly larvae, or maggots, develop in decaying organic material, including chicken waste. As they move and feed, they can spread disease-causing organisms. If these pathogens are present in large enough numbers, they can cause health problems for your chickens, such as diarrhea or respiratory issues.

The presence of a large fly population can also cause stress and disturbances to your flock. Chickens, like most animals, don't enjoy being pestered by flies. The incessant buzzing can cause distress, disrupting their normal behaviors like feeding and laying. This can lead to decreased egg production, slower growth rates in young chickens, and overall decreased health and happiness. If flies become too much of a nuisance, your chickens might even start to refuse to use certain areas of their coop or run, which can lead to crowding and additional stress.

Now that we've got a grasp of why flies are a problem let's discuss how to manage their population. Fly population management revolves around two main strategies: making your coop less attractive to flies and taking measures to reduce the existing fly population.

Making your coop less attractive to flies involves managing the things that attract them in the first place. Flies are drawn to the coop by food, water, and suitable breeding sites. Ensuring that food and water sources are clean and well-maintained can significantly reduce fly attraction. This might involve regularly cleaning and refilling food and water containers and removing any spilled food promptly.

Flies also love to breed in chicken waste. Regularly removing and properly disposing of chicken waste can go a long way in reducing fly populations. Depending on the size of your flock and the design of your coop, this might mean daily clean-ups or a more extensive weekly cleaning. It's also beneficial to ensure that the coop is dry, as flies are attracted to damp environments. Fix any leaks, ensure the coop has good drainage, and consider using absorbent bedding materials.

As for reducing the existing fly population, there are several approaches you could take. One is to use traps or fly zappers. These can be effective in reducing adult fly numbers, but remember that they should be used in conjunction with good sanitation practices. Without addressing the things that are attracting and breeding flies, you'll just end up with a never-ending cycle.

Natural predators can also play a role in managing fly populations. Birds, bats, spiders, and certain types of insects are all natural predators of flies. Encouraging these species to make a home near your coop can provide a natural and sustainable form of fly control. This could involve putting up bird or bat houses, planting gardens to attract insect-eating birds, or avoiding the use of broad-spectrum pesticides that could harm beneficial insects.

The importance of managing fly populations in your coop can't be overstated. Flies are more than just a nuisance. They can cause significant issues for the health and happiness of your flock. However, with a good understanding of what attracts flies and how to reduce their numbers, you can keep the situation under control. It might take a bit of work and vigilance, but it's well worth it for the well-being of your chickens. Armed with the understanding that flies can cause significant issues for our chickens, it becomes even more critical to explore every possible method for controlling their population in your coop. This is where the beauty of nature, and more specifically, the power of herbs comes into play. There are numerous herbs that are remarkably effective for fly control, and adding these to your arsenal can dramatically help in keeping your chicken coop fly-free.

Starting with Basil. This culinary favorite, beloved for its aromatic appeal in many a kitchen, is also a potent deterrent for flies. Its strong smell is found unattractive by flies, which makes it an effective fly repellent. To use Basil, you can plant it around the coop or hang dried bouquets inside the coop. As the basil plants grow, they emit an aroma that repels flies, adding an aromatic ambiance to your coop and acting as a first line of defense against those pesky flies.

Next on our list is Bay Leaves. Bay leaves are a gift that keeps on giving. Not only do they elevate the flavor profiles in our kitchens, but their strong, distinctive smell is also an effective fly deterrent. Like basil, you can hang dried bunches of bay leaves around your coop or scatter the leaves in areas where flies are particularly problematic. As an added bonus, bay leaves are also known to repel other pests such as mice and cockroaches.

Let's not forget about Citronella. This perennial clumping grass is well-known for its insect-repelling properties, especially against mosquitoes. But it's equally effective against flies, too. The smell of citronella is incredibly off-putting to flies. Planting citronella around your chicken coop or even using citronella oil in a diffuser can help keep those irritating flies at bay.

Lavender, with its soothing scent and beautiful purple flowers, can also play a role in your fight against flies. It's known to be a natural insect repellent, deterring flies, mosquitoes, and even moths. Lavender is especially effective when planted around the coop, but you can also use dried lavender inside the coop. Plus, your chickens will likely appreciate the calming aroma!

Marigolds are another excellent herb to consider. These bright, cheerful flowers can repel a variety of pests, including flies. The secret lies in the pyrethrum, a compound found in marigolds that many insects find undesirable. Planting marigolds around the perimeter of your chicken coop can provide a colorful, effective barrier against flies.

Lemongrass, similar to citronella, produces a strong aroma that flies don't particularly enjoy. This tall, tropical grass can be planted around your coop to create a fragrant, fly-free zone. Or, you can use lemongrass essential oil, dilute it in water, and spray it around the coop.

Incorporating these herbs into your chicken coop environment can significantly aid in the control and prevention of flies. Using herbs for fly control is a natural, safe, and effective approach, devoid of chemicals that could potentially harm your flock. Furthermore, many of these herbs offer other benefits, including improving the smell of the coop, providing shade, and even offering health benefits if consumed by your chickens.

It's also worth noting that variety is beneficial here. Different types of flies may be more deterred by different herbs, so don't be afraid to use several of these herbs in combination. Similarly, the effectiveness of these herbs may vary depending on your specific situation and local fly species, so feel free to experiment and find what works best for you and your flock.

We've looked at some wonderful herbs that can serve as formidable weapons in our war against flies. Now, it's time to delve deeper into how we can craft effective, natural, and non-toxic fly deterrents using these herbs. While simply growing these herbs around your coop or hanging dried bunches can be beneficial, we can take things a step further by making targeted herbal treatments. So, let's get our hands dirty and explore the art of crafting herbal fly deterrents.

One of the simplest and most versatile ways to use herbs for fly control is by creating an herbal coop spray. This is nothing more than a diluted solution of herbs that you can spray around the coop and on the chickens themselves. To make a basic herbal coop spray, all you need is a handful of your chosen herbs, some water, and a little bit of dish soap to help the solution stick to surfaces. Simply steep the herbs in boiling water for about 20 minutes, strain the solution, add a drop or two of dish soap, and voila! You have a homemade, all-natural coop spray. Not only does it deter flies, but it can also make the coop smell amazing. Apply this spray generously around the coop, focusing on problem areas where flies tend to congregate.

Next, consider crafting herbal bundles. These are essentially bunches of dried herbs tied together that you can hang around the coop. They work on the principle that as the herbs dry, they release essential oils into the air, which deter flies. To create an herbal bundle, gather a bunch of your chosen herbs, tie them at the stem end using a string, and hang them upside down to dry in a cool, dry place. Once they're dried, these bundles can be hung in the coop. They are a simple, easy-to-make, and aesthetically pleasing way to keep flies at bay.

If you're feeling a bit more adventurous, herbal-infused bedding can be a fun and effective project. This entails infusing your chicken's bedding material with herbs that repel flies. There are many ways to do this, but one of the easiest methods involves simply scattering dried herbs over the bedding material and mixing them in. Over time, as the chickens move around the coop, they'll naturally distribute the herbs, helping to release their aromatic oils. Not only can this help deter flies, but it can also create a calming, pleasant environment for your chickens.

You can also create herbal sachets. These small bags filled with dried herbs can be hung in various places around the coop, tucked into corners, or even placed in nesting boxes. To make a sachet, simply fill a small cloth bag with a combination of dried herbs, close it tightly, and hang or place it in the coop. The advantage of sachets is that they're portable, easy to replace, and can be placed in areas where it might not be practical to spray or scatter herbs.

One final idea to consider is herbal oil or vinegar infusions. These involve steeping herbs in oil or vinegar to extract their essential oils and then using the resulting infusion to deter flies. Infusions can be sprayed around the coop, added to cleaning solutions, or even used to treat specific problem areas.

In creating these herbal fly deterrents, don't forget to let your creativity shine. Feel free to experiment with different herbs, combinations, and application methods to find what works best for your particular situation. Remember, the key is to create an environment that's unappealing to flies but comfortable and safe for your chickens.

These are just a few ideas to get you started. The beauty of using herbs is that there are so many ways to incorporate them into your fly control regimen. Whether it's a coop spray, an herbal bundle, infused bedding, sachets, or infusions, each of these methods leverages the power of herbs to help keep your coop fly-free. By incorporating these strategies into your regular coop maintenance routine, you'll not only help reduce the fly population but also create a healthier and more pleasant environment for your flock.

Having discussed the art of crafting herbal fly deterrents, we now move to the next crucial aspect of managing the fly problem: the strategic implementation of these control measures. This involves carefully considering where and how we apply our herbal treatments, maintaining coop cleanliness, and effectively managing waste to reduce fly attraction.

First, let's consider strategic placement of our herbal deterrents. Placement plays a vital role in the effectiveness of these treatments. The goal is to distribute the scent of these herbs in areas that flies frequent, as well as in spaces where your chickens spend most of their time. This could mean hanging herbal bundles near windows and entrances to the coop, spraying the herbal solution around feeding and roosting areas, and scattering infused bedding in the nesting boxes. For sachets, consider hanging them near your chicken's favorite roosting spots, tucking them in corners, or hiding them in nesting boxes. Remember, the aim is to create an environment that's comfortable for your chickens, yet unattractive to flies.

Coop hygiene is another key aspect of controlling flies. A clean coop is less likely to attract flies and provides fewer breeding grounds for them. Cleaning the coop involves regularly removing old bedding, scraping out droppings, and sweeping up any leftover feed. This not only minimizes the smells that attract flies but also helps prevent diseases that could make your chickens vulnerable to fly attacks. A deep clean of the coop, including scrubbing down surfaces with a vinegar solution, should be performed every few weeks. Don't forget to reapply your herbal deterrents after each cleaning.

A clean coop also includes managing waste effectively. Chicken waste is one of the primary attractions for flies. Having a good waste management plan can significantly reduce the number of flies your coop attracts. This might involve regularly cleaning out the coop's droppings tray if it has one, or installing a droppings board under roosting bars to make cleaning easier. Some keepers compost their chicken waste, turning a potential problem into a resource. If you choose to compost, remember to do it correctly. A well-managed compost heap should not smell or attract flies.

Another waste product to consider is leftover food. If you're feeding your chickens kitchen scraps or wet feed, be sure to remove any leftovers promptly. Rotting food is a major attractor for flies and can quickly lead to a population boom if not managed correctly. Ideally, only provide as much food as your chickens can consume in one day.

We can also look at the coop's design to help combat flies. Good ventilation is key. Flies prefer stagnant, humid environments, so a well-ventilated coop can be a significant deterrent. Including features such as screened windows or vents can keep air moving and reduce the coop's attractiveness to flies. At the same time, ensuring that the coop is secure and doesn't have any gaps or holes where flies can easily enter is essential.

Water sources can also be a magnet for flies. Ensure waterers are clean and fresh, changing the water regularly. If possible, consider using a poultry nipple system for watering. These systems reduce spillage and eliminate the standing water that can attract flies.

By carefully considering the placement of our herbal deterrents, maintaining rigorous coop hygiene, and managing waste effectively, we can significantly reduce the fly problem. All these strategies tie into one overarching principle: create an environment that's comfortable and healthy for chickens but unappealing and inhospitable to flies. It's a delicate balancing act, but with a bit of effort, dedication, and the aromatic power of herbs, it's an act that any chicken keeper can master.

Now, having talked about all the strategies to keep flies at bay, we must understand that fly control isn't a one-time job. It requires a continuous process of monitoring and adjusting, based on observations, effectiveness, and the need for modifications. This ongoing vigilance is what will truly ensure the well-being of your flock.

Observations are our first step to maintaining control over the fly problem. Watch your chickens and their behaviors. Are they scratching more often? Are they displaying discomfort, such as shaking their heads, feather ruffling, or signs of stress? Noticing an increased fly activity in the coop or around the run? These can all be indications that your fly control methods may need some tweaking. It's all about learning to read the signs your chickens and the environment are giving you.

Just as important as watching your chickens is regularly inspecting the coop. Check corners, roosting bars, and under nesting boxes for fly larvae or pupae, which look like tiny, wriggling grains of rice. Keep an eye on areas around feeders and waterers, as well as any wet or damp areas in the coop. These spots tend to be hotspots for fly activity. If you notice a rise in the number of flies or larvae, this might be a signal that your current methods aren't cutting it and it's time to step things up.

That brings us to effectiveness. Every coop, every flock, and every situation is unique. The herbs and methods that work wonders for one might not be as effective for another. Perhaps you've tried basil and lavender but still see a significant number of flies buzzing around. Maybe it's time to introduce citronella or bay leaves into your arsenal. The key to effectiveness is experimentation. Don't be disheartened if the first thing you try doesn't immediately solve the problem. Fly control is more of a marathon than a sprint, requiring persistence and patience.

Then there's the consideration of modifications. Maybe you've noticed that your herbal spray is effective, but its scent doesn't linger long enough. You might need to adjust the remedy to include more potent, longer-lasting herbs, or you may need to apply the spray more frequently. Perhaps the herbal bundles are working well, but they're not deterring the flies from the nesting boxes. In that case, infusing the bedding with herbs could be a useful addition to your strategy.

Modifications can also involve changes to your coop management practices. If you've tried all the herbs in the book but are still struggling with flies, it might be time to examine the coop's hygiene and waste management. Could you be cleaning the coop more frequently or managing waste more effectively? Is there a damp spot in the coop that's attracting flies, which you could address by improving ventilation or fixing leaks?

In all of this, remember that every small victory is progress. Celebrate when you see fewer flies, when your chickens seem more comfortable, or when that new herb you tried appears to be making a difference. There's no one-size-fits-all solution, but with a dash of persistence, a sprinkling of observation, and a good measure of aromatic herbs, you can tailor a fly control strategy that fits your unique situation.

Remember, the goal here isn't to eliminate every single fly. A few flies are a part of life, particularly in a rural or semi-rural setting. Instead, our aim is to keep the fly population at a manageable level, where they pose minimal risk and disturbance to your chickens. By doing this, we not only create a healthier environment for our flock but also contribute to a more harmonious and natural balance between our chickens and the world around them.

Successful fly control comes down to vigilant observation, assessing the effectiveness of our methods, and being open to making modifications as needed. It's about being in tune with your flock, understanding their environment, and being responsive to their needs. Keep these principles in mind as you continue your journey in chicken keeping, and you'll be well-equipped to maintain a comfortable, healthy, and fly-controlled coop for your happy, contented flock.

Part IV: Worm Wisdom: Herbal Parasite Prevention

Having discussed how to naturally deal with external pests like fleas and flies, we're going to dive into a topic that might make your skin crawl a little – internal parasites in chickens. Yes, we're talking about worms. Unpleasant though it may be, understanding these unwelcome guests is crucial to maintaining the health and happiness of your feathered friends.

Chickens, just like any other animals, are susceptible to various types of internal parasites. Among the most common are worms, including roundworms, tapeworms, and gapeworms, each of which poses its unique challenges and health risks to your flock. Here, we will focus on understanding these different types of worms, how they can affect your chickens, and signs you need to be vigilant for in order to identify an infestation.

Roundworms are probably the most common type of worm to affect backyard chickens. These long, spaghetti-like worms live and reproduce in the chicken's gut, feeding off the contents. Adult worms release their eggs in the chicken's intestines, which are then passed out of the chicken through their droppings. From there, the eggs can end up in the soil or be ingested by other members of the flock, perpetuating the cycle.

In small numbers, roundworms may not cause significant problems, but a heavy infestation can lead to severe health issues. These can include reduced egg production, weight loss, dull feathers, and lethargy. In severe cases, a blockage of the intestines can occur, which can be fatal.

Tapeworms, on the other hand, have a more complex life cycle. They require an intermediate host, typically a small invertebrate like a slug, snail, or earthworm. When a chicken eats the infected host, the tapeworm eggs develop into adults in the chicken's gut. These flat, segmented worms attach themselves to the gut lining and feed off the nutrients the chicken consumes.

Again, in small numbers, tapeworms may not cause significant harm, but a heavy infestation can lead to malnutrition and weakness. You might also notice segments of the tapeworm, which look like small grains of rice, in your chicken's droppings.

Gapeworms are a bit different. These worms get their name from their preferred location – the trachea, or windpipe, of birds. Chickens can pick up gapeworm larvae from the soil or from eating infected earthworms or snails. The larvae then travel to the chicken's trachea, where they mature and reproduce.

Gapeworms can cause a chicken to gasp for air, stretch their neck and make a distinctive 'gaping' motion, hence their name. This can be particularly distressing for both the chicken and the keeper, and in severe cases can lead to suffocation.

So now that we have an understanding of the types of worms your chickens might encounter, it's essential to talk about signs of a worm infestation. As previously mentioned, a drop in egg production, weight loss, dull feathers, lethargy, and changes in droppings can all be signs of worm trouble. For gapeworms, the key sign is respiratory distress.

But here's the tricky part – chickens can carry a worm burden without showing any outward signs. That's why regular monitoring and preventative measures are crucial. Worms are a normal part of the environment, and a healthy chicken can usually handle a small worm burden. But a heavy infestation, particularly in younger, older, or otherwise stressed birds, can lead to serious health problems and even death.

The silent nature of worm infestations makes prevention so much more critical. For that, we're going to explore one of the most effective and natural methods – using herbs. You'll be amazed to discover how many common herbs can help prevent and controlling worm infestations in chickens. Some of these include garlic, pumpkin seeds, thyme, and many more.

Let's start with the mighty garlic. Garlic is truly a superstar when it comes to natural health boosters for chickens. But it's not just its strong odor that makes it an excellent choice for parasite prevention. Garlic contains sulfur compounds that have antimicrobial properties. These compounds can help to create an internal environment in the chicken's digestive system that is less hospitable to worms. Additionally, garlic has immune-boosting properties that can help the chickens fight off the parasites naturally. Fresh garlic cloves can be chopped up and added to the chickens' food or drinking water. Although it might take a while for your chickens to acquire a taste for it, the health benefits are well worth the effort.

Pumpkin seeds are another fantastic natural remedy for worms. They contain a compound called cucurbitacin, which has been found to have anti-parasitic properties. Cucurbitacin paralyzes the worms, making them lose their grip on the chicken's intestinal walls and eventually being expelled from the body. Feeding your flock raw pumpkin seeds regularly can help control worm infestations and boost their overall health. Plus, chickens love them, making this a treat as much as a medicinal supplement.

Moving on to thyme, it's not just a flavorful herb for cooking but also a potent natural dewormer for chickens. Thyme contains thymol, a compound known for its antiseptic, antifungal, and antimicrobial properties. This makes it a formidable adversary for internal parasites. You can incorporate thyme into your chickens' diet by adding fresh or dried thyme to their feed. Alternatively, a strong thyme tea can be made and added to their drinking water.

There are other herbs too that have been known for their worm-fighting capabilities. Wormwood, for instance, has been used for centuries as a natural dewormer. It's potent stuff and should be used with care – a small amount of dried wormwood can be sprinkled in the chicken feed periodically. Diatomaceous earth, though not an herb, is a natural product that can be mixed with feed to help control worms.

Cloves, fennel, and oregano are other herbs that can be beneficial for worm control. They can be added to the chicken feed in their dried form. Just remember, variety is key. Don't be afraid to try different herbs and see which ones your chickens prefer and which ones seem to have the best effects.

Remember, each herb works differently and may not be effective against all types of worms. It's not about finding a silver bullet that will eliminate all worms forever but about creating an environment in your chickens' guts that discourage worms from setting up shop. The beauty of using herbs is that they provide a wide range of health benefits beyond just parasite control. They can boost the immune system, improve digestion, and even increase the nutritional value of the eggs your chickens lay.

It's essential to use these herbs as part of a comprehensive worm control strategy that includes good coop hygiene, regular health checks, and rotational grazing if possible. Remember, the goal is not to eliminate all worms – a few worms are normal, and a healthy chicken can handle them. But by being proactive with natural preventative measures, you can help ensure that a minor worm burden doesn't turn into a full-blown infestation.

By employing the correct preventative measures, you can control the worm population and maintain the health and productivity of your flock. Herbal parasite preventatives come in various forms, like feeds, tinctures, and additions to water. You'll be glad to know that preparing these remedies is straightforward and, in most cases, can be done using ingredients you have at home or can easily grow in your garden.

Let's talk about herbal feeds first. The easiest way to incorporate herbs into your chickens' diet is by adding them directly to their feed. You can use fresh herbs from your garden, dried herbs from your pantry, or even herbal supplements from a health food store. Some chicken keepers like to create their own custom blend of herbs, mixing and matching based on their chickens' needs and preferences. For example, you might make a mix of garlic powder, dried thyme, and crushed pumpkin seeds. This not only adds variety to your chickens' diet but also provides them with a broad spectrum of health benefits.

Herbs can also be added to your chickens' water. This can be done in two ways - either by steeping the herbs to make a sort of 'herbal tea' or by adding a few drops of an herbal tincture. To make the tea, simply add a handful of herbs to boiling water, let it steep until it cools, and then add it to your chickens' waterer. The tincture method involves soaking herbs in alcohol for a few weeks, then straining out the herbs and using the liquid as a concentrated herbal extract. A few drops of this tincture can be added to the chickens' water. Remember to clean the waterer thoroughly before adding the herbal tea or tincture to prevent any bacterial growth.

Making your own herbal tinctures might sound intimidating, but it's actually quite simple. You'll need a clean glass jar, your chosen herb (fresh or dried), and a high-proof alcohol like vodka or brandy. Fill the jar about halfway with the herb, then pour in the alcohol until the jar is full. Make sure the herbs are completely covered by the alcohol. Seal the jar tightly and store it in a cool, dark place for about 4 to 6 weeks, shaking it every few days. Once the tincture is ready, strain out the herbs and store the liquid in a clean, dark bottle. Use a dropper to add the tincture to your chickens' water or feed.

Creating herbal infusions for bathing or for use in the chicken coop can also be beneficial in controlling parasites. You might want to try a lavender infusion, which can help repel mites, or a rosemary infusion, which can help deter lice. To make an infusion, you'll again steep herbs in hot water, much like making tea, but this time, you'll use a larger quantity of herbs and let it steep longer, often several hours to overnight. The resulting liquid can be used to spray in the coop or added to your chickens' bath water.

A more unconventional method that some chicken keepers swear by is fermenting feed with herbs. Fermentation not only makes the feed more digestible but also enhances the availability of nutrients. Simply soak the feed in water, add your chosen herbs, and leave it to ferment for a few days. The process is complete when the feed has expanded and smells slightly sour. Remember to start with a small batch until you get the hang of it and observe how your chickens react to it. Fermentation is a fantastic way to not only make the feed more nutritious but also to ensure that the herbs' active components are well-absorbed.

Now, once you've prepared your herbal preventatives, the next big question is: how do you administer them? This process involves figuring out correct dosages, setting up a schedule, and ensuring that your chickens actually consume these herbal preparations.

First, let's talk about dosages. Determining the right amount of herbs to give your chickens can be a bit of a balancing act. Too little, and it might not be effective. Too much, and it could potentially be harmful. A general rule of thumb is to start with small amounts and gradually increase until you find the right balance. For instance, if you're adding herbs to your chickens' feed, you might start with a tablespoon of herbs per pound of feed and adjust as necessary based on your observations of your chickens' health and behavior. Thoroughly study the appendix to understand the importance of correct dosage.

As for tinctures, remember that they are concentrated extracts, so a little goes a long way. A few drops per chicken per day is typically enough. However, the exact amount can vary depending on the specific herb and the size and health status of your chickens. It's always best to consult with an experienced herbalist or a holistic vet if you're unsure.

When it comes to scheduling, consistency is key. Parasites are persistent, so your efforts to control them should be as well. While it's not necessary to give your chickens herbs every day, a regular schedule can help ensure that the herbs have the desired effect. You might decide to add herbs to their feed once a week, give an herbal bath once a month, or add a tincture to their water every other day. Again, the exact schedule can vary depending on your specific circumstances and the herbs you're using. The important thing is to establish a routine and stick to it.

The final challenge, and perhaps the biggest, is ensuring that your chickens actually consume these herbal preventatives. Chickens, like all creatures, have their own likes and dislikes. Just because something is good for them doesn't mean they'll eat it. However, there are a few tricks you can use to encourage them. One is to mix the herbs thoroughly with their feed. This makes it harder for the chickens to pick out and discard the herbs. Another is to introduce the herbs gradually. Start with small amounts and increase slowly over time. This gives your chickens a chance to get used to the new flavors.

If you're having trouble getting your chickens to accept a particular herb, you might try offering it in a different form. For example, if they turn up their beaks at dried thyme in their feed, they might be more willing to peck at a fresh thyme plant in their run. Or, if they're refusing to drink water with a tincture, try making a strong herbal tea instead. It's all about finding what works for your flock. The goal here is not to force your chickens to consume something they clearly dislike but to find ways to make these health-promoting herbs a palatable and routine part of their diet. However, you do want to ensure that the chickens consume these herbs willingly as a natural part of their diet. By being creative, patient, and observant, you'll find ways to make these herbal preparations palatable and even enjoyable for your flock. Now, as we journey further into the world of natural parasite prevention, let's discuss another essential component - regular parasite checks.

Parasite checks are just as they sound: routine examinations to ensure that your flock is not harboring unwanted guests. As mentioned earlier, chickens can carry a certain amount of parasites without showing any outward signs of distress. However, a heavy infestation can quickly lead to health problems and even mortality. Regular parasite checks can help you catch an infestation early and take appropriate action before it becomes a serious issue.

Now, you might be wondering, how do you check your chickens for parasites? The most obvious signs of infestation are changes in behavior or physical appearance. Chickens with a heavy worm burden may appear lethargic, lose weight, produce fewer eggs, or have diarrhea. You might also notice changes in the appearance of their comb and wattles - they may become pale or shriveled. If you observe any of these signs, it's a strong indication that something is amiss and that further investigation is needed.

Another effective method of checking for parasites is through fecal exams. This involves taking a sample of your chicken's droppings and examining it under a microscope for the presence of worm eggs. This is a fairly straightforward procedure that can be done at home with a bit of training and the right equipment, or you can send the sample to a vet or a lab that specializes in fecal exams.

The frequency of these checks can vary depending on the health status and age of your chickens, your local climate and parasite prevalence, and other factors. As a rule of thumb, performing a fecal exam every 3-6 months is a good starting point. For chickens that are more susceptible to parasites - such as chicks, older birds, or birds under stress - more frequent checks may be needed.

What do you do if you discover that your chickens have a parasite problem? The first step is not to panic. Remember, a certain level of parasites is normal, and a healthy chicken can handle a small worm burden. The goal is not to completely eliminate all parasites but to keep their numbers in check so that they don't cause harm.

Depending on the severity of the infestation, you may need to intervene with herbal or conventional treatments. But before you reach for the wormer, take a moment to consider your options. If the infestation is mild, increasing the use of preventative herbs, improving coop hygiene, or adjusting your flock's diet may be sufficient. In cases of severe infestations, more aggressive treatments may be needed.

Remember, herbs can be potent allies in the fight against parasites. They work best as part of a comprehensive parasite prevention strategy that includes regular health checks, good coop management, and a balanced diet.

For those interested in more detailed information on herbal preparations, be sure to check out the appendix. This appendix contains a wealth of remedies and instructions for creating your own herbal parasite preventatives.

Chapter 8: Herbal Routines for the Changing Hen

Part I: From Chick to Hen: Herbs for Growing Birds

We are going to turn our attention to the different stages of life our feathered friends go through and how we can support them with herbs at each turn. Let's kick things off by looking at the journey from a chick to a fully grown hen.

Imagine a fluffy chick, just a day or two old. It's incredibly small and delicate, but don't be fooled – this little creature is about to embark on a rapid and incredible transformation. Over the next several weeks and months, this chick will grow into a full-fledged hen, going through several distinct developmental stages along the way.

In the first few days of life, chicks are completely dependent on their mother – or, in the case of chicks raised by humans, their surrogate parent and heat source. During this time, they're mostly eating, sleeping, and growing, with a special focus on developing their primary feathers. These are the long, stiff feathers that will eventually allow them to fly, although they're not yet ready to take to the skies.

Around the second week of life, things start to change rapidly. Chicks start to sprout their secondary feathers, which are the smaller feathers that cover the body and provide insulation. You might notice that your chicks are becoming more active, exploring their surroundings, and establishing their pecking order – that is, figuring out who's the boss.

By the third and fourth weeks, the chicks are no longer tiny fluff balls. They're growing at a fast pace and developing their personalities. This is also the time when you might start to see the first signs of their adult plumage, including the characteristic color patterns of their breed. Depending on the temperature, chicks may also be ready to spend some time outside, under close supervision, of course.

From the fifth week onwards, the chicks will continue to grow and mature, with their physical development largely following the rhythm of their breed. Some breeds mature faster than others, so don't be alarmed if your chicks are growing at a different pace than what you read in the books.

By the time they reach around 16-20 weeks of age, the chicks are no longer chicks – they're now young hens. At this point, they're nearly fully grown and are getting ready to lay eggs or fulfill their roles in the flock. You might also notice that their behavior is changing. They're becoming more independent, exploring further from the coop, and interacting more with each other and with you.

This rapid development from chick to hen is an exciting journey, but it's also a challenging one. At each stage, the chickens have different needs, from the heat and nutrition they require to the social and physical challenges they face. As chicken keepers, it's our job to provide them with the support they need to navigate these stages successfully. And one of the ways we can do this is through the strategic use of herbs.

Whether it's using herbs to support healthy growth, prevent disease, promote feather development, or ease the transition into adulthood, these natural remedies can be a valuable tool in our chicken-keeping toolkit. But it's not just about throwing a bunch of herbs into the coop and hoping for the best. It's about understanding the specific needs and challenges of each developmental stage and using herbs in a targeted way to support our chickens' health and well-being. So, how can we use herbs to support our chickens as they grow from adorable little chicks into magnificent hens?

At the heart of our approach is a thoughtful selection of herbs, each with specific benefits for growing birds. One of these star performers is nettle, a common plant that's often overlooked due to its stinging leaves. But when it comes to chicken health, nettle is nothing short of a powerhouse. Its high levels of iron, calcium, and other essential minerals make it a fantastic supplement for young birds. Furthermore, nettle contains a considerable amount of protein, a key nutrient for feather development and growth. Nettle can be fed fresh, but to avoid the stinging aspect, it's often better to offer it dried or as tea in the water.

Another herb that deserves recognition is alfalfa. Often found in livestock feed, alfalfa is no stranger to the world of farming. Its bright green leaves are teeming with nutrients, including vitamins A, C, E, and K, along with calcium, potassium, and magnesium. When chickens consume alfalfa, they're not just filling their bellies; they're fueling their bodies with the nutrients they need to grow and thrive. Alfalfa can be served fresh, dried, or even as sprouts. Plus, its pleasant flavor tends to be a hit with chickens.

Let's not forget about the wonders of parsley. This herb is often relegated to garnish status in human cuisine, but for chickens, it's a nutritional hero. Packed with vitamins and minerals, including a hefty dose of vitamin K, parsley supports bone health – an essential factor as chicks grow into full-sized birds. Plus, parsley's high vitamin C content helps bolster the immune system, promoting overall health. Chopped fresh parsley can be added to feed or scattered around the coop for a bit of foraging fun.

Garlic is another herb that's beneficial for growing chickens. It might seem a little odd to feed garlic to chickens, but it's actually a fantastic natural remedy for various health issues. Garlic contains allicin, a compound known for its antibacterial and antifungal properties. It can help protect chickens against a range of common diseases, supporting their immune systems. Garlic can be added to the chickens' water or crushed and mixed into their feed.

Mint, particularly peppermint and spearmint, can also be beneficial. In addition to its refreshing taste that chickens seem to enjoy, mint can help deter pests in the coop. Its strong aroma can mask the scent of chickens, making it less likely for pests to find their way into your flock. Plus, the cooling properties of mint can be particularly beneficial in hot weather, helping chickens stay comfortable as they navigate the challenges of growth.

Dandelions might be seen as a pesky weed in your lawn, but for chickens, they're a nutritional gold mine. Rich in vitamins A, C, and K, as well as calcium and potassium, dandelions can support growth in multiple ways. The leaves can be served fresh or dried, and even the flowers are safe – and enjoyable – for chickens to eat.

By incorporating herbs like nettle, alfalfa, parsley, garlic, mint, and dandelions into your chickens' diet, you can support their development in a natural and holistic way. Including these powerful herbs into a chick's diet doesn't have to be complicated. With a few key steps, you can create a nutrient-dense, herbal-enriched feed that your young birds will love.

Start with a good-quality chick feed. This forms the base of their diet and provides the essential nutrients that chicks need for healthy growth. The next step is to select the herbs you wish to include. For growing chicks, focus on nutrient-dense herbs like nettle and alfalfa, as well as immune-boosting herbs like garlic and parsley.

Herbs can be incorporated into chick feed in various forms. Fresh herbs can be finely chopped and mixed into the feed. However, remember to introduce fresh herbs gradually as the high water content can affect the consistency of the feed and might require some getting used to for the chicks.

Dried herbs are a convenient option as they can be stored for a long time and are easy to mix into the feed. A simple way to prepare dried herbs is to chop fresh herbs and spread them out in a single layer on a baking sheet. Leave them to dry in a warm, airy space. Once dry, the herbs can be stored in airtight containers. To use, simply crumble the dried herbs into the feed.

Fermented feed is another fantastic way to incorporate herbs. It's a process that not only enriches the feed with probiotics but also enhances the digestibility and availability of nutrients in the feed. Here's a basic remedy: Start by soaking the chick feed in water in a clean, airtight container. Add your chosen herbs, cover the container loosely to allow gas to escape, and leave it in a warm place. Stir the mixture daily. Within a few days, the feed will have fermented and be ready to use. Start by replacing a small amount of their regular feed with the fermented version and gradually increase the quantity as they get used to it.

Herbal teas or infusions can also be used as a way to introduce herbs to chicks. Steep your chosen herbs in hot water for about 15 minutes, strain the mixture, and let it cool. The herbal infusion can be added to the waterer or mixed into the feed. A popular choice for this method is nettle, given its impressive nutrient content.

Creating an herbal feed blend can be a bit of an experiment. For instance, a simple blend for young chicks might include equal parts of dried nettle, alfalfa, and parsley, with a smaller amount of crushed garlic added for its immune-boosting benefits. Start with small amounts and observe how the chicks react to it. They may pick out some herbs and leave others, or they might dive right in and eat everything up. Don't be discouraged if they're a bit hesitant at first. Keep trying, perhaps changing the form or the blend of herbs. By providing your chicks with an herbal-enhanced diet, you're not just giving them a treat. You're supporting their growth, bolstering their health, and setting them up for a vibrant, productive life.

Monitoring the health of your chicks as they consume an herb-enriched diet is a vital part of their care. By paying close attention to their behavior, growth, and overall health, you can better understand their needs and make necessary adjustments to their diet and care.

Let's start by discussing what healthy development looks like in growing chicks. It's a joy to watch these tiny beings transform into full-fledged chickens, but it's also essential to know what to look for during each stage to ensure they're on the right track.

Initially, chicks should be alert, active, and display a healthy appetite. Their eyes should be clear and bright, and their feathers should start coming in neatly without any bald patches. As they grow, their development should include steady weight gain, robust feathering, and an increase in activity levels. Their droppings should be firm and well-formed, not too loose or too dry.

Regular weight checks can provide useful insight into how well your chicks are growing. A steady increase in weight indicates that they're consuming enough food and absorbing the nutrients properly. However, remember that growth rates can vary among different breeds.

As part of your regular health checks, observe your chicks' behavior. Healthy chicks are generally active, curious, and sociable. They should show interest in their environment, be quick to explore new additions to their space, and interact positively with their flockmates.

Now, while it's great to know the signs of healthy development, it's equally important to be aware of potential red flags. Any deviation from their regular behavior or growth pattern could be a cause for concern and warrants further investigation.

For example, a chick that is less active or more lethargic than usual might be feeling under the weather. Changes in appetite, such as eating less or more than usual, can also indicate a potential health issue. Poor feathering, weight loss or lack of weight gain, and changes in droppings are additional warning signs that something might be amiss.

Additionally, watch for changes in their interactions with the other chicks. If a chick becomes withdrawn or if it's being bullied by the others, it could be a sign of illness. Remember, the sooner a potential health issue is addressed, the better the outcome is likely to be.

As a chicken keeper, your role doesn't stop at observing. Based on your observations, you may need to make adjustments to ensure your chicks continue to thrive.

If you notice that your chicks are not eating the herbal feed, you might need to tweak the remedy. Maybe the herbs are too coarse, or the mix contains an herb they don't like. Try grinding the herbs into a finer powder or changing the mix of herbs. I always run the herbs I feed my chicks through a single-serve blender or even a coffee grinder would work.

If a chick appears undernourished or is not gaining weight as expected, consider increasing the protein content in their feed or adding nutrient-dense herbs like nettle or alfalfa. If a chick seems overstimulated or anxious, consider introducing calming herbs like chamomile or lavender.

Remember, monitoring and adjusting are ongoing processes, not one-time events. By keeping a close eye on your chicks and adjusting their care as needed, you're setting them up for a healthy and happy transition from chick to adult hen. And this, my friend, is one of the most rewarding aspects of raising chickens. So keep observing, keep learning, and enjoy the journey!

Part II: Laying Low: Supporting Hens During Molting

Molting! If you're a first-time chicken keeper, this term may be new to you. If you're a seasoned veteran, the mention of it might make you wince, bringing back memories of your chickens looking a little worse for wear. Whether it's your first or fifth time, the molting process can seem a bit alarming, but fear not, it's a completely natural part of a chicken's life cycle.

Molting is the process where chickens shed their old, worn-out feathers and grow new ones. This isn't a vanity project for the chickens, though. Replacing old feathers is crucial for their health and survival. Feathers are not just for show; they're a chicken's first line of defense against the elements, providing insulation against the cold, protection from the sun, and even waterproofing. They're also crucial for flight - okay, chickens might not soar through the sky, but those little flaps can help them escape danger or reach a tasty treat hanging just a little too high.

Molting usually happens once a year, typically in late summer or early fall, when the days start getting shorter. But don't mark your calendar just yet. The timing can vary depending on factors like the breed of the chicken, their age, and their overall health.

The entire molting process can take anywhere from two to six months. It doesn't happen overnight, and it doesn't happen all at once. It's a gradual process, starting from the head and neck, moving down the back, breast, and thighs, and finally, reaching the tail. The new feathers don't just pop out fully formed, either. They start as 'pin feathers', which are essentially feather shafts filled with blood vessels. These pin feathers grow and eventually burst open, revealing the new feather inside.

The molting process can be a bit uncomfortable for your chickens. Imagine having a head full of tiny, new, growing feathers - it's akin to having a scalp full of tender new hair after shaving your head. The newly forming feathers can be sensitive, and chickens may be less tolerant of being handled during this time. This sensitivity is another reason why chickens require a little extra TLC during molting.

You'll also notice that your hens may stop laying eggs during this period. This might seem concerning, but it's a completely normal part of the molting process. Producing feathers and eggs are both protein-heavy activities, and it's hard for a chicken's body to do both at the same time. So when molting starts, egg production takes a backseat.

One important point to note is that not all feather loss is due to molting. If you see your chickens losing feathers outside the usual molting season or if the feather loss doesn't follow the typical head-to-tail pattern, it might be due to other issues like lice, mites, or nutritional deficiencies.

Molting is an essential, natural process that every chicken goes through. It may look a bit alarming, and it can be a bit tough on your chickens, but with the right understanding and care, they'll come out the other side sporting a fabulous new set of feathers. The aim is to support them through this period and ensure they have everything they need to grow a healthy, new coat of feathers.

So, how can we support our feathery friends during this feather-filled period? The answer, unsurprisingly, lies in the power of herbs. But before we jump into the specifics, it's worth noting that the foundation of feather regrowth, like all things in the chicken world, starts with a balanced diet. Ensuring your chickens are getting enough protein is crucial. Since feathers consist of about 85% protein, it's easy to see why.

Once we've ensured the fundamentals are in place, we can look at how herbs can support the process. Let's start with Comfrey. This humble plant might not be on your radar yet, but it's about to become a major player in your chicken herb repertoire. Comfrey is high in protein, making it an excellent herb to support feather regrowth. It's also packed with vitamins and minerals, including calcium, potassium, phosphorus, and Vitamin B12, all of which contribute to overall chicken health.

You can offer fresh Comfrey leaves to your chickens directly, or you can dry them and mix them into their feed. If you're feeling adventurous, you can even make a Comfrey 'tea' by steeping the leaves in hot water, then cooling it down before offering it to your chickens.

Next up on our herb roster is Calendula. You may know Calendula for its bright, cheery flowers that bring a pop of color to any garden. But did you know that this plant is also a boon for your molting chickens? Calendula is high in lutein and other carotenoids, compounds that promote feather color vibrancy. Not only will Calendula help your chickens grow their new feathers, but it will also make those feathers look better than ever. You can offer Calendula flowers fresh or dried, mixed into their feed, or as a treat on their own.

Let's not forget Alfalfa. This herb is a protein powerhouse, making it another excellent choice for supporting feather regrowth. But its benefits don't stop there. Alfalfa is also packed with vitamins and minerals that contribute to overall health, including vitamins A, C, E, and K, calcium, potassium, and iron. Offer Alfalfa fresh or dried, mixed into the feed or as a standalone snack.

Last but certainly not least, let's talk about Nettle. This herb may have a bit of a sting in the wild, but it's a chicken's best friend when it comes to molting. Nettle is high in both protein and iron, two key components for feather regrowth. It's also a great source of vitamins A, C, and K, as well as calcium, magnesium, and selenium.

Feeding Nettle to your chickens might seem like a prickly proposition, but it's quite simple once you know how. Always wear gloves when handling fresh Nettle to avoid the sting. You can then blanch the Nettle leaves to remove the sting, or you can dry them out completely. Once the sting is gone, you can offer the Nettle leaves to your chickens directly, or you can mix them into their feed.

By incorporating herbs like Comfrey, Calendula, Alfalfa, and Nettle into your chickens' diet during molting, you can support the feather regrowth process, bolster their overall health, and help them come out the other side looking better than ever. Your chickens will thank you for it, and you'll get the joy of watching them strut around the coop sporting their shiny new set of feathers. Including these herbs into your chickens' diet isn't just about tossing them into the coop and hoping for the best. It's about crafting a balanced, nutritious, and palatable diet that meets the specific needs of your molting chickens. A little bit of creativity and culinary experimentation can go a long way in this regard. Let's take a look at some remedies you can make to give your chickens a tasty and nutritious treat during their molting phase.

A favorite is the Herbal Protein Scramble. This treat is not only delicious but it's also packed with the protein and nutrients your chickens need to support feather regrowth. To make it, start with a dozen eggs. Yes, chickens can safely eat eggs, and they're an excellent source of protein. Scramble the eggs and cook them without any added fat or seasoning. Once the eggs are cooked, mix in a handful of fresh or dried Comfrey, Alfalfa, and Nettle. If you have them available, throw in some Calendula flowers for an extra dose of nutrients and color. Serve the scramble to your chickens once it's cool enough to eat. They'll love pecking at the colorful mix, and you'll love knowing they're getting a nutrient-packed treat.

For a quick and easy treat, try the Herbal Layer Mix. This is essentially a blend of dried herbs that you can mix directly into your chickens' regular feed. To make it, combine equal parts dried Comfrey, Alfalfa, Nettle, and Calendula flowers. If you want to get fancy, you can also add other beneficial herbs like Parsley and Dandelion. Store the mix in an airtight container and sprinkle it on top of their feed each day.

If you're looking for a refreshing treat for hot days, the Herbal Ice Pop is a must-try. This is a fun way to keep your chickens hydrated and give them a nutrient boost at the same time. Start with an ice cube tray or a similar container. Fill each compartment with chopped fresh herbs – any combination of Comfrey, Alfalfa, Nettle, Calendula, and others will do. Then, fill the tray with water and freeze it. Once the ice pops are frozen, pop them out and give them to your chickens. They'll have a blast pecking at the ice, and they'll get a nice dose of herbs in the process.

Lastly, there's the Herbal Mash, a comforting treat that's perfect for colder days. To make it, start with a base of cooked grains. This could be quinoa, barley, or a similar grain. Then, mix in a handful of fresh or dried herbs. Again, Comfrey, Alfalfa, Nettle, and Calendula are excellent choices. You can also add other ingredients like chopped vegetables or cooked eggs. Serve the mash to your chickens warm for a cozy treat.

These remedies are just a starting point. Feel free to experiment and adjust based on what you have available and what your chickens seem to prefer. The important thing is to provide a variety of herbs that can support their health during molting. Whether it's in the form of a scramble, a mix, an ice pop, or a mash, your chickens will appreciate the tasty and nutritious treats.

Nourishing your molting hens with beneficial herbs and concocting delicious treats for them is only one side of the coin. Equally crucial is keeping a vigilant eye on their health throughout the molting period. After all, molting can be quite stressful for your feathered friends, and their bodies have to work overtime to produce a new set of feathers. Therefore, it's our responsibility to ensure their health doesn't take a hit during this challenging time.

So, what signs should you look out for? Well, a healthy molting chicken will still be active, maintain its appetite, and exhibit no signs of distress or illness other than the obvious loss of feathers. Their new feathers, called pinfeathers, should start to appear after a short time. These look like small, pointy quills pushing through the skin. You should see a steady regrowth of new feathers throughout the molting period.

But sometimes, things don't go quite as smoothly. Certain signs could indicate that a chicken is having a harder time with molting. These include prolonged loss of feathers with no signs of regrowth, loss of appetite, lethargy, weight loss, or any signs of distress or discomfort. In these cases, it's essential to take swift action to support your chicken's health.

For instance, a prolonged loss of feathers could suggest a nutritional deficiency. Here, you might want to increase the quantity or variety of herbs in your chickens' diet. Herbs like Comfrey and Alfalfa, which are rich in proteins, could be especially helpful in promoting feather growth.

A loss of appetite during molting, while not uncommon, should be addressed to prevent weight loss. If a chicken isn't eating its regular feed, try enticing it with some of the herbal treat remedies discussed earlier. Warm mashes or protein-rich scrambles could be particularly appealing. You can also add appetite-stimulating herbs like garlic to their diet.

Lethargy or noticeable weight loss in a molting chicken could be signs of underlying health issues. While a bit of sluggishness can be normal during molting, excessive lethargy is a cause for concern. It's worth consulting with a vet or a chicken health expert in these cases. In the meantime, you can support your chicken's energy levels by providing nutrient-dense foods and herbs.

One crucial thing to remember is to handle your molting chickens gently, if at all. Pinfeathers are sensitive, and rough handling can cause discomfort or even injury. Therefore, routine health checks during molting should be done with extra care.

It's also wise to limit any unnecessary stress during this period. For example, introducing new flock members, making significant changes to the coop or feeding routines, or other stressful events should be avoided if possible.

Monitoring your chickens' health during molting is all about being observant, responsive, and proactive. The key is to look out for any changes in behavior or appearance that could indicate a problem. In most cases, supportive actions like adjusting their diet, providing herbal supplements, or creating a stress-free environment can help your chickens navigate through molting successfully.

The joy of keeping chickens, after all, isn't just in the fresh eggs or the natural pest control. It's in the connection we form with these delightful birds and the satisfaction we get from seeing them thrive. Supporting them through molting with attentive care and herbal aids is one way we can give back to our chickens for all the joy they bring into our lives.

Part III: Golden Girls: Herbs for Senior Hens

Chickens, like us humans, have a life cycle, and there comes a time when they transition from being the productive layers we've known into their golden years. As a chicken keeper, it's our responsibility to recognize the signs of aging in our chickens and ensure they continue to live comfortable and happy lives even as they slow down a bit.

Recognizing the signs of aging in chickens starts with understanding what is considered typical for their age group. The average lifespan of backyard hens can vary considerably, typically ranging from 5 to 10 years, but some breeds can live even longer. It's important to note that a chicken is considered 'old' not so much by its age in years but by its physical and behavioral changes.

One of the most prominent signs of aging in hens is a decrease in egg production. While some hens can lay eggs well into their golden years, many begin to slow down their laying as early as 2 to 3 years of age. You may also notice changes in the eggs themselves. Older hens' eggs tend to be larger with thinner shells. Sometimes, they may lay shell-less eggs. This is all part of the natural aging process.

Physical changes are another key sign of aging. Just like in people, the aging process in chickens often brings about changes in posture and mobility. You may notice your older chickens moving a bit slower, taking more time to rise from sitting or having difficulty reaching higher perches. Some may develop arthritis, which can further impact their mobility.

Feather condition can also provide clues about a chicken's age. While feathers are replaced annually during molting, older chickens may have feathers that appear dull, ragged, or thin even outside of the molting season. This isn't a cause for alarm but just another sign of the natural aging process.

Other signs of aging can include changes in weight and muscle mass. Some older chickens may become thinner despite maintaining a good appetite. On the other hand, some may gain weight, particularly if their decreased activity levels are not accompanied by a reduction in feed intake.

Behavioral changes are common as chickens age. Older chickens might become less social, preferring to spend more time alone rather than with the flock. They may also sleep more, both during the day and at night. It's also worth noting that older chickens are often lower in the pecking order, so it's important to ensure they're not being bullied or deprived of food and water by younger, more assertive flock members.

Aging is a natural process, and while we can't stop the march of time, we can make our chickens' golden years comfortable and fulfilling. This involves understanding and recognizing the signs of aging, making necessary adjustments to their care, and most importantly, providing them with lots of love and attention. Our aim is to support these wise old birds, helping them age with grace and dignity while providing them with the best quality of life in their golden years.

Supporting your elderly hens naturally can be achieved with the help of certain herbs. Herbs like Milk Thistle and Echinacea are not just beneficial for us humans, but they also have tremendous benefits for our feathered friends, especially those who are entering or enjoying their golden years.

Let's talk about Milk Thistle first. This vibrant herb with its purple flowers and prickly leaves is a powerhouse of liver support. The liver plays a pivotal role in a chicken's overall health and vitality. It aids in digestion, processes nutrients, eliminates toxins, and even plays a role in the production of yolk for the eggs laid by your hens. As chickens age, their liver function can naturally slow down. Milk Thistle, specifically the compound silymarin that it contains, is known for its liver-protective qualities. It helps in detoxifying and regenerating the liver cells, thereby enhancing the liver's functionality and overall health.

Incorporating Milk Thistle into your chickens' diet can be as simple as sprinkling dried, ground Milk Thistle seeds over their regular feed. You can also make a warm infusion with the seeds and add it to their water. The flavor is typically well-received by chickens, and you'll have the peace of mind of knowing you're supporting their liver health in a natural and gentle way.

Next up is Echinacea, a herb renowned for its immune-boosting properties. Elderly hens, just like aging people, can have weakened immune systems, making them more susceptible to infections and diseases. Echinacea can help boost their immune system, thanks to its rich content of phenols, which are potent antioxidants. It also contains alkylamides, which can stimulate the immune system, enhancing the body's defense mechanisms.

Echinacea can be given to chickens in various forms. Fresh or dried leaves and flowers can be mixed directly into the feed, or you can prepare a tea infusion to add to their water or moisten their feed. As an occasional treat, consider planting some Echinacea in your garden or in pots around the chicken run. Chickens naturally enjoy foraging and will benefit from access to fresh Echinacea.

Along with these two powerhouse herbs, there are several others that can support the well-being of your aging chickens. For instance, Turmeric, which contains curcumin, a compound known for its anti-inflammatory and antioxidant properties, can be beneficial, especially for chickens suffering from arthritis or other inflammatory conditions.

Garlic, a favorite among many chicken keepers, is also an excellent addition to the diet of elderly chickens. Its antibacterial and antiviral properties can help boost their immune system, while its sulfur compounds can support respiratory health.

Ginger, another common kitchen herb, can aid in digestion and offer anti-inflammatory benefits, while herbs like Parsley and Sage can offer a nutritional boost, being rich in vitamins and minerals essential for overall health.

By incorporating these herbs into your senior chickens' routine, you're not just adding a variety to their diet but also naturally supporting their health, ensuring they remain comfortable and happy during their golden years. The use of these herbs is to provide overall support and enhance their quality of life.

Caring for senior hens goes beyond providing a diet enhanced with beneficial herbs. As your chickens age, their needs change, and it becomes necessary to make certain adjustments in their coop conditions, nutrition, and overall care to ensure they continue to live comfortably and happily.

Let's start with the coop conditions. An ideal chicken coop is safe, clean, dry, well-ventilated, and, of course, comfortable. For older hens, comfort takes on an even more significant role. Make sure their roosting bars are low enough to prevent any potential injury from jumping or flying down. If you have noticed your older birds are having difficulties getting up onto the roost, you may need to install a "chicken ladder" or a ramp to help them.

The bedding should be soft and thick, providing ample cushioning for older birds, some of whom may prefer to rest on the ground instead of roosting. Wood shavings or straw can be ideal for this. Additionally, ensure there's plenty of space for each bird in the coop. Overcrowding can lead to stress, especially for older birds, which can have a negative impact on their health and well-being.

Next, let's talk about nutrition. Nutritional needs for chickens change as they age. Laying hens, for instance, require a diet rich in calcium for egg production. However, as hens age and their egg production decrease, their dietary needs shift. Too much calcium, for instance, can lead to kidney problems in non-laying hens. For this reason, it's essential to switch older hens to a lower-calcium diet.

A well-balanced senior feed should include a good protein source, fiber, and a variety of vitamins and minerals to support overall health. Don't forget about greens. Fresh, leafy vegetables not only add variety to their diet but are also a good source of essential nutrients.

Remember, hydration is as crucial as nutrition. Ensure your chickens always have access to clean, fresh water. In colder months, check regularly to make sure the water hasn't frozen over.

When it comes to care, older chickens may require more attention. Regular health checks are essential to detect any potential issues early on. Pay attention to their weight, feather condition, behavior, appetite, and droppings.

Older chickens can be more prone to parasites, both internal and external, so a good parasite management routine is critical. This could include regular dust baths for your flock, which not only help in parasite control but also seem to be quite enjoyable for the chickens.

Older hens might not be as quick or agile as their younger flock mates. They might have trouble competing for food or may be more susceptible to bullying. Monitor the flock dynamics carefully and make any necessary adjustments, such as providing separate feeding areas for your older birds or separating any particularly aggressive birds.

Caring for senior hens can be a little more demanding, but it's also incredibly rewarding. You want to make their golden years comfortable and stress-free, ensuring they continue to enjoy a good quality of life.

One of the most important aspects of caring for senior hens is to be observant. Regular monitoring of your chickens' behavior, physical condition, and comfort levels can provide invaluable insights into their health. Being aware of common issues that can affect elderly hens can also help you identify problems early so you can address them before they become serious.

Starting with behavior, chickens are creatures of habit. They have routines they stick to every day. A change in these routines can often be the first sign that something is amiss. Perhaps you've noticed your previously voracious hen showing disinterest in her food. Maybe their egg-laying patterns have changed, or their clucking sounds are different. All these changes in behavior warrant a closer look.

Observing physical condition is equally important. The state of a chicken's feathers can tell you a lot about their health. Good, shiny, and well-preened feathers indicate good health. On the other hand, dull, broken, or missing feathers could suggest the bird is unwell or stressed. Check for changes in weight, too. Both sudden weight loss and weight gain can be signs of health problems.

Examining the comb and wattle, the fleshy, brightly colored protuberances on the top of the head and underneath the chin, respectively, can provide insights. In healthy birds, these should be bright and vibrant. If they look pale, dry, or shriveled, it could indicate a health issue.

Checking the eyes and the beak can also be useful. The eyes should be bright and clear, with no discharge or swelling. The beak should be strong and well-formed, with no cracks or discoloration.

Now, let's talk about comfort. Elderly hens may have more difficulty moving around than their younger counterparts. They might develop arthritis, which can make walking painful. Watch for any signs of discomfort when they walk, such as limping or reluctance to move. Look out for hens who prefer to sit or lie down most of the time, as this could be a sign they're in pain.

There are several common health issues that can affect elderly hens. These include arthritis, as mentioned above, respiratory problems, parasites, and various reproductive issues in hens, such as egg-binding or ovarian cancer. By keeping a close eye on your birds and catching these issues early, you can greatly improve the quality of life for your senior hens.

Remember, just like humans, each chicken ages differently. Some might remain spry and active well into their senior years, while others may start showing signs of aging earlier. Your role as a caregiver is to understand these individual differences and provide care tailored to each bird's specific needs.

Observation is a powerful tool in chicken care. By spending time with your flock every day and getting to know their habits and personalities, you become finely attuned to what's normal for each bird and what's not. This sensitivity allows you to pick up on the subtle signs that something might be wrong so you can act quickly to address the issue.

Part IV: Broody Brilliance: Herbal Care for Mother Hens

A broody hen is one of the most fascinating phenomena in the chicken world. It's the point when a hen decides she's ready to hatch a clutch of eggs and raise chicks. This phase can occur at any time but is often triggered by a variety of factors, including the number of daylight hours, the availability of a suitable nesting site, the presence of fertilized eggs, and the hen's individual hormonal rhythms. Let's delve into what the broody stage is, what it entails, and its implications for your hens and your flock as a whole.

At its core, the broody stage is a hormonal shift. It's when a hen's body tells her it's time to reproduce. It is interesting how, regardless of whether the eggs are fertilized or not, the hen's biological instinct will kick in, prompting her to sit on her eggs to incubate them. This desire to hatch eggs and mother chicks is so strong that it will completely alter the hen's behavior, turning her into a fiercely protective and sometimes surprisingly aggressive mother-to-be.

A broody hen's behavior changes in many ways. She'll stop laying new eggs and instead focus all her attention on the eggs in her clutch. She'll rarely leave the nest, only doing so briefly to eat, drink, and poop. She'll sit on the eggs constantly, fluffing her feathers to create an insulating layer that helps maintain the temperature and humidity levels needed for the eggs to develop.

One clear sign of a broody hen is the unique clucking noise she makes, a sort of low, throaty, repetitive sound quite different from the usual clucking sounds hens make. She may also become aggressive if you try to approach her or her nest, pecking at you or trying to scare you away. This is entirely normal; it's her way of protecting her unborn chicks.

The physical changes a broody hen undergoes are equally dramatic. She will lose feathers on her chest and belly, an adaptation that allows her body heat to better warm the eggs. This process, known as 'brood patch' formation, helps ensure the eggs receive the correct level of heat for optimal development.

From an owner's perspective, a broody hen presents a unique set of challenges and opportunities. On one hand, a broody hen will stop laying eggs, meaning your egg production will drop. On the other hand, if you want to expand your flock naturally, a broody hen is your best friend. She'll do all the work of incubating and hatching the eggs, and once the chicks are born, she'll teach them how to be chickens, showing them what to eat, where to find food, how to scratch, and more.

It's important to note that not all hens will go broody. Some breeds are more prone to broodiness than others. Silkies and Cochins, for example, are famous for their strong broody tendencies, while Leghorns and Rhode Island Reds rarely go broody. Even within breeds that commonly go broody, not all individuals will do so. It's largely a matter of individual genetics and temperament.

As fascinating as the broody stage is, it can also be a physically taxing period for the hen. She spends most of her time on the nest, rarely eating or drinking, resulting in weight loss and sometimes a drop in overall condition. In this demanding period of a hen's life, it's crucial to offer nutritional and calming support to her. The use of herbs can provide both these elements, helping to make the broody stage a less stressful and more healthful experience for your mother-to-be hen. Two standout herbs in this respect are Raspberry Leaf and Chamomile, both offering unique benefits to your broody hens.

Raspberry Leaf, a plant known for its beneficial effects on reproductive health, is an excellent herb to support a broody hen. Its leaves are rich in iron, which can help replenish the hen's iron stores, often depleted due to the physical demands of the broody period. The leaves also contain calcium, necessary for eggshell strength for any new eggs she might lay post-broodiness.

But Raspberry Leaf is not only beneficial for its nutritional content. It also has properties that can help the hen's body cope with the stress of broodiness. Its natural compounds have been known to soothe and relax smooth muscle tissue, offering a calming effect, which is a boon for a hen in the broody stage, which can be a period of heightened stress and agitation.

Chamomile, on the other hand, is a well-loved herb renowned for its calming properties. It's a gentle herb that can help reduce stress and anxiety in your broody hen. The act of sitting on eggs around the clock can be a bit anxiety-inducing for a hen, as she might be on high alert for any potential threats to her clutch. A regular dose of chamomile can help soothe these natural anxieties and create a more peaceful brooding experience for her.

Chamomile also has other benefits, including promoting good digestion and helping with inflammation. Given that broody hens eat less, it's essential to ensure that what they do eat is easily digestible, and Chamomile can help with this. It's also beneficial if your hen is suffering from a bit of inflammation due to constant sitting.

Now, Raspberry Leaf and Chamomile are just two examples. There are many other herbs you can use to support your broody hens. Nettle, for instance, is packed with essential nutrients like calcium, magnesium, and iron. It can help bolster your hen's nutrition during this time of less eating. Lavender can provide a calming effect, much like Chamomile, reducing the hen's stress levels. Calendula can boost the immune system and provide antioxidants, both crucial during this physically demanding stage.

These herbs can be provided in various forms. Fresh, dried, or powdered herbs can be mixed directly into your hens' feed. Some herbs, like Chamomile and Lavender, can be brewed into a tea, which can then be added to your chickens' water supply for a soothing and hydrating treat. You can also scatter herbs around the coop and nesting areas, where the hens can peck at them as desired.

The goal is to make the broody stage as stress-free and healthful as possible for your hen. The use of these and other herbs can provide the much-needed nutritional support and calming effects your hen needs during this demanding time.

While herbs are amazing they should not be the only form of care you provide to your broody hens. It's also important to monitor your hen's physical condition and behavior closely during this time. Look for signs of excessive weight loss, dehydration, or unusual behavior. At times, with a broody hen, you may need to make sure that she has food and water accessible very close to her nest. It all depends on how committed she is to sitting on and hatching her eggs.

Looking after your broody hen is not just about herbs. It also involves providing an ideal environment for her to lay, brood, and hatch her eggs. A key part of this is her nest box. The right nest box, tailored with the right herbs, can go a long way in supporting your hen through her broody period. So, let's dig into how to create an herbal nest box that is both comfortable and healthful.

The first step in preparing an herbal nest box is to choose the right herbs. You'll want to select herbs that offer comfort and health benefits to your broody hen. We've already talked about a few herbs that can be beneficial during the broody stage, such as Raspberry Leaf, Chamomile, and Lavender. These can also be great additions to your nest box.

Raspberry Leaf can provide a nice soft layer for the hen to sit on and has the added benefit of being full of nutrients that she can peck at throughout the day. Chamomile can help keep her calm and relaxed while she's brooding. Lavender, with its lovely fragrance, can create a serene environment for her.

Another good herb to include in the nest box is Lemon Balm. Its citrusy fragrance is known to be a natural insect repellent, which can help keep annoying pests away from the brooding hen and her eggs. It can also promote relaxation, adding to the calming environment in the nest box.

Peppermint is another herb you might consider. This herb has cooling properties, which can be beneficial if your hen is brooding during the warmer months. It can help keep the nest box a little cooler, making it more comfortable for your hen.

Now, you might be thinking - How do I put all this together? It's easier than you might think! Simply layer the bottom of the nest box with a mix of these herbs. You can use fresh or dried herbs, depending on what's available to you. You'll want to layer them thick enough to provide a soft, comfortable surface for your hen to sit on. But not so thick that it becomes a tangled mess that traps eggs or droppings.

But that's not all! You can add extra comfort to the nest box by including other natural materials along with the herbs. Straw or wood shavings, for example, can provide additional padding and help to insulate the box. They also absorb any droppings, helping to keep the box clean.

Just remember, cleanliness is key. You'll need to check the nest box daily for any droppings or soiled materials. If you find any, remove them promptly to keep the nest box clean and hygienic. Replace any removed materials with fresh ones to maintain a comfortable and healthful nest box for your broody hen. An herbal nest box is a wonderful way to support your hen during her broody stage. By choosing the right herbs and other materials, you can create a nest box that is not only comfortable for her to sit in but also provides beneficial herbs for her to peck at during this crucial period. Cleanliness does not just stop at the nest box, though. It extends to all aspects of hen care, especially during the broody period. This is the time when your hens are more prone to health issues due to the physical stress of laying, brooding, and hatching eggs. As such, it becomes even more critical for you to keep a close eye on your hens' health, the progress of the hatch, and the care of the chicks post-hatch.

Monitoring your hen's health during the broody stage is vital. You want to ensure she remains healthy so she can successfully hatch her eggs and take care of her chicks. Daily checks are in order. Look for signs of illness, such as loss of appetite, lethargy, or abnormal behavior. Also, ensure she is eating and drinking enough. While broody hens tend to eat less, it is crucial that they still receive adequate nutrition to sustain them through this physically demanding period.

On the flip side, observe for any signs of broodiness ending prematurely. If your hen leaves her nest for prolonged periods or seems disinterested in her eggs, she might be ending her broody phase. This requires immediate action, like moving the eggs to an incubator to ensure they continue to develop.

Next up is keeping tabs on the hatch's progress. As the hatching date approaches, you might notice a change in your hen's behavior. She might become more protective of her nest or start to cluck softly - these are signs that her chicks are about to hatch. Once the chicks start to hatch, avoid disturbing the nest. It can take up to 24 hours for a chick to fully emerge from its egg.

Post-hatch care is just as important as care during the broody and hatching stages. Once the chicks have hatched, they will stay in the nest with their mother for 24-48 hours until they are dry and strong enough to leave the nest. Ensure the mother hen has easy access to food and water, which she will teach her chicks to eat and drink.

As for the chicks, they'll need a heat source for the first few weeks. While the mother hen will provide warmth, if you're raising the chicks without a hen or if the weather is particularly cold, you might need to provide additional heat.

In addition to heat, chicks require a nutritious diet to support their rapid growth. You'll need to provide chick starter feed, a type of feed specifically designed for young chicks. This will typically be your chicks' primary food source for the first 6 weeks. Fresh water should be available at all times as well.

As we round out this chapter, I want to note that herbs can play a significant role in all stages of a hen's life - from the spry young chick to the beautiful hen and the seasoned elder of the flock. They offer an array of benefits, from boosting general health and well-being to addressing specific issues that may arise.

Remember the value of observation, the power of herbs, and the importance of providing a comfortable and healthy environment for your chickens at all stages of life. Herbal care, in conjunction with good husbandry practices, can contribute greatly to a vibrant and thriving flock.

Chapter 9: Power to the Rooster

Part I: Rooster Boosters: Vitality Herbs for Males

Let's shift our attention from the laying and brooding hens to the gallant roosters of our flock. Understanding the unique physiological needs of roosters is crucial in ensuring their optimal health and well-being.

Roosters, while part of the same species as hens, have distinctive physiological traits and health needs due to their role as the protectors and procreators of the flock. For instance, one of the first things you might notice about a rooster, apart from their stunning plumage, is their size. Roosters are typically larger than hens, with more muscle mass. This physical robustness is essential for their role in the flock. They must be strong and agile to protect the hens and maintain order in the flock.

The rooster's larger size and increased muscle mass mean that their nutritional requirements are slightly different from those of hens. While they also need a balanced diet of proteins, carbohydrates, fats, vitamins, and minerals, the ratios might be different. For instance, because of their higher muscle mass, roosters might require more protein in their diet.

The rooster's comb and wattles, those fleshy, lobed appendages on their heads and necks, are more prominent than those of hens. While these features enhance the rooster's attractiveness to hens, they also serve a vital physiological function. The comb and wattles are rich in blood vessels, and by altering the blood flow to these areas, the rooster can regulate his body temperature. This feature is important for roosters who must endure the elements to keep a watchful eye over their flock.

Moreover, roosters are equipped with sharp, curved spurs and long, sturdy legs, both of which are used in defending their flock against predators or rival roosters. These limbs need to be strong and healthy for the rooster to effectively fulfill his protector role.

Additionally, a rooster's vocal cords are more developed than those of a hen, which allows him to sound the familiar crowing call at the break of dawn or at various other times throughout the day. This crowing serves multiple purposes, from alerting the flock to potential dangers to asserting his dominance.

Understanding the rooster's physiology also includes knowledge of their reproductive system. As the primary procreator in a flock, a healthy rooster ensures the continuation of the flock through the fertilization of the hens' eggs. A rooster's reproductive health, therefore, is crucial. Any issues, such as reduced fertility or problems with their physical ability to mate, can have significant implications for the flock's future.

Lastly, like all creatures, roosters are prone to various health issues. These can range from infections, parasites, injuries, and age-related conditions. It's crucial to be aware of the common health problems that roosters can face and to monitor your rooster regularly for any signs of illness. Early detection often makes treatment easier and more successful.

Given their unique physiological and health needs, roosters require careful attention and specialized care. Understanding their specific requirements and characteristics enables you to provide optimal care, ensuring that your roosters remain healthy, active, and capable of performing their vital roles within the flock. Just like hens, roosters too can significantly benefit from herbal supplements, providing them with the vitality and strength they need to rule the roost.

There are several beneficial herbs that boost vitality and promote overall health. One of the standouts in this category is Ginseng, a root that has been used for thousands of years in traditional medicine for its array of health benefits.

Ginseng is known for its energy-boosting properties. It is a natural adaptogen, which means it can help the body resist different types of stress, physical or mental. Roosters, being the guardians of the flock, can face a variety of stressors. Adaptogens like Ginseng can be particularly beneficial in helping them manage these stressors without hampering their overall health. Additionally, Ginseng can support a healthy appetite and immune system, contributing to the overall vitality of your rooster.

Another herb that's a boon for roosters is Turmeric. Known for its bright yellow color, this root is packed with curcumin, a powerful antioxidant and anti-inflammatory compound. Roosters, being more active, might occasionally suffer from inflammation or minor injuries. Turmeric, when included in their diet, can help in the management of inflammation and speed up the recovery process. It's also known to support cardiovascular health, a beneficial feature given a rooster's active lifestyle.

Nettles are another excellent herb to include in your rooster's diet. Rich in essential nutrients like iron, calcium, magnesium, and vitamins A and C, Nettles can provide a natural boost to your rooster's nutritional intake. These nutrients support various bodily functions, including the production of red blood cells, muscle function, and the immune system, all of which contribute to the overall vitality of your rooster.

Milk Thistle is also worth mentioning. Primarily known for its liver-supportive properties, Milk Thistle can assist in the detoxification process, helping to keep your rooster's liver healthy and functioning optimally. As the liver plays a vital role in digestion and the removal of waste from the body, maintaining its health is crucial for your rooster's overall well-being.

Garlic, though not technically an herb, is another natural supplement that can do wonders for your rooster's health. It's a natural antimicrobial, helping to fend off a variety of infections. It also has immune-boosting properties, making it a valuable addition to your rooster's diet, particularly during periods of stress or during the colder months when the risk of respiratory infections is higher.

To add these herbs, a balanced diet enriched with proteins, healthy fats, and a variety of fruits and vegetables is essential. Remember, while these herbs can significantly contribute to the overall health and vitality of your rooster, they should not replace a balanced diet but rather supplement it. Supplementing your rooster's diet with herbs doesn't mean just tossing a few leaves into their feed and calling it a day. You can and should get creative with how you serve these beneficial plants. Combining them with other nutritious foods can make them more appealing and can maximize their health benefits. Here are a few suggestions for creating rooster-boosting remedies that your boys are sure to enjoy.

First, consider making herbal-infused grains. Start with a base of whole grains like oats, barley, or quinoa. Grains are an excellent source of carbohydrates, providing your roosters with the energy they need for their active lifestyles. Steep some Ginseng and Turmeric in water until the water is colored and fragrant. Use this herbal water to cook the grains, infusing them with the beneficial properties of the herbs. Once cooled, this can be served as a hearty meal for your roosters.

You can also use these herbs to create an invigorating herbal tea for your roosters. While chickens, including roosters, get the majority of their hydration from their food, providing them with water infused with herbs like Ginseng, Turmeric, or Nettles, can offer them additional health benefits. Just steep the herbs in hot water for a few minutes, let it cool, then serve it in their water dish.

When thinking about how to prepare these herbs for your roosters, remember that they enjoy variety. Mixing herbs into their regular feed, adding them to grains, or even using them to create herbal tea, all offer different ways for your roosters to consume these beneficial plants.

Grit treats are another way to introduce herbs to your roosters. Grit is essential for poultry as it aids in their digestion. Mix a variety of herbs like Ginseng, Nettles, and Milk Thistle with grit and shape them into small, bite-sized treats. You can bind these treats with a bit of molasses, which also serves as a good source of iron and other essential nutrients.

Garlic is a potent addition to your rooster's diet, but remember, a little goes a long way. A great way to include garlic in your rooster's diet is by adding fresh, minced garlic to their water or food. Start with a small amount and increase gradually, observing your rooster's reaction to ensure he is comfortable with the taste and aroma.

One more way to incorporate these herbs into your rooster's diet is through an herbal salad. This is a great way to introduce a variety of herbs in a fresh, raw form. Combine leafy greens like lettuce or spinach with chopped Nettles, Turmeric root, and a sprinkle of crushed Milk Thistle seeds. Remember to chop the herbs finely enough for your roosters to consume comfortably.

In all these preparations, it's essential to ensure the herbs are fresh and free from pesticides or other harmful chemicals. Whether you're growing these herbs in your backyard or sourcing them from a trusted supplier, quality is key.

Creating these rooster-boosting remedies is an enjoyable process, allowing you to cater to the specific needs of your roosters while also providing them with tasty and nutritious meals. A well-fed rooster is a happy and active rooster, so take the time to prepare meals that they will enjoy and benefit from.

With these herbal remedies in your poultry care toolbox, the next important step is knowing how to monitor your roosters' health and watch for signs of common male poultry issues. Regular health checks are vital for maintaining a robust rooster population and for early detection of potential health problems. Remember, a proactive approach is always better than reactive when it comes to poultry health.

A healthy rooster displays a number of physical attributes. Their feathers are shiny and full, devoid of any gaps or irregularities. The comb and wattles—those characteristic, fleshy, brightly colored growths on their heads and necks—are firm, bright red, and free of spots or discoloration, indicating proper circulation and overall vitality.

The eyes should be clear, bright, and alert. Cloudy eyes or discharge can indicate illness or infection. The beak should be intact, with no cracks or unusual coloration. Check the nostrils as well; they should be clear and free from any signs of discharge.

A healthy rooster has a robust appetite, so sudden changes in eating habits can be a red flag. If a rooster is consuming less feed or not showing interest in food, it could indicate discomfort or illness.

Roosters should have a steady gait, and any limping or favoring of one leg could be a sign of injury or arthritis. Observe your rooster's mobility and posture. Changes in either can signal various issues, including nerve problems or issues with internal organs.

When it comes to behavior, a rooster should be active and alert. Lethargy, withdrawal from the flock, or unresponsiveness are all cause for concern. An important sign of a healthy rooster is their crowing. A strong, regular crow is a good indication of a rooster's vitality. Changes in their crow, or lack of crowing altogether, could suggest health issues.

Roosters are naturally protective of their hens, so they should respond if they feel their flock is threatened. A lack of protective behavior may indicate that a rooster isn't feeling well or is suffering from some form of stress.

Don't forget to check the rooster's droppings. Healthy droppings should be firm, well-formed, and consistent in color. Variations in color, texture, or frequency might indicate dietary issues or internal parasites.

Also, monitor your rooster's weight regularly. Sudden weight loss can be a sign of illness. To check a rooster's weight, you can pick them up and feel their breastbone. If it's prominent and there's not much muscle on either side, your rooster might be underweight.

Finally, be aware of any changes in your rooster's breathing. Wheezing, coughing, or labored breathing can be signs of respiratory diseases, which can be severe if not addressed quickly.

While this might seem like a lengthy checklist, it's actually a routine you can easily incorporate into your poultry care schedule. Remember, early detection is key to addressing potential health issues, and your roosters depend on you for their well-being. Armed with these tips and your understanding of how vital herbs like Ginseng, Turmeric, and others can support your roosters, you're well on your way to ensuring a healthy and harmonious flock.

Part III: Crow Proud: Vocal Health Herbs

Let's take a moment to appreciate one of the most iconic sounds on the farm—the crow of a rooster. "Cock-a-doodle-doo!" or "cock-a-doodle-dawn!" or however you choose to mimic it in human speech, is undeniably associated with the break of day on the farm. The importance of this sound, this rooster crowing, stretches far beyond its romantic association with rural life. It's a sound that carries weight, meaning, and health implications for the rooster and the flock at large.

Roosters don't crow simply because the sun is rising, contrary to what those old cartoons would have you believe. They crow to communicate, establish dominance, and maintain the social structure of the flock. They also crow in response to disturbances or perceived threats to protect their flock. Each crow is a statement, a declaration of their territory, and a vocal testament to their fitness and vitality.

The crowing of a rooster is a marker of his health and well-being. A strong, robust crow reflects a healthy and confident rooster, while changes or disruptions in a rooster's crow can be the first sign of stress, disease, or injury.

Crowing involves the coordination of several bodily systems. It requires good respiratory health to produce a powerful crow. The muscles of the chest and neck also contribute to the process, and even the digestive system plays a role. When a rooster crows, it's almost as if it's undergoing a quick health check. A successful crow indicates that all systems are functioning well.

Just as human voices are unique, so too are rooster crows. Each rooster has a unique crow, and this distinct sound plays a crucial role in its identity within the flock. It can also provide you, the poultry keeper, with insight into the individual rooster's health and well-being.

For a poultry keeper, learning to recognize the different crows of your roosters and being attentive to changes can help in the early detection of potential health issues. A rooster that is usually loud and confident might suddenly crow less frequently or not at all, while changes in the sound of the crow could indicate a respiratory infection.

Listening to your roosters and understanding the importance of their crowing is an essential aspect of keeping a healthy flock. It's not just about the sound echoing across the yard at dawn; it's about communication, health, and the social order of your flock.

So, the next time you hear a rooster crowing, pause and appreciate not just the call of the farm waking up but also the complex communication and health check happening right in front of you. Recognize the crow for what it is—a vital aspect of rooster behavior and health. Crowing is not just an arbitrary behavior but a meaningful and insightful aspect of rooster life.

By understanding and respecting the importance of rooster crowing, you're taking a significant step toward holistic poultry care. To further amplify your efforts, let's delve into herbs that can specifically support rooster vocal health.

When it comes to maintaining vocal health, two stand-out herbs come to mind - marshmallow root and licorice. These may not be the first herbs you think of when you consider poultry health, but both are known for their soothing and healing properties, particularly for the throat and respiratory system.

Marshmallow root, with its slippery, mucilaginous texture, coats and soothes the throat, reducing irritation and inflammation. This property can be particularly beneficial for roosters who are enthusiastic crowers, as it can help protect their throat from potential strain or damage. Additionally, marshmallow root has anti-inflammatory properties, which can be beneficial in the event of a respiratory infection or irritation. Including marshmallow root in your rooster's diet can contribute to vocal longevity, supporting them in maintaining their assertive, melodic crows.

Licorice, on the other hand, is a powerhouse herb with a wide range of benefits. Beyond its sweet flavor that chickens seem to enjoy, licorice has anti-inflammatory, immunomodulatory, and even mild antimicrobial properties. Like marshmallow root, licorice is also demulcent, meaning it can soothe irritated tissues. Given these properties, licorice can be an excellent addition to your rooster's diet to maintain good respiratory and throat health, which in turn, supports their crowing.

While these two herbs can be the stars of the show, there are a host of other herbs that can complement their actions and provide additional benefits for your roosters. Lemon balm, for instance, can provide an uplifting effect, potentially stimulating more frequent and enthusiastic crowing. Sage, thyme, and oregano, all well-known culinary herbs, have potent antimicrobial properties and can help maintain a healthy respiratory tract, which is essential for effective crowing.

When it comes to using these herbs, you have several options. They can be added to the feed, provided fresh, or brewed into a tea. One practical approach is to incorporate dried herbs into the rooster's regular feed. Alternatively, you can create a special treat by combining the herbs with other foods your rooster enjoys, like fruits, vegetables, or mealworms.

If you prefer to make an herbal tea, simply steep the chosen herbs in boiling water for 15-20 minutes, strain, and allow it to cool before offering it to your rooster. Some roosters may even enjoy pecking at the spent herbs! Be creative, experiment with different combinations, and observe your rooster's preferences.

While herbs are excellent tools for promoting health, regular monitoring of your rooster's behavior, vocalizations, and overall health is key. Changes in crowing behavior or sound should always prompt a closer examination to identify any potential problems early.

Dedicated poultry keepers like you understand that herbs can be incredibly beneficial for the health of your roosters, particularly when it comes to their vocal health. You're well versed now in the importance of rooster crowing and some herbs that can support this aspect of their health. However, knowing which herbs to use is just the beginning. The next step is to understand how to prepare these herbs in a way that your roosters will enjoy and benefit from. In this section, we'll delve into the exciting world of herbal mix remedies that can help maintain a healthy and strong crow.

Let's start with the basics - the key herbs. From our previous discussion, we have identified several important herbs, including marshmallow root, licorice, lemon balm, sage, thyme, and oregano. A simple but potent herbal mix for crowing can include these ingredients. Remember, every rooster has different preferences and dietary needs, so feel free to modify this remedy as necessary.

The base of your herbal mix can be a combination of marshmallow root and licorice. These two herbs provide the main throat-soothing properties. You might choose to use two parts of each for every ten parts of your rooster's feed. Next, add one part each of lemon balm, sage, thyme, and oregano. These herbs will not only add a variety of flavors to stimulate your rooster's appetite but also offer additional health benefits, including support for the immune and respiratory systems.

Preparing the herbal mix is straightforward. Start by sourcing quality, preferably organic, dried herbs. It's essential to ensure that they are free from pesticides and other chemicals that could be harmful to your roosters. Once you have your herbs, mix them together in the appropriate proportions and store the mixture in an airtight container in a cool, dark place to maintain their potency.

When it's feeding time, simply sprinkle the herbal mix onto your rooster's regular feed. Be sure to mix it in thoroughly to distribute the herbs evenly. Observe your rooster as he eats. Some roosters might be hesitant about the new addition to their feed, while others may take to it immediately. Adjust the quantity and types of herbs based on your rooster's preferences and tolerance.

You can also offer these herbs as a special treat. For example, you could steep a teaspoon of the herbal mix in hot water to make an herbal tea, cool it down, and mix it with their favorite treats such as chopped fruits, vegetables, or mealworms. This not only provides the benefits of the herbs but also offers a bit of dietary enrichment, giving your roosters something new and exciting to enjoy. Making herbal mixes for your roosters is an engaging process, and experimenting with different herbs can yield fascinating insights into your roosters' preferences and health.

Our journey so far has made it clear that taking care of your roosters involves more than just feeding them well—it's about keen observation, understanding their behaviors, and meeting their unique health needs. Having explored the importance of rooster crowing and various herbs that can support their vocal health, let's now focus on an equally important task: monitoring your roosters' crowing habits and identifying signs of potential vocal health issues.

Crowing is more than a wake-up call for the farm—it's a significant behavior that communicates a rooster's well-being, position in the pecking order, and overall health. A change in a rooster's crowing habits can be one of the first indicators of potential health issues, particularly those related to their vocal cords or respiratory system. Understanding what to look for and how to interpret these signs can help you identify problems early and provide your rooster with the necessary care and attention.

Your daily farm routine should include some time devoted to observing your roosters as they crow. Pay attention to the volume, clarity, frequency, and duration of their crows. Each rooster has its unique crowing pattern—some may crow only at dawn, while others may crow sporadically throughout the day. Over time, you'll become familiar with each rooster's normal crowing behavior, which will help you notice any changes.

Volume and clarity of the crow are key indicators of a rooster's vocal health. A strong, clear crow suggests good vocal and respiratory health. If a rooster's crow suddenly becomes hoarse, weak, or if they struggle to crow, these may be signs of vocal strain or respiratory issues. Similarly, if a rooster typically crows frequently but suddenly becomes silent, this is cause for concern and warrants further investigation.

Crowing frequency and duration can also indicate health or behavioral issues. An increase in crowing can be a sign of heightened stress or disturbance in the flock, such as changes in the pecking order or a perceived threat. On the other hand, a decrease in crowing or shorter crows can suggest weakness or illness.

Observation goes beyond just listening. Watch your roosters as they crow. Do they appear to struggle or gasp for air? Are they extending their necks unusually high? Are there any noticeable changes in their posture or behavior during crowing? Visual cues can sometimes offer more insight into potential issues than auditory ones.

Also, don't forget to monitor your roosters' appetite and overall behavior. Are they eating and drinking normally? Have their droppings changed in consistency or color? Are they active and engaging with the flock as usual, or are they retreating and showing signs of lethargy? All of these observations can provide a fuller picture of their health status.

If you notice any changes in your roosters' crowing habits or other behaviors, consider consulting with a poultry veterinarian. While some changes might be due to minor issues that can be addressed with simple interventions—like adding more herbs to their diet or providing them with a quiet space to rest—others might indicate serious conditions that require professional intervention.

Monitoring rooster crowing and identifying potential vocal health issues is an essential part of maintaining a healthy, happy, and harmonious flock. With patience, practice, and a keen eye (or ear!), you'll become adept at understanding and responding to the subtle cues your roosters offer through their crows. Enjoy the symphony of crows on your farm, knowing that each crow tells a unique story of rooster life!

Part III: Rooster Rendezvous: From Crowing Casanovas to Galant Guardians

Roosters have a critical role to play in a chicken flock. They're not just the crowing Casanovas but also the gallant guardians, and their demeanor towards the hens is a vital part of their role. Teaching your roosters to respect the hens is key to a harmonious flock. This practice goes beyond ensuring peace among your chickens—it aids in creating an environment where each bird feels safe and can thrive.

Roosters naturally have a drive to mate. It's part of their role in the flock—to maintain the population and contribute to the next generation of chickens. However, sometimes, a rooster may be too aggressive in his approach, leading to stress among the hens.

The first step to teaching roosters to respect the hens is understanding chicken behavior and hierarchy. The pecking order is real, and both hens and roosters have their places in the order. A healthy balance of power can lead to respectful behavior. Roosters need to understand that while they're the protectors of the flock, they're not tyrants ruling over the hens.

Observation is your best tool here. Spend time watching how your rooster interacts with the hens. A respectful rooster performs a dance, also known as "tidbitting," when he finds a tasty morsel, calling over the hens to eat first. He also stands guard while the hens are eating or drinking.

On the other hand, if you notice that your rooster is overly aggressive, chasing the hens incessantly, or causing physical harm, it's time to intervene. In such cases, the rooster might need a time-out—a separate space where he can calm down and the hens can have some peace. This action isn't a punishment but a way to disrupt undesirable behavior and give the rooster time to reset his behavior.

It's also worth mentioning that younger roosters, or cockerels, tend to exhibit more aggressive behavior as they reach sexual maturity and figure out their place in the flock. Patience is required during this phase as they navigate their hormones and hierarchies.

Another approach to teaching roosters to respect hens is through training. You can establish your dominance in a non-aggressive way by gently but firmly holding the rooster on the ground until he calms down. This technique, known as "taming," can help in reducing aggressive behavior. However, use this method with caution as it might cause stress to the bird if not done correctly. Many chicken keepers will pick up their rooster and carry him around while they are tending to their chicken chores. This helps to establish your dominance in a gentle way.

In addition to these hands-on strategies, herbs can be utilized to influence rooster behavior. Certain herbs, like lavender and chamomile, are known for their calming properties. Incorporating these herbs into the flock's diet or housing can promote a more peaceful and less aggressive environment.

Creating a safe, spacious, and engaging environment for your flock also contributes to respectful rooster behavior. Overcrowding can cause stress and lead to increased aggression. Provide plenty of space for your chickens to roam, peck, and rest. Additionally, keeping your roosters engaged with things like dust baths, perches, or treat-dispensing toys can reduce the likelihood of aggressive behavior.

Building upon the idea of fostering a balanced environment for your roosters, it's crucial to acknowledge their innate role as protectors of the flock. These natural guardians often take their jobs very seriously, scanning the sky for predators, alerting the hens of any dangers, and sometimes even sacrificing their own lives to protect their flock. Training your rooster for flock protection, therefore, is about enhancing their inherent instincts and skills to ensure the safety of your entire flock.

Recognizing danger is a primal instinct for roosters. However, the type of threats they face can vary depending on their environment. For instance, a rural setting might present threats from raccoons, foxes, or hawks, while urban environments might involve stray cats or dogs. Understanding these risks and exposing your rooster to safe simulations can help improve their response to such dangers.

Mock drills can be an effective way to train your rooster for flock protection. Using audio recordings of predators, or even predator decoys, can help your rooster learn to identify threats. Remember, the goal of this training is not to scare your rooster, but to equip him with the skills to identify threats and react appropriately.

One thing to keep in mind is that you are part of your rooster's world, and you should be recognized as a friend, not a foe. Spend time with your flock, let your rooster see you often, and ensure he associates your presence with safety. A rooster who knows you well will be less likely to view you as a threat and more likely to focus on real predators.

While training your rooster for flock protection, it's equally important to equip your coop for the task. A sturdy coop that's predator-proof is the first line of defense against threats. Regularly check the coop for any weak spots, ensure it's well-lit around the perimeter at night, and keep it clean to prevent attraction of pests and predators.

The diet of your rooster also plays a crucial role in his ability to protect the flock. A well-nourished rooster will have the strength and alertness to fend off threats. Herbs like rosemary, thyme, and oregano can boost your rooster's immunity, making him less susceptible to diseases and more fit to fulfill his duties.

Behavioral cues are crucial in rooster training. It's important to reward your rooster's positive behaviors to reinforce them. For example, if your rooster successfully alerts the hens about a threat, a reward of his favorite treat could be in order. This positive reinforcement encourages the repetition of the desired behavior.

But remember, no amount of training can make your rooster invincible. While they can deter smaller predators, they are not a match for larger ones. This is why having a safe, secure coop is indispensable.

It's also crucial to ensure your rooster isn't becoming overly aggressive in his role as a protector. Overly assertive roosters might become a threat to the hens they're supposed to protect or even to the poultry keeper. Training for protection should be balanced with the teachings of respect discussed earlier in this chapter.

Training your rooster for flock protection is about recognizing and respecting his natural instincts and guiding those instincts in a way that benefits the entire flock. It requires a solid understanding of chicken behavior, careful observation, patience, and consistent, gentle training methods. The goal isn't to create a super-rooster but to foster a healthy, safe environment where every bird, rooster, and hen alike can thrive.

The goal of fostering a safe and thriving environment extends beyond the chicken coop and includes the relationship between roosters and their human caregivers. Just as you're training your rooster to protect the flock from external threats, it's equally vital to ensure your rooster sees you as a friend rather than a threat.

Aggression in roosters can manifest in various ways, such as lunging, pecking, or flying towards people. It's not unusual for roosters to become protective of their territory, including the hens. However, it becomes a problem when they start displaying these behaviors towards the human caregivers, who are there to ensure their well-being.

First and foremost, it's important to remember that a rooster's aggressive behavior is not a personal attack but a response driven by their instincts. They're naturally programmed to guard their flock, and if they perceive you as a threat, they might react defensively. Therefore, the key to curbing aggression towards humans is to build trust and establish yourself as a non-threatening presence.

Building trust with a rooster takes time, patience, and consistency. Regular, peaceful interaction is the starting point. Spend time near your rooster without making any abrupt movements. Let him observe you and become accustomed to your presence. This passive interaction allows the rooster to see you as a regular part of his environment, not an intruder.

Another vital part of this trust-building process is respecting the rooster's space. While it's essential for you to be near your rooster, avoid encroaching upon his personal space aggressively. Instead, approach him slowly and respectfully, taking care not to corner him or make him feel threatened.

One practical strategy to build trust with an aggressive rooster is feeding by hand. This method requires patience as the rooster might not immediately accept food from your hand. Start by leaving treats near him and slowly work your way up to hand feeding. This process allows the rooster to associate your presence with positive experiences, further solidifying trust.

Maintaining a calm demeanor is key when handling an aggressive rooster. Chickens can pick up on tension and may react defensively if they sense stress or fear. So, even if a rooster shows aggression, remain calm, move slowly, and speak softly. In time, the rooster will learn that you pose no threat.

Training a rooster using these methods is not about dominating them but about communication and mutual respect. Always remember that aggressive behavior is often a sign of fear or uncertainty, so responding with aggression will only exacerbate the problem.

Herbs can also play a supportive role in managing aggression in roosters. For example, herbs like chamomile and lavender are known for their calming effects and can be included in the rooster's diet to promote tranquility. Furthermore, lemon balm has been noted to help reduce aggressive behavior in poultry, making it another worthy addition to the rooster's diet.

Curbing aggression in roosters towards humans is a process that requires understanding, patience, consistency, and a whole lot of love. Remember, you're dealing with a creature that's guided by instinct, not malice. Respond with calm, steady, and compassionate actions, and you'll gradually see a change in your rooster's demeanor toward you.

Part IV: Herb Heros: Maintaining Rooster Health & Temperament

Let's dive deeper into the subject of herbs and how they can play a significant role in maintaining rooster health and temperament. After all, who would have thought that the garden's peaceful greenery might just be the secret to fostering harmony in the coop?

When we talk about 'herb heroes,' the list is quite extensive. But let's focus on some key players, shall we? In addition to chamomile, lavender, and lemon balm, which we have mentioned, there are a few more herbs that deserve attention for their beneficial impacts on rooster health and behavior.

Garlic is a known powerhouse, an allium that works wonders for the immune system. It's known to be a potent natural antibiotic, antifungal, and antiparasitic agent. Regularly including garlic in your rooster's diet can help keep him robust, helping to fight off diseases and parasites that could otherwise compromise his health and performance.

Next up, let's talk about nettle. This herb may not be the first one to come to mind, mainly due to its stinging reputation. However, once dried or cooked, nettle loses its sting and offers an abundance of nutrients, including iron, calcium, magnesium, and a range of beneficial vitamins. It's a superb herb for ensuring your rooster's overall health and vitality.

Thyme is another herb to consider. It's an excellent respiratory aid and can help keep those vibrant crows sounding clear and strong. Respiratory health is paramount for a rooster, as a congested rooster may struggle to communicate effectively, which can lead to stress and potential conflicts within the flock.

Oregano is often regarded as a 'natural antibiotic' for poultry. It's known to promote gut health, boost immunity, and help to ward off several common poultry diseases. Plus, most chickens, roosters included, enjoy the taste, making it an easy addition to their diet.

Calendula is a wonder herb that deserves special mention. Aside from its bright, uplifting appearance, Calendula has potent healing properties and can aid in wound recovery – handy for those incidental scrapes and cuts roosters might incur while protecting their flock. It's also known to boost coloration in yolks, so while that doesn't directly benefit the rooster, it's a nice bonus for the hens and your breakfast table!

Let's explore some specific herbs known to help calm an aggressive rooster. It's important to note that while these herbs may aid in calming your rooster, they should be used in conjunction with proper training and handling techniques to effectively manage aggression.

Chamomile is a well-known calming herb often used in teas to promote relaxation in humans, and it can have similar effects on roosters. It has been observed that incorporating chamomile into your rooster's diet or roosting area could potentially help reduce his stress levels and, in turn, lower aggressive behaviors.

Lavender is an aromatic herb that is also known for its calming properties. The scent of lavender is considered relaxing, and its essential oil is often used in aromatherapy to reduce anxiety and promote calmness. For roosters, dried lavender can be added to their roosting areas to create a more peaceful environment.

Lemon balm has been observed to reduce aggressive behavior in some poultry. This herb has calming properties that can help ease anxiety, making it a great addition to your rooster's diet or living area.

Vervain (Verbena) is an herb that has a long history of use in calming nervous system disorders and could be used to help manage an overly aggressive rooster. Its tranquilizing effect helps to reduce anxiety and hyperactivity.

Hops, yes, the same plant used to brew beer has sedative properties. Chickens, including roosters, can benefit from the calming effects of hops. Scatter some dried hops in their coop to promote a calmer environment.

Ashwagandha is not a traditional herb for poultry. Some backyard chicken enthusiasts have had success using this Ayurvedic herb to reduce stress and aggression in their roosters. It's often available in powdered form, which can be easily mixed into feed.

Passionflower is an herb used for its calming effects in many traditional medicines, and some chicken owners have used it to help reduce aggression and promote calmness in their birds. As with any new addition to your rooster's diet, introduce it gradually and monitor for any changes.

Remember that while these herbs can help, they're not a magic fix for an aggressive rooster. It's vital to ensure that your rooster's aggression isn't due to other issues, like illness, overcrowding, or dominance disputes within the flock. Observing your rooster and understanding the cause of his aggression will make your interventions much more effective.Also, they're not a substitute for a balanced diet, a clean environment, and proper care. Herbs should be used as a complement to these fundamental aspects of rooster care, not a replacement. A happy, healthy rooster requires a multifaceted approach, and these herbs are just one piece of the larger puzzle.

Incorporating herbs into your rooster's routine can be as simple as adding fresh or dried herbs to their feed, scattering them around their enclosure for them to peck at, or brewing herbal infusions for them to drink. The beauty of using herbs as natural remedies is that they allow you to work in tandem with nature. It's a gentle approach that respects the rooster's biology while benefiting from the healing power of plants.

Part V: Hen Harmony: Fostering Respectful Relationships in Your Flock

The rooster is an essential part of a flock. Understanding his role and providing him with the support he needs to fulfill it is a vital part of chicken keeping. After all, a healthy, well-adjusted rooster contributes to a harmonious, thriving flock.

One crucial aspect of supporting your rooster is ensuring a suitable hen-to-rooster ratio in your flock. Generally, the recommended ratio is around eight to ten hens for each rooster. This balance allows the rooster to fulfill his protective and procreative instincts without causing undue stress to the hens or himself. If you have too many roosters and not enough hens, the competition can lead to fights and injuries. Conversely, too few hens for a rooster can result in over-mating, causing stress and physical harm to the hens.

Space is another crucial factor in maintaining peace and balance. Ensure your chickens have enough room to roam, forage, and engage in natural behaviors without crowding. Overcrowding can lead to stress, which can trigger aggressive behavior in roosters. In addition to outdoor space, each bird should have enough room in the coop for roosting and nesting comfortably.

Ensuring a balanced and nutritious diet for your rooster is also paramount. A diet deficient in essential nutrients can lead to health problems that can affect a rooster's ability to perform his duties. Incorporate a good quality layer feed into their diet and supplement it with fresh fruits, vegetables, and herbs to ensure they're getting a well-rounded diet. Herbs like oregano and thyme are not only enjoyed by chickens but also have the added benefit of supporting their immune system.

Roosters, like any other bird in your flock, require clean, fresh water daily. Dehydration can quickly lead to health issues and can increase stress levels, potentially causing conflict within your flock. Make sure your roosters have constant access to clean water, and consider adding herbs like parsley or mint to their water, which can aid digestion and provide extra nutrients.

Just as herbs can support a rooster's health, they can also contribute to a calm and balanced flock. Calming herbs such as chamomile and lavender can be added to nesting boxes or scattered in the coop to create a soothing environment. This can help reduce stress levels, making for a more peaceful flock.

Regular health checks are crucial to catch any potential problems early. Keeping a close eye on your rooster's behavior, comb color, weight, and overall demeanor can alert you to issues before they become serious. If your rooster is acting out of character, it may be a sign he's unwell.

Providing opportunities for natural behaviors like dust bathing, foraging, and perching can also improve the overall mood of your flock. Activities like these allow your rooster to express his natural behaviors, reducing stress and potentially aggressive behaviors.

While it's normal for roosters to occasionally assert their dominance, excessive aggression should not be overlooked. Training can be an effective method to curb aggressive tendencies. Simple actions, like not backing away when your rooster postures or gently but firmly pushing him away when he's too aggressive, can help establish your dominance.

Last, but not least, remember that each rooster has a unique personality. Understanding your rooster's individual quirks and tendencies can go a long way in supporting him and ensuring a peaceful flock. Patience and a gentle approach are key. Celebrate your rooster's instincts and unique behaviors and provide a caring, supportive environment for him to thrive.

By implementing these methods and using supportive herbs, you can support your rooster in his many roles, from protector and leader to mate and father. This doesn't just benefit your rooster; it contributes to the overall health, productivity, and harmony of your entire flock. Remember, a happy rooster leads to a happy flock. And a happy flock makes for a happy chicken keeper.

In the kaleidoscope of a chicken flock, the rooster is a vibrant splash of color and sound, a figurehead that guides the swirling patterns of the flock dynamics. Understanding these dynamics and how the rooster fits into them is the key to resolving conflicts and maintaining harmony.

One of the first steps to understanding flock dynamics is simply to observe. Watching your flock can provide valuable insights into how your rooster interacts with his hens and other roosters if you have more than one. It's a fascinating spectacle of social maneuvers, filled with displays of dominance, intricate mating dances, and sometimes, confrontations.

In observing, you'll notice that your rooster, if he's a mature and responsible sort, doesn't just randomly chase after hens for mating. Instead, he'll perform a unique dance known as "tidbitting," where he makes specific sounds while picking up and dropping a piece of food to attract a hen's attention. It's not only an invitation to share a meal but also a courtship ritual that shows the rooster is a provider.

Conflicts within a flock are often quick and decisive, typically over as quickly as they began. Roosters will confront each other, often over access to food, mates, or space. While these confrontations can seem intense, they are usually harmless and necessary for establishing a social hierarchy within the flock.

Yet, not all conflicts are resolved quickly or peacefully. If you notice ongoing, unresolved aggression, this is where your role as a chicken keeper becomes crucial. If a rooster is consistently bullying a particular hen or another rooster, or causing serious harm, it may be necessary to separate them for a time. In some instances, rehoming may be the best solution for the sake of the flock's overall peace.

While separation should be a last resort, there are preventive measures to help maintain harmony. As mentioned previously, a proper hen-to-rooster ratio can help reduce conflicts. Providing plenty of space and resources - like food, water, and nesting spots - can also lessen the chances of disputes.

Watching the flock dynamics closely can help you pick up on any issues early. A sudden change in behavior can often signal a problem. For instance, if a rooster who is usually active and dominant becomes quiet and withdrawn, he could be sick or injured. Quick intervention is critical to prevent further health decline or an upheaval in the flock's social structure.

Keep in mind that flock dynamics are not set in stone. They will shift and change over time as chickens age, new birds are introduced, or others pass away. Being adaptable and ready to manage these changes is part of keeping a flock.

Herbs can be a valuable ally in maintaining harmony. Herbs with calming properties like chamomile, lavender, and lemon balm can help ease tensions and reduce stress. Sprinkling these herbs around the coop or adding them to nesting boxes can create a soothing environment for your birds. They smell wonderful, and the act of pecking at them can also serve as a welcome distraction for a rooster who may be a little too focused on asserting his dominance. In more serious cases of ongoing aggression, calming herbs like valerian can be added to the rooster's diet to help curb his aggressive tendencies.

Consideration and understanding of flock dynamics require patience and observation. Yet, the rewards of a balanced, harmonious flock are worth the effort. Not only does it make for happier, healthier birds, but it also makes your job as a chicken keeper a whole lot easier and more enjoyable. No one wants a coop full of conflict. With a strong, supportive rooster at the helm and a chicken keeper willing to step in and smooth out any ruffled feathers when needed, a peaceful flock is entirely achievable.

The essential role of a rooster within a flock becomes evidently clear. He's not merely a barnyard figurehead, his crowing echoing off the farm buildings in the morning light. No, he's an integral part of the flock's fabric, his roles as protector, leader, mate, and father woven into the daily rhythm of the chicken community.

Imagine a flock without a rooster. There'd be no morning fanfare, no strutting guardian looking out for his ladies, and no dance and call of courtship during feeding times. Roosters bring a unique dynamic that enlivens the flock. They add vigor, color, and an element of stability to the poultry society. In essence, they give the flock its 'flock-ness,' its communal character.

Yet, understanding the rooster's role is only part of the equation. As a chicken keeper, you also need to support the rooster in these roles. This involves a measure of patience and love, ensuring that he matures into a gentleman and not a tyrant. Nurturing a young rooster requires a gentle hand, understanding, and a readiness to implement measures that can help him develop into a respectable flock leader.

In dealing with a rooster, remember that patience is key. Young roosters, just like young dogs or young humans, can be a bit feisty. They're eager, brash, and quick to assert themselves. However, with time, they learn to temper their energy to harness their vigor into constructive channels. Give your rooster time to grow, to mature, and you'll likely see that wild, young bird mellow into a fine, noble gentleman of a rooster.

It's essential to recognize that an aggressive rooster isn't a 'bad' rooster. He's just a rooster doing his job, protecting his flock as his instincts tell him to. Even if that aggression is directed towards you, the chicken keeper, remember it's not personal. The rooster doesn't harbor any ill will towards you. He's merely doing what he believes is necessary to keep his ladies safe.

With an aggressive rooster, culling should never be the first option. Every effort should be made to tame the rooster, to teach him that you're not a threat but a friend. There are plenty of methods to help you achieve this, from handling techniques to dietary supplements, including the use of herbs.

Implementing these remedies into your rooster's diet can significantly aid in curbing aggression and promoting peaceful coexistence. In the grand scheme of things, it's about finding the balance, the harmony within your flock. It's about understanding the vital role your rooster plays and supporting him in fulfilling his duties. It's about learning to interact with him respectfully and lovingly, guiding his youthful energy in the right direction, and allowing him the time and space to mature into the rooster he's meant to be.

The relationship between a rooster and a chicken keeper can be a fulfilling one, filled with mutual respect and cooperation. Yes, there may be bumps along the way. Yes, there may be times when your patience is tested. But stick with it, work with your rooster, and soon enough, you'll have a gallant gentleman strutting about your yard, watching over his hens, fulfilling his duties, and adding that unique, dynamic touch that only a rooster can bring to a flock.

"Until one has loved an animal, a part of one's soul remains unawakened."
— Anatole France

Chapter 10: Herbs for Egg Quality

Part I: Golden Yolks: Herbs for Nutrient-Dense Eggs

In the world of chicken keeping, there's nothing quite like the joy of cracking open an egg to find a rich, golden yolk staring back at you Every chicken keeper, no matter how small or large their flock, delights in the sight of a nutrient-dense, richly colored egg yolk. A robust yolk suggests a healthy chicken that's been well-fed and well-cared for. It's a testament to your efforts and care as a chicken keeper, a tangible reward for the love and attention you pour into your flock.

So, what makes a yolk nutrient-dense? What goes into the making of that golden orb that we so prize in our breakfast plates? Understanding this is akin to appreciating a work of art; hence, we call it the 'Art of the Yolk.' It involves a fascinating journey into the biology of chickens, their nutritional needs, and how those needs translate into the eggs they lay.

At the heart of a nutrient-dense yolk is, unsurprisingly, nutrition. What a chicken eats significantly influences the quality of the eggs it lays. Feed your hens a balanced, nutritious diet, and they're more likely to lay eggs with robust, nutrient-rich yolks.

The diet of a laying hen needs to include a balance of proteins, carbohydrates, vitamins, and minerals. Proteins provide the building blocks for egg production. They help form the albumen or egg white and contribute to the yolk's overall nutrient content. Carbohydrates give your hens the energy they need to lay eggs, while vitamins and minerals play various roles in the overall health of your hens and the quality of their eggs.

Herbs can be a valuable addition to your hens' diet. Many herbs are rich in vitamins, minerals, and other nutrients that can contribute to the quality of egg yolks. For example, herbs such as parsley, dill, and oregano are known for their high vitamin and mineral content, including calcium, an essential nutrient for eggshell formation.

Yet, there's more to a nutrient-dense yolk than meets the eye. It's not merely about stuffing your hens with nutrients and hoping they'll produce golden yolks. The health of your hens plays a significant role in the quality of their eggs. A stressed, unhealthy hen is unlikely to lay nutrient-rich eggs, regardless of the quality of her diet.

This is where herbs shine. Not only do they offer nutritional benefits, but they also contribute to the overall health and well-being of your hens. Herbs like lavender and chamomile can help reduce stress in your flock, promoting a calm, serene environment that's conducive to laying high-quality eggs.

The quality of your hens' environment can also influence the nutrient content of their yolks. Chickens need plenty of sunshine to produce vitamin D, an essential nutrient for calcium absorption. They also need ample space to exercise and forage. Exercise helps keep your hens healthy and reduces stress, while foraging allows them to supplement their diet with a variety of foods, contributing to the richness of their egg yolks.

So, the 'Art of the Yolk' is a delicate balance of nutrition, health, and environment. It's about providing your hens with a balanced, nutritious diet, ensuring they're healthy and stress-free, and giving them a conducive environment in which they can thrive. It's an ongoing process, a labor of love that yields tangible rewards every time your hens lay eggs.

Our goal isn't to produce the 'perfect' yolk. There's no such thing. The goal is to ensure your hens are healthy and happy. A nutrient-dense yolk is a sign that you're on the right track and that your hens are flourishing under your care. So pay attention to those golden orbs, appreciate the art that goes into their creation, and continue nurturing your flock to the best of your ability. The eggs they lay are a reflection of your care, and each one is a work of art in its own right.

One of the most intriguing aspects of chicken keeping is identifying and using specific herbs known for their yolk-enhancing properties. Let's learn about some of the herbs that can help enrich your hens' yolks with the nutrients that make them so prized.

Consider alfalfa, for instance. This herb is a favorite among many chicken keepers and for a good reason. Alfalfa is packed with vitamins and minerals, including calcium, which is crucial for strong eggshells. It's also rich in protein, which contributes to the overall nutritional content of the egg. Furthermore, alfalfa contains xanthophylls, a class of carotenoids that give yolks their rich, golden color. Offering your hens alfalfa in their diet can, therefore, significantly enhance the nutrient content and color of their yolks.

Nettle is another yolk-boosting herb that deserves mention. It's a powerhouse of nutrients, including iron, calcium, magnesium, and a host of vitamins. Adding nettle to your hens' diet can not only boost the nutrient content of their yolks but also improve their overall health and productivity. What's more, nettle has been used traditionally for its blood-purifying properties, which can further contribute to the health of your hens and the quality of their eggs.

Moving on, we have oregano, a herb famous in the culinary world for its aromatic and flavorful qualities. Yet, oregano is much more than a kitchen staple. It's packed with antioxidants and has natural antimicrobial properties. By adding oregano to your hens' diet, you're not only enriching their yolks with nutrients but also helping to bolster their immune systems, keeping them healthier and more resilient to diseases.

The herb list doesn't end there, though. Marigold petals, while not technically an herb, can do wonders for your hens' yolks. They're rich in xanthophylls, much like alfalfa, and can give your yolks that coveted golden color. Marigolds also contain lutein and zeaxanthin, two antioxidants that are beneficial for eye health. Therefore, by feeding your hens marigolds, you're enhancing the nutritional value of their eggs and contributing to the health of anyone who eats them.

The benefit of using herbs to enhance yolk quality is two-fold. On one hand, you're providing your hens with a variety of nutrients that can improve the nutritional content of their yolks. On the other hand, you're also supporting their overall health, which in turn influences the quality of their eggs. Healthy hens are likely to lay healthier eggs, after all.

Adding these yolk-enhancing herbs to your hens' diet can be as simple as mixing dried or fresh herbs into their feed, offering them separately as a treat, or even growing them in your yard for your hens to forage. Be creative, have fun, and experiment to see what your hens prefer.

How do we incorporate these amazing herbs into your chicken's diet effectively? It's one thing to have the knowledge about these herbs and their benefits, but another altogether to apply them practically in a way that your chickens will enjoy and benefit from.

One of the easiest ways to incorporate these nutrient-boosting herbs into your flock's diet is by mixing them directly into their feed. Dried herbs can easily be ground up into a fine powder and mixed thoroughly with your flock's regular feed. This method is great because it ensures that every bite your chickens take is enriched with the goodness of these herbs. It also has the added benefit of requiring minimal extra effort on your part once the initial grinding and mixing are done.

If you prefer using fresh herbs, or if you have an abundance of fresh herbs growing in your garden, then by all means, use them! Chickens love the taste of fresh greens. What better way to treat them than with fresh, nutrient-rich herbs? You can chop these up into small, manageable pieces and mix them into their feed or even offer them separately as a treat. Chickens are naturally curious creatures and will peck at anything that piques their interest. So, a bunch of fresh, fragrant herbs is sure to grab their attention.

Another excellent way to provide these herbs to your hens is through a method called 'deep litter.' This method involves scattering a mix of herbs, grass clippings, leaves, and compost over the floor of your chicken coop. The chickens will naturally turn over the litter in search of bugs and seeds, in the process mixing the herbs into the litter. The deep litter method not only helps enrich your flock's diet but also contributes to a healthier, cleaner, and more odor-free coop.

Speaking of coops, why not make your chicken's home a haven of herbs? Plant these herbs around and within the enclosure. It's a great way of providing your chickens with a steady supply of fresh herbs. Not to mention, certain herbs like lavender and mint can help keep pests at bay, making the coop a more pleasant and safer place for your flock.

Remember that free-ranging chickens are natural foragers. Given the opportunity, they'll roam around, pecking at all sorts of greens and bugs. Why not make the most of this by growing these herbs right in your backyard? This way, your chickens can have their fill of fresh, nutritious herbs right from the source. And let's be honest, there's a certain joy in seeing your chickens happily foraging around, their heads bobbing up and down as they peck at their newfound treats.

Creating an herbal 'dust bath' can be another unique and fun way to get these herbs into your chickens. Chickens love to dust bathe - it's their way of keeping clean and pest-free. Adding herbs like lavender, mint, or rosemary to the dust bath can not only provide their benefits but also help keep your flock smelling fresh and fragrant.

Finally, as we have discussed in previous chapters, think about making herbal tea for your chickens. Yes, you read that right! Making a mild herbal infusion and adding it to your chickens' water can be a great way to get these herbs into their system. Just make sure the tea is cooled before you offer it to your chickens.

And now that we've got the herbal menu all sorted out for our ladies, the next crucial step in our quest for golden, nutrient-rich yolks is learning how to identify them. Understanding what a nutrient-dense yolk looks like and how to monitor yolk quality is vital to ensuring your efforts are paying off.

Let's start with a question. What does a healthy, nutrient-dense egg yolk look like?

Well, the first indicator is the color. Conventionally raised, store-bought eggs often have pale yellow yolks, a sign of a diet low in variety and nutrients. In contrast, eggs laid by hens that have a diet enriched with herbs, greens, and a variety of other nutrient sources tend to have yolks that are a rich, deep orange color. This vibrant color is an indicator of higher levels of carotenoids, a type of antioxidant that not only enhances yolk color but also contributes to the overall nutritional value of the egg.

However, color isn't everything. While a deep orange yolk is a good sign, it doesn't necessarily guarantee a nutrient-dense yolk. Other factors play into this as well, such as the chicken's overall diet and health and the freshness of the egg.

Another indicator of a nutrient-rich yolk is its size. When an egg has a larger yolk in proportion to its white, it often suggests the hen has a diet rich in proteins and fats, vital nutrients for egg production. A small, overly pale yolk, in contrast, could suggest dietary deficiencies.

The texture of the yolk can also tell us a lot about its quality. A healthy yolk should hold its shape when the egg is cracked open, with a thick, viscous outer layer surrounding a more fluid inner core. If the yolk spreads out thin and flat immediately upon cracking the egg, it could indicate a lack of freshness or a lower nutritional value.

Even the eggshell can give you clues about the egg's internal quality. A strong, thick eggshell often means the hen's diet is adequately rich in calcium, an essential nutrient for eggshell production. Thin, brittle eggshells could signal a calcium-deficient diet or possibly an unhealthy hen.

Now that we know what signs to look for in a nutrient-rich yolk, let's discuss how to monitor yolk quality. Keeping a record might seem like an unnecessary chore, but it can be a valuable tool in your chicken-keeping arsenal. It helps you spot changes over time, note any improvements or decline in quality, and gauge the effectiveness of your interventions, like the inclusion of herbs in their diet.

A simple way to do this is to keep an egg journal. Whenever you collect eggs, take a moment to examine a few of them. Note down the hen's name, color, size, and texture of the yolks and the thickness of the shells. Over time, you will have a log that can provide a valuable overview of your flock's egg production quality. You can also take photographs of the yolks. A visual record can sometimes be more impactful than a written one, allowing you to compare eggs from different periods easily. Occasional odd eggs or variations in yolk quality are normal and not always a cause for concern. However, if you notice a persistent decline in yolk quality or other consistent issues with your eggs, it might be time to reevaluate your hens' diet and health.

The yolk is the heart of the egg - its quality directly reflects the care you provide for your chickens. Understanding what contributes to a nutrient-dense yolk and learning to identify and monitor it is an essential skill for anyone aiming to raise a healthy, productive flock. So, as you crack open each egg your hens gift you, take a moment to appreciate the art of the yolk. Each one is a testament to the magic of chickens and the nurturing environment you've created for them.

Part II: Hard as a Hen's Beak: Herbs for Strong Eggshells

Let's talk eggshells. Often seen as the protective packaging for the yolk and egg white, the humble eggshell contributes a lot more than just physical security. The quality of the eggshell plays a crucial role in the health of the hen that laid it, the freshness of the egg, and even the health of potential chicks that might emerge from it. So, let's crack the case wide open and delve into understanding the importance of eggshell quality.

When we discuss eggshell quality, we're really talking about three key aspects: thickness, strength, and texture. A good-quality eggshell is thick enough to withstand reasonable handling without cracking, strong enough to resist penetration by bacteria, and has a clean, smooth texture devoid of abnormal bumps or ridges. Achieving this trifecta of eggshell perfection is a balancing act involving the hen's diet, age, and overall health.

First up is thickness. The thickness of the eggshell is primarily determined by the amount of calcium in the hen's diet. Eggshells are about 94% calcium carbonate, so if a hen is deficient in calcium, her body will pull the necessary calcium from her own bones to form the eggshell, leading to long-term health problems for the hen and thinner, more fragile eggshells.

Eggshell strength, on the other hand, is determined by the amount of protein matrix present. This matrix, formed by proteins in the hen's body, binds the calcium carbonate crystals together and gives the shell its strength. Adequate levels of protein in the diet are thus just as important as calcium for eggshell strength.

Then there's texture. A smooth, clean eggshell is an indicator of a well-functioning shell gland in the hen. The shell gland is the part of the hen's reproductive tract that deposits the shell around the egg. Issues with the shell gland can lead to shells with abnormal shapes, rough textures, or unusual bumps or ridges.

So, why is eggshell quality so important?

Well, for one, the quality of the eggshell directly affects the egg's freshness and food safety. A thick, strong eggshell prevents bacteria from penetrating the egg, keeping the yolk and egg white safe from contamination. This is especially important if the eggs aren't going to be refrigerated immediately or if they're going to be stored for a while before consumption.

But the importance of eggshell quality goes beyond just human food safety. If you're hatching your eggs, the quality of the eggshell can significantly impact the success of the hatch. A shell that's too thin could break during incubation, while a shell that's too thick could make it difficult for the chick to break through when it's time to hatch.

For the hens themselves, consistently laying eggs with poor-quality shells can be an indicator of health issues. It could mean they're not getting enough calcium or protein in their diet, that they're stressed, or that they're experiencing issues with their reproductive tract. This makes monitoring eggshell quality an important part of keeping your hens healthy. Eggshells are more than just nature's packaging for eggs. They're a crucial factor in the quality and safety of the eggs, the success of hatching chicks, and the health of the laying hens. Understanding the importance of eggshell quality helps us make better choices for our flock, whether it's about their diet, their environment, or their care.

So, now we know that ggshells are more than just a protective shell, we now know that they are an indicator of a hen's overall health and the diet they are on. Armed with this knowledge, the question then arises: how can we encourage our hens to produce strong, healthy eggshells? While providing a balanced chicken diet with sufficient calcium and protein is key, there's another secret weapon you can employ to promote robust eggshells: herbs. Yes, the same plants that add flavor to your meals can also be used to help your hens lay eggs with strong, healthy shells.

Let's start with a classic: Oregano. This herb, known for its robust flavor and aromatic scent, also has plenty of health benefits. For chickens, it serves as a natural antibiotic, enhancing their immune system and helping them fight off diseases. But more pertinent to our discussion here, oregano is a good source of calcium. Adding fresh or dried oregano to your hens' diet can help ensure they have the calcium they need to produce thick, strong eggshells.

Next on our list is Parsley. This herb is packed with nutrients beneficial to chickens. It's rich in vitamins A, C, and K, and also contains trace amounts of calcium and iron. These nutrients support overall hen health, which can translate to the production of high-quality eggshells. Additionally, Parsley has been known to stimulate egg-laying in hens. More eggs mean more opportunities for those shells to strengthen and improve.

Other herbs that promote strong eggshells include Comfrey, Dill, and Mint. Comfrey is high in calcium and promotes bone and muscle health. Its leaves can be dried and added to chicken feed or grown in the chicken run for them to peck at. Dill, on the other hand, not only enhances eggshell strength but also improves the taste of the eggs. It's a source of calcium, manganese, and iron, all crucial elements for eggshell formation. Mint is an excellent stress reliever for chickens. A stress-free hen is more likely to lay healthy eggs with robust shells. Behind every great egg is a hen who's been given the chance to thrive, and that's what it's all about.

There's a symphony of herbs out there that can be beneficial for your hens and, in turn, for the quality of their eggshells. Now that we've identified these eggshell-strengthening herbs, how do we go about incorporating them into our hens' diets? You can sprinkle chopped fresh or dried herbs onto their feed. Alternatively, consider creating a dedicated herb garden for your hens to forage in. They'll appreciate the greenery and the opportunity to pick at fresh herbs. Just be sure to research each herb thoroughly before offering it to your chickens, as not all herbs are chicken-safe.

Let's discuss some concrete, practical ways to integrate these powerhouse plants into your chickens' diets. We know that simply sprinkling them onto feed or allowing your hens to forage in an herb garden are effective methods, but if you're in the mood for something a bit more fun and interactive, why not try your hand at making some herbal treats? Not only do these treats serve as a way to supplement your hens' diet with the shell-strengthening benefits of herbs, but they also provide an engaging activity for your flock, promoting their natural foraging behaviors.

Firstly, let's discuss 'Herb Cubes'. This is an incredibly simple yet effective way to incorporate a variety of herbs into your chickens' diet. To make Herb Cubes, simply chop up a mixture of fresh herbs — remember to focus on the ones high in calcium and beneficial to eggshell strength, like oregano, parsley, dill, and comfrey. Then, distribute the chopped herbs evenly into an ice cube tray, pour water to fill each compartment, and then freeze. Once frozen, these Herb Cubes can be given to your chickens, providing a refreshing and nutrient-rich treat. And, as they peck away at the cubes, they'll be getting those beneficial herbs into their system, which contributes to the production of strong eggshells.

Next, let's talk about a 'Herbal Layer Mash'. This treat combines your regular layer feed with a mixture of beneficial dried herbs and a few other key ingredients to promote shell strength. Here's a simple remedy to get you started:

- 4 cups of layer feed
- 1 cup of mixed dried herbs (oregano, parsley, dill, comfrey)
- 1 cup of old-fashioned oats
- 1/4 cup of diatomaceous earth (food grade)
- 1/4 cup of dried crushed eggshell

Mix these ingredients together and serve to your hens in their feeders. The layer feed ensures they're getting their usual balanced diet, the oats add a bit of diversity and extra fiber, the diatomaceous earth aids in parasite control, and the crushed eggshell gives an extra calcium boost. The dried herbs are the star of the show, providing the necessary nutrients for strong eggshells.

Lastly, let's explore the concept of 'Herbal Forage Cakes'. These cakes are designed to be hung in your chicken run, promoting natural pecking and foraging behaviors while delivering the herbal goodness that strengthens eggshells. Here's a simple forage cake remedy:

- 4 cups of scratch grains
- 1/2 cup of molasses
- 1/4 cup of coconut oil
- 1 cup of mixed fresh herbs (oregano, parsley, dill, comfrey)

Mix the scratch grains and freshly chopped herbs. Heat the molasses and coconut oil until runny, then pour over the grain and herb mixture. Mix well until everything is coated. Press the mixture into a Bundt or ring cake pan and let it set in the fridge. Once set, it can be unmolded and hung in the chicken run.

These remedies are just a starting point. You're welcome, and indeed encouraged, to play around with these ideas. Maybe your hens have a favorite herb not mentioned here, or perhaps there's a local plant you've researched and found to be chicken-safe and beneficial. Use what's available to you, always with an eye on providing the best diet for your hens. Through these fun and nutritious treats, you're not only improving the quality of your hens' eggshells but also enriching their environment and day-to-day life.

While crafting these treats and observing your chickens enjoying them brings great satisfaction, it's also crucial to keep an eye on the tangible results – the eggs themselves. Regularly checking the eggshells laid by your hens is an important aspect of chicken care and one that gives you direct feedback on the success of your herbal interventions. This regular 'Shell Check' is about understanding what to look for in an eggshell, how to interpret different signs, and how to respond if potential issues are detected.

What should you look for during a shell check? Firstly, consider the thickness of the shell. A well-formed eggshell should have a certain level of firmness. It shouldn't feel overly delicate or brittle. If you notice that your hens are laying eggs with thin or easily cracked shells, this could indicate that their diet is lacking in certain nutrients, especially calcium, even with your herbal additions. In such instances, you might want to increase the portion of shell-strengthening herbs in their diet or consider other forms of calcium supplementation.

Next, pay attention to the eggshell's surface. It should generally be smooth, with a slight natural graininess. Bumps, wrinkles, or rough patches on the eggshells could point to various issues. Stress, aging, or an interruption during the egg formation process can cause these irregularities. On the other hand, you might find that the shells are too smooth or glossy, which could indicate a lack of protein. Again, while herbs contribute to a healthy diet, they may not be sufficient to address all nutritional needs, so additional adjustments may be necessary.

Lastly, don't overlook the color of the eggshell. While different chicken breeds lay different colored eggs – from white to brown to blue – each hen will usually lay eggs of consistent color. If you notice a significant change in shell color, this could be a sign of disease or nutritional deficiency. But remember, slight variations in color are normal and can even reflect changes in diet, light exposure, or the hen's age.

So you've been keeping a keen eye on your chickens' eggshells. But what happens when you detect potential issues? Firstly, don't panic. Chickens, like all creatures, can have off days, and a single misshapen or thin-shelled egg is not a cause for immediate alarm. However, if you're noticing a consistent pattern of poor-quality shells, it's time to play detective.

Look at the overall picture of your hens' health and happiness. Are they behaving normally? Are they eating and drinking regularly? Have there been any changes in their environment that could be causing stress? Are they getting enough exercise and sunlight? All of these factors can influence eggshell quality.

On the nutritional side, consider the balance of their diet. Herbs are a powerful tool for boosting eggshell strength, but they're only one piece of the puzzle. Ensure your hens are getting a balanced diet with plenty of protein, calcium, and other essential nutrients. You might need to adjust the ratio of herbs to feed or supplement with additional calcium or vitamins.

Don't forget to consult a poultry expert or veterinarian if issues persist. Sometimes, eggshell irregularities can be a symptom of more serious health issues that require professional attention. But remember, you're already one step ahead by conducting regular shell checks and taking proactive steps to optimize your hens' diet with beneficial herbs.

In the journey of rearing chickens, constant learning and adaptation are key. Just as you've learned to whip up Herbal Layer Mash or Forage Cakes, you'll also become proficient in interpreting the stories that eggshells tell. This practice will only deepen your connection with your hens and further your appreciation of the intricate process of egg formation.

Part III: Frequent Layers: Herbs for Egg Production

Whether you're a seasoned chicken keeper or just starting your journey with backyard chickens, one question probably pops up now and then: "How often should my hens lay?" This is a pretty critical question, especially if egg production is one of your main goals for raising hens. Understanding the egg production cycle can help you manage your expectations, identify potential issues early, and ensure your hens are as healthy and productive as possible.

Let's start with the basics. Once a hen reaches maturity, typically around five to six months of age, she'll start laying eggs. However, keep in mind that breed plays a considerable role in this – some breeds start laying earlier than others, and some lay more frequently than others. On average, a healthy and well-cared-for hen will lay an egg almost every day. That's right, almost every day.

The egg-laying cycle of a chicken is dictated by light. Hens need about 14 to 16 hours of daylight to lay regularly. That's why egg production often dips in winter when daylight hours are fewer. Chickens have a special gland behind their eyes, the pineal gland, which reacts to light and sends signals to their ovary to release an egg. Fascinating, isn't it?

However, laying an egg every day is quite a taxing process for a hen's body. After a few days of constant laying, most hens will take a break. This usually happens after five to seven eggs, so it's normal to have a day with no egg every week or so. This is the hen's way of resting and recharging.

As your hens age, their egg production will start to slow down. The majority of hens are most productive in their first two years of laying. After that, they may lay fewer and fewer eggs each year. By the time they're five or six, many hens stop laying entirely. However, this doesn't mean they're not valuable members of your flock. Older hens often serve as calm and wise leaders among your birds.

Your hens' laying patterns can also be influenced by their overall health and comfort. Stress, illness, molt (when chickens shed and regrow their feathers), poor diet, or unsuitable living conditions can all cause hens to lay fewer eggs or stop laying altogether. If you notice a sudden drop in egg production, it's crucial to find the cause and address it as quickly as possible to ensure your hens' well-being.

Diet plays a vital role in egg production. Laying hens need a well-balanced diet packed with protein and calcium to keep up with the demands of egg production. That's where the magic of herbs comes in. Certain herbs can boost your hens' health and potentially enhance their egg-laying abilities.

It's completely normal for egg production to vary a bit from hen to hen and from season to season. Regular egg production indicates that your hen is healthy and content, while any changes can serve as a useful barometer of her health and happiness. Understanding the egg production cycle of your hens gives you a foundation of knowledge to build on as we explore how different herbs can be used to encourage regular laying in the next sections. Take some time to observe your hens and their laying patterns. You'll find it not only informative but also a rewarding way to connect with your flock.

Now that you have a solid understanding of the egg production cycle, let's discuss some herbs that can potentially enhance your hens' egg-laying abilities. Two herbs, in particular, stand out in this regard: Red Raspberry Leaf and Fennel. Let's explore why these herbs are so lauded in the world of backyard chicken keeping.

Starting with Red Raspberry Leaf, this herb is a powerhouse for your laying hens. It's been used for centuries in herbal medicine to support reproductive health in humans, and it turns out it's beneficial for chickens, too! Rich in vitamins and minerals, it provides essential nutrients your hens need for egg production.

Red Raspberry Leaf is high in calcium, which is critical for producing strong eggshells. But what makes it truly special is its high magnesium content. Magnesium aids in the absorption of calcium, making sure your hens get the maximum benefit from their food. This can lead to more frequent laying of eggs with stronger shells.

What about Fennel? This sweet, licorice-flavored herb is a favorite in culinary circles, but it's also a blessing for your hens. It's packed with vitamins and minerals that can support your hens' health and potentially boost egg production.

Fennel is rich in iron, which can help hens produce more and better quality eggs. It also contains essential vitamins like Vitamin C and A, known to support overall health and immunity. And just like Red Raspberry Leaf, Fennel is also a great source of calcium and magnesium, key nutrients for eggshell formation.

You may wonder how to incorporate these herbs into your hens' diet. It's easier than you might think. Fresh or dried, these herbs can be mixed into your hens' feed. You can also brew a mild herbal tea with these herbs and offer it to your hens in their waterer. Alternatively, consider growing these herbs in your backyard for your hens to forage. They'll not only benefit from the nutrients but also enjoy the process of foraging, which is a natural behavior for them.

There are also other herbs known for their potential to boost egg production. Nettle, for instance, is high in calcium and other essential nutrients that can support egg production. Mint, particularly spearmint, is believed to stimulate the hen's reproductive system, possibly leading to more frequent laying. Alfalfa, while not technically an herb, is packed with nutrients that can contribute to egg production.

Remember that while herbs can support your hens' health and potentially boost egg production, they're not a miracle cure. They're a supplement to a balanced diet and proper care, not a replacement. Factors like breed, age, light exposure, and general health have a considerable impact on egg production. If you're concerned about a drop in egg production, it's essential to look at the big picture and consider all potential contributing factors.

With this new knowledge about Red Raspberry Leaf, Fennel, and other egg-boosting herbs, take some time to consider how you might incorporate these into your flock's diet. These herbs aren't just potential egg boosters, they're also an excellent way to add variety to your hens' diet and stimulate their natural foraging behavior. That's a win-win in my book!
Now that you're armed with a list of egg-boosting herbs, it's time to roll up our sleeves and dive into creating some herbal feed blends that could potentially maximize your hens' laying frequency.

Creating an herbal feed blend for your chickens is a lot like cooking. You want a mix of ingredients that each bring their own benefits to the table (or the feed dish, as the case may be). It's about finding a balance of flavors and nutrients that work together. And just like with cooking, it's always a good idea to keep your diners' preferences in mind.

Let's start with a simple blend that I like to call "The Layer's Delight". This blend is designed to be mixed directly into your hens' regular feed, adding a punch of herbal goodness to their daily diet.

You will need:

• 2 parts dried Red Raspberry Leaf
• 2 parts dried Fennel seeds
• 1 part dried Nettle leaves
• 1 part dried Mint leaves
• 1/2 part dried Alfalfa leaves

This blend combines the egg-boosting powers of Red Raspberry Leaf and Fennel with the added benefits of Nettle, Mint, and Alfalfa. Each herb brings a unique benefit to your hens' diet, from the calcium in the Nettle to the refreshing and potentially stimulating effect of Mint. Alfalfa, while not technically an herb, adds a dose of rich, leafy green nutrients.

To prepare the blend, simply mix the dried herbs together thoroughly. You can then add a small amount of this mixture to your hens' regular feed each day. Start with a small amount and gradually increase it, observing how your hens react to the new addition to their diet.

Next, let's explore a remedy that introduces the herbs in a different way through a soothing herbal tea. I call this remedy "The Herbal Hen Hydrator".

You will need:

• 2 tablespoons of dried Red Raspberry Leaf
• 2 tablespoons of dried Fennel seeds

- 1 tablespoon of dried Nettle leaves
- 1 tablespoon of dried Mint leaves
- A handful of fresh Alfalfa leaves

To prepare this herbal tea, add all the dried herbs to a teapot or large jar. Pour a liter of boiling water over the herbs and let them steep for 15 to 20 minutes. Once the tea has cooled down, strain out the herbs and add the herbal infusion to your chickens' waterer. Add the fresh Alfalfa leaves to the waterer for an extra nutrient boost.

These are just two examples of how you can incorporate egg-boosting herbs into your hens' diet. Feel free to experiment with these remedies and adjust them to suit your hens' taste and your available resources.

The key to success in using herbs to potentially enhance egg production lies in consistency and balance. Regularly providing your hens with these beneficial herbs while ensuring they also receive a balanced diet and proper care can potentially lead to an increase in egg production over time. Using herbs in your flock's diet not only potentially boosts egg production but also adds variety to their diet and encourages natural foraging behavior. Now that's a triple win if you ask me!

With herbs thrown into the feed mix, your chickens dining experience is much more exciting, and their health potentially boosted. However, the proof of the pudding is in the eating, right? So, how do you measure the success of your herbal intervention? That's where egg counting and tracking come into play.

Counting eggs might seem like a no-brainer. After all, how hard can it be to count the number of eggs your hens lay each day? Yet, there's more to tracking egg production than simply tallying up daily totals. It involves understanding the natural rhythms of your flock and being alert to any changes.

Egg-laying isn't a constant process, nor is it identical for every chicken. Some hens are champion layers, producing an egg almost every day. Others lay less frequently, with breaks between egg-laying days. This variety is normal and is part of what makes each hen unique.

Your job as a backyard farmer is to establish the baseline laying patterns of your flock. This baseline will serve as a reference point, allowing you to detect any changes or irregularities. Start by recording the number of eggs laid each day, noting down any observations, such as changes in weather, diet, or behavior. Over time, you'll be able to identify patterns and rhythms in your hens' egg-laying habits.

Now, you might ask, "Why bother tracking egg production? Isn't it enough to know that the hens are laying?" Well, monitoring egg production does more than just give you bragging rights at the local farmer's market. It's a vital tool in managing the health and well-being of your flock.

A sudden drop in egg production can signal a number of potential issues. Stress, disease, mite infestations, or dietary deficiencies can all lead to a decrease in laying. By keeping an eye on your hens' output, you're more likely to catch these problems early when they're easier to address. A consistent increase in egg production, on the other hand, might be a sign that your herbal supplements or dietary changes are having a positive effect.

While the number of eggs laid is important, don't forget to consider the quality of those eggs too. Healthy layers usually produce eggs with sturdy shells, bright yolks, and a generous size. Irregularities in egg shape, shell texture, or color could indicate potential health issues. Remember, quantity never trumps quality when it comes to egg production.

In addition to tracking egg production, keep an eye on your hens' behavior. Healthy layers are typically active, alert, and exhibit natural behaviors such as foraging, dust bathing, and roosting. Any changes in behavior can provide early signs of potential issues. By keeping a close eye on your flock and their egg output, you can better manage their health and respond more effectively to their needs.

It's crucial to note, however, that using herbs should not replace a balanced, nutritious diet for your hens. Think of herbs as a supplement, a way to add variety and extra nutrients to your hens' meals. Ensure your flock gets a proper diet composed mainly of balanced poultry feed, complemented by healthy kitchen scraps, foraging opportunities, and, of course, our nutrient-boosting herbs.

"In every walk with nature one receives far more than he seeks."
— John Muir

Bonus Chapter: Clucking Around the Seasons

Develop Seasonal Herbal Rituals

Part I: Spring Cleaning: Herbal Detox for Your Flock

Let's turn our attention to the changing of seasons and how they impact our chickens' health. It's no secret that each season brings with it unique challenges and opportunities. In the case of chickens, we often see a shift in their behavior, diet, and overall health as they adapt to the changing environment. As we're about to discover, this transition can be especially notable in the leap from winter to spring.

Take a moment to consider the life of a chicken during the winter months. Winter, as we all know, is a period of slow-down and, for many animals, a time of hibernation. Chickens don't hibernate, of course, but they do go through their version of slowing down - most notably, they often stop or reduce their egg-laying and go through a molt, losing old feathers and growing new ones.

Chickens also change their dietary habits in winter. Their bodies crave more energy to keep warm, so they tend to eat more grain and fewer fresh greens, insects, and other delicacies that are hard to come by in the cold months. This shift in diet can lead to a buildup of toxins in their systems over the winter. Come spring, it's time for a detox.

Why a detox, you ask? Well, detoxification is all about helping the body to eliminate toxins and waste products that have built up over time. In the case of chickens, these toxins can come from a variety of sources: pesticides or other chemicals in their feed or bedding, internal parasites, bacteria, fungi, or simply the metabolic waste products from their winter diet.

Detoxification is a normal and healthy process that chickens, like all animals, do naturally. Their liver and kidneys are designed to filter out toxins from the blood and excrete them through urine and feces. But sometimes, especially after a long, hard winter, their systems can use a little help.

This is where the concept of a spring detox comes in. Just as humans often feel the need for a health kick or cleanse after a period of indulgence, so too can chickens benefit from a detox at the end of winter. A good detox can help to clear out their systems, improve their digestion, boost their immune systems, and get them ready for the busy egg-laying season ahead.

There are several ways to go about a chicken detox, but as you might guess, we're going to focus on the herbal approach. Herbs can offer a gentle and natural way to support your chickens' health and help their bodies eliminate toxins. Certain herbs are known for their detoxifying properties, including their ability to stimulate the liver and kidneys, support digestion, and boost the immune system.

But before we dive into the specifics of which herbs to use and how to use them, let's take a moment to consider what a detox will look like in practical terms. The goal here isn't to put your chickens on a strict cleanse or fasting regime (which wouldn't be healthy or even feasible for them). Rather, it's about adding certain beneficial herbs to their diet and making a few simple changes to their environment to promote better health.

With that concept of a gentle, supportive detox in mind, we can now turn our attention to the specific herbs that can play a starring role in this process. Two herbs stand out in particular when it comes to detoxification: dandelion and milk thistle. Now, you might be thinking, "Aren't those weeds?" And indeed, they are! But as we're about to discover, these humble plants are also powerful allies when it comes to supporting your chickens' health.

Dandelion, a common sight in yards and fields, is a powerhouse of nutrition. Every part of this plant – from its sunny yellow flowers to its deep taproot – is edible and packed with vitamins and minerals. But beyond its nutritional profile, dandelion has some special properties that make it particularly useful in a detox.

Firstly, dandelion is a diuretic, meaning it helps to stimulate the kidneys to produce more urine. This can aid in flushing toxins out of the body. Secondly, it's a bitter herb. Bitter herbs stimulate the production of digestive juices, helping to improve digestion and the absorption of nutrients. They also stimulate the liver, the body's main detoxification organ.

Milk thistle, with its distinctive spiky leaves and purple flowers, is another weed-turned-medicine. Its active compound, silymarin, is a potent antioxidant that can help to protect the liver from damage and enhance its detoxification processes. Milk thistle has been used for centuries to treat liver and gallbladder disorders in humans, and it can offer similar benefits to chickens.

Incorporating dandelion and milk thistle into your chickens' diet can be as simple as allowing them access to areas where these herbs grow naturally. If that's not possible, or if you want to provide a more concentrated dose, both herbs are available in dried form from herbal suppliers. They can be added to your chickens' feed or brewed into a tea and added to their water.

Beyond dandelion and milk thistle, there are several other herbs that can play a supportive role in a spring detox. Nettle is a nutrient-dense herb that can support overall health and vitality. Garlic has antibacterial and antiparasitic properties and can help support the immune system. Burdock root, another bitter herb, can support digestion and liver health.

Creating a detox blend for your chickens can be a fun and rewarding process. Start with a base of regular chicken feed, then add a handful of dried herbs – perhaps a mix of dandelion, milk thistle, nettle, and burdock. Garlic can be added fresh or in powdered form. So, there you have it – a closer look at how the humble dandelion, milk thistle, and a few of their friends can help your chickens shake off the winter blues and step into spring with vitality and good health.

Now, let's talk about crafting a spring cleaning menu that integrates all these wonderful herbs into your chickens' diet. We will provide remedies and feed adjustments that are simple yet effective in promoting detoxification. You'll find that these are easy to prepare and, more importantly, delightful for your hens.

Let's start with a simple, nutritious blend we can call the "Detox Delight". For this, you need your regular chicken feed as the base. You'll also need dried dandelion (leaves, stems, and flowers), milk thistle seeds, nettle leaves, burdock root, and garlic powder. It's important to note that while the quantities of these ingredients will depend on the size of your flock, a good rule of thumb is to aim for about 5% to 10% of the total feed volume as your herbal mix. Mix these ingredients well and serve as a daily ration. Remember, consistency is key here. So, plan to offer this Detox Delight blend for a good month at the onset of spring.

For a wet feed option, let's consider a "Herbal Mash". Wet feeds can be a nice change for your hens, and they offer a great way to include fresh or dried herbs in a tasty, easy-to-digest format. To prepare this, you'll need a base of regular chicken feed and the same herbs we've discussed: dandelion, milk thistle, nettle, burdock root, and garlic. Start by soaking the feed in water for 15-30 minutes or until it has absorbed most of the water and achieved a porridge-like consistency. Then, add your mix of finely chopped fresh or dried herbs. The herbal mixture should constitute about a quarter of the total volume. Serve this mash a couple of times a week as a treat alongside their regular feed.

Then we have the "Spring Sipper", a detoxifying drink that helps keep your hens hydrated and supplies them with additional nutrients. Prepare an herbal tea by steeping a mix of dried dandelion leaves and flowers, milk thistle seeds, nettle leaves, burdock root, and a few crushed garlic cloves in boiling water for about 15 minutes. After it cools, add this herbal infusion to your chicken's water. This blend is not only refreshing, but it also carries the detox benefits we've discussed. Offer this herbal water a few times per week, alternating with their normal fresh water.

To add variety and ensure all these herbs are accepted and eaten by your hens, alternate between these remedies. These detox remedies, while aimed at the spring season, can be used whenever you feel your chickens need an extra boost.

Alright, we have the herbs. We have the remedies. Now, let's turn our attention to monitoring the effects of our springtime detox on the health of our flock. Just as you would with any new addition to your chicken's diet, it's vital to keep a keen eye on your flock during this detox period.

Watching your chickens isn't just about counting the eggs they produce (though that's certainly important). It's about taking in the whole picture of their health and happiness. You're looking for signs that they're thriving, not just surviving.

The first thing to observe is their behavior. Are your chickens active, curious, and alert? These are good signs. On the other hand, a chicken that's sluggish, isolated, or behaving unusually may not be feeling well. Each chicken is an individual with their own unique behaviors and quirks. As their caretaker, you're well-positioned to notice any changes, whether they're subtle or obvious.

A healthy chicken will also have bright, clear eyes and a red comb and wattles that are vibrant but not excessively dark or swollen. Their feathers should be sleek and smooth, not ruffled or dull. A chicken that's in good health will have a good appetite and will maintain a stable weight. They should be enthusiastic about foraging, scratching, and pecking at their food.

Next, take a close look at the quality of the eggs they're producing. Are the shells hard and smooth? Are the yolks a vibrant yellow or orange, and the whites clear and firm? These are signs of good egg health and, therefore, good chicken health. Conversely, soft or thin shells, pale yolks, or runny whites could indicate a nutritional deficiency or other health issues.

One aspect that is often overlooked is their droppings. While not the most glamorous part of chicken keeping, droppings can give us a wealth of information about a chicken's health. Healthy droppings should be firm but not hard, with white uric acid on top. An unusual color, consistency, or smell could be an early warning sign of a health issue.

During the detox period, you might see some changes in your flock. A detox is to rid the body of toxins, so it's not unusual for a chicken to seem a bit under the weather as their body processes and eliminates these substances. This might manifest as a slightly lower energy level, a minor drop in egg production, or changes in droppings. As long as these changes are mild and temporary, there's no need for concern. However, if you observe severe or persistent changes, it might be best to consult with a veterinarian.

So, after you've introduced the spring detox menu, continue to observe your chickens closely for the next several weeks. Are they more active? Do their feathers seem shinier and healthier? Are their eyes brighter? Are they laying consistently? How is the quality of their eggs? These observations will help you evaluate the effectiveness of the detox.

This "chickens in bloom" phase, as I like to call it, is all about giving your chickens the best possible start to the year. It's about clearing away the old and making way for the new, just as nature does every spring. It's a time of rejuvenation and renewal, both for your flock and for you as a chicken keeper. So take the time to enjoy it, to celebrate the end of winter and the arrival of spring.

Part II: Summer Spritzes: Herbal Hydration and Cooling

I like to think of summer as a sunny, celebratory time on the farm. The hens are busy laying, the garden is bursting with life, and everything seems to be in full swing. But while summer brings plenty of positives, it also brings its share of challenges for backyard chicken keepers. The heat, in particular, can be tough on our feathery friends.

You see, chickens aren't designed for hot weather. They're essentially little feathered ovens with a normal body temperature that ranges from 105 to 107 degrees Fahrenheit. Unlike us, they don't have sweat glands to help them cool down. Instead, they rely on panting, spreading their wings, and seeking shade to keep their body temperature in check.

Heat stress in chickens is no joke. It can lead to a decrease in egg production a decrease in food intake, and in severe cases, it can even be fatal. Therefore, it becomes essential to understand the importance of hydration and cooling for your chickens during the summer months.

Hydration is critical for chickens in hot weather. Water helps regulate their body temperature, carries nutrients to their cells, and aids in digestion. If a chicken gets dehydrated, it can't cool itself effectively, which can lead to overheating.

To ensure your chickens stay hydrated, they should always have access to clean, fresh water. On very hot days, you may need to refill their water several times. Adding ice cubes to the water can help keep it cool and make it more appealing to your chickens.

Also, remember that hens require more water when they're laying. A large portion of an egg is water, so hens laying regularly will need to drink more. Dehydration can cause a hen to stop laying, so make sure your laying hens always have plenty of water.

Cooling is just as important as hydration in the summer months. Chickens will naturally seek shade when the sun is at its peak, so make sure your coop and run provide plenty of shaded areas. If natural shade isn't available, you might need to get creative. A tarp, a patio umbrella, or even a few strategically placed garden plants can create much-needed shade.

Ventilation in the coop is also critical. Good airflow can help reduce the temperature and keep your chickens comfortable. If your coop gets hot, consider adding more ventilation or even installing a fan.

Providing a dust bath area is another great way to help your chickens cool down. Chickens will naturally dig shallow pits in the dirt or sand to bathe in, which helps them cool down and keeps their feathers in good condition.

So, understanding the need for hydration and cooling during the summer months is a must for any backyard chicken keeper. Keeping your chickens comfortable during the hot weather will help ensure they stay healthy, happy, and productive.

The understanding of hydration and temperature regulation for chickens during the hot months is fundamental. Now, let's give our feathered friends an herbal boost to combat the heat. The world of herbs is vast and varied, and certain herbs can serve a multitude of purposes. When it comes to dealing with heat, two herbs come to mind: Mint and Lemon Balm.

Let's start with mint. This aromatic herb is well known for its cooling properties. Mint leaves contain a compound called menthol, which gives them that distinctive, refreshing flavor. This menthol has a cooling effect on the body, both when ingested and when applied externally. Mint is a powerhouse of a plant that comes with a whole host of benefits. Not only does it have cooling properties, but it also aids digestion and has anti-inflammatory properties, which can be especially beneficial during the hot summer months.

Feeding mint to your chickens can be as simple as scattering some fresh leaves in their run or mixing dried leaves into their feed. You could also make mint-infused water for your chickens to drink. Just steep a bunch of fresh mint leaves in their waterer for a few hours and then remove the leaves before giving it to your chickens. The result is a refreshing, cooling drink that your chickens will love.

Now, let's talk about Lemon Balm. This herb is a member of the mint family and shares many of its cooling and digestive benefits. But Lemon Balm has an added bonus: it has a calming effect. It's been used for centuries in traditional medicine to relieve anxiety and promote sleep. This calming effect can be particularly beneficial during the summer when the heat can make your chickens more irritable. Lemon Balm can be fed to your chickens in much the same way as mint. Fresh or dried leaves can be added to their feed, or you can make a Lemon Balm-infused water.

But the use of herbs in your chicken's summer care routine doesn't stop there. Other herbs, such as Lavender and Chamomile, have calming properties that can help your chickens deal with the stress of the heat. Basil and Oregano are rich in antioxidants and can support their immune system. Parsley is packed with nutrients and can help keep your chickens healthy.

All these herbs can be used to create a summer herbal blend for your chickens. Start with a base of mint and Lemon Balm, then add in smaller amounts of other herbs based on your chickens' needs and preferences. This blend can be mixed into their feed, scattered in their run for them to peck at, or steeped in their water for a refreshing summer drink.

Using herbs like mint and Lemon Balm in your chicken care routine during the summer can make a big difference in how well your chickens deal with the heat. Not only do these herbs help keep your chickens cool and hydrated, but they also offer a range of other health benefits. Plus, they add variety to your chickens' diet and help stimulate their natural foraging behavior.

Herbal drinks and misters can be valuable tools in our chicken care arsenal, offering a creative way to deliver the benefits of these plants.

Creating an herbal drink for your chickens is relatively simple. The primary goal is to infuse water with the beneficial properties of herbs. Let's look at a simple remedy using mint, a favorite cooling herb. Take a handful of fresh mint leaves and place them in a jug of water. Allow this to steep for several hours, much like making iced tea. The result is a refreshing herbal drink that your chickens can access throughout the day. The mint-infused water will help keep your chickens hydrated while also providing a pleasant cooling effect, perfect for those hot summer days.

To add a bit of variation and additional benefits, you can create a blend of herbs for your chicken's drink. For instance, adding Lemon Balm to the mint infusion can provide calming effects, while a bit of parsley will deliver a nutrient boost. The key is to experiment with different combinations and observe your chickens' responses. Remember to thoroughly wash all herbs before adding them to the water to ensure they are free from any chemicals or pests.

Next, let's explore the concept of an herbal mister. The idea is similar to the herbal drink, but instead of drinking the herbal infusion, you'll be spritzing it onto your chickens. This provides immediate cooling and can also help deter pests. Here's a straightforward way to create your own herbal mister.

Start by choosing herbs that your chickens enjoy and that have cooling properties. Mint and Lemon Balm are excellent options but feel free to get creative. You might want to try chamomile for its calming effects or lavender for its delightful scent and soothing properties. Once you've chosen your herbs, you'll need to create a strong infusion. To do this, simply add a generous amount of herbs to boiling water and let it steep until it cools.

After the infusion has cooled, strain the herbs out, and you're left with an aromatic herbal water. Put this water in a spray bottle, and voila, you have a homemade, natural chicken mister. On those really hot days, lightly mist your chickens with this herbal infusion. They'll benefit from the cooling properties of the herbs, and the spray can help deter bugs and pests. Please be sure not to mist this mixture into their eyes or nostrils. The beauty of these herbal tools is not just in their practical benefits but also in their versatility. Feel free to mix and match herbs, experimenting with what works best for your flock.

While creating these herbal drinks and misters, it's also important to ensure you're providing fresh, cool water for your chickens at all times. These herbal additions should not replace their regular water source but rather supplement it. Hydration is of utmost importance, especially during the hot summer months.

With the fundamentals of creating herbal drinks and misters in place, it becomes critical to shift our focus on the art of observation and ensuring your chickens' comfort during hot weather. Observing your chickens' behavior and physical state is a crucial part of maintaining their wellbeing. Particularly during the hot summer months, keen observation and quick response can make the difference between happy chickens and a flock suffering from heat stress.

To start, understanding your chickens' normal behavior is key. Chickens have a natural rhythm to their day, with periods of activity and rest. On hot days, chickens tend to slow down and seek out cooler areas, such as shady spots under trees or in the coop. While reduced activity is normal during high temperatures, it's essential to watch for signs of heat stress, which can include panting, spreading their wings away from their body, lethargy beyond the normal heat-induced slow down, or in severe cases, seizures and other physical signs of distress.

With these signs in mind, being proactive about your chickens' comfort can go a long way. Apart from the refreshing herbal drinks and misters, consider other practical steps to help them beat the heat. Provide access to shady areas, whether it's under trees, an overhang, or a specially designed area within their run. Ventilation in the coop is another essential aspect. Ensure there's a good airflow to help keep the environment cool and fresh.

Experiment with frozen treats, a surefire way to help your chickens cool down. Fruits like watermelon or berries can be frozen and offered as a chilly snack. You can also freeze herbal infusions into ice cubes for a peckable cooling treat. These treats not only help lower their body temperature but also encourage natural pecking behavior, which can be a nice distraction on hot days.

One important observation tool is checking the color and condition of your chickens' combs and wattles. Healthy chickens combs and wattles should be bright and vibrant. During heat stress, they might appear darker and even bluish. If you notice this, it's time to take immediate action, as this is a sign of severe heat stress.

A consistent supply of clean, fresh water is vital. Chickens drink more in hot weather, and being even slightly dehydrated can affect their egg production and overall health. Hydration sources should be in shady spots, as chickens prefer cool water. The herbal drinks can supplement the water supply, providing added nutrients while encouraging your chickens to drink more.

Temperature regulation is also critical in maintaining your chickens' comfort during hot weather. This goes beyond just providing shade. Consider the location of your coop; is it directly in the sun for most of the day, or does it get some relief? If it's in a particularly sunny spot, can you add a shade cloth or move it to a better location? Similarly, consider the materials your coop is made from. Certain materials, such as metal, can absorb and retain heat, making the coop uncomfortably hot.

Lastly, keep a keen eye on the vulnerable ones. Younger birds and older ones, as well as heavier breeds or those with large combs and wattles, are more susceptible to heat stress. These birds may need extra care and attention during hot weather to ensure they remain comfortable and healthy.

As you can see, maintaining your chickens' comfort during hot weather is an active process requiring observation, quick action, and, of course, a good understanding of your flock. With these tools in your arsenal, your chickens can weather the summer heat, staying happy, healthy, and productive.

Part III: Autumn Adjustments: Preparing Your Flock for Winter

Falling into the heart of autumn, a chicken keeper's keen observation skills get called upon once again. But this time, it's not the stifling heat we're countering, but the increasingly cooler weather and the changes it brings to our flock's routines and needs. This is the autumn shift – a time of transition, and understanding this change is an integral part of keeping your chickens healthy and happy.

As the weather cools, the habits and needs of your chickens start to change. Daylight hours decrease, temperatures drop, and chickens' behaviors and habits adjust to match these changes. Knowing what to expect can help you prepare and keep your flock thriving.

One of the most noticeable changes in autumn is the reduction in daylight hours. Chickens, particularly layers, are sensitive to light. They need a certain amount of daylight to keep up their egg production. As the days grow shorter, don't be surprised if your egg count starts to decrease. This is a natural response, not a cause for alarm. Chickens may also begin to molt in autumn, replacing their old feathers with new ones in preparation for the winter. During this time, their energy goes into growing new feathers, which may further reduce egg-laying.

The drop in temperature is another significant aspect of the autumn shift. Chickens are pretty robust and can handle cold weather quite well, but sudden changes or extremely cold temperatures can cause stress. It's essential to monitor the weather and your chickens to ensure they are adjusting well.

Changes in diet are also part of the autumn shift. As temperatures drop, chickens need more calories to help them maintain their body temperature. While your chickens will naturally start to eat more, you may need to adjust their feed to ensure it's energy-rich. The lush greenery of summer may also start to dwindle, limiting the availability of fresh forage. You might need to supplement their diet to ensure they are getting all the nutrients they need.

Autumn is also a time when many plants and trees produce seeds and fruits, some of which can be harmful to chickens. Be aware of what's growing in and around your chicken run and ensure they don't have access to anything toxic.

An increase in pest and parasite activity is another aspect of the autumn shift. Many pests lay their eggs in the fall, leading to a surge in numbers. Regularly checking your chickens for parasites and keeping their coop and run clean can help keep any unwanted visitors at bay.

As you can see, the autumn shift is a time of significant change for your chickens. It's a time of preparation for the coming winter, with changes in behaviors, dietary needs, and potential challenges. But, with understanding and preparation, you can help your chickens navigate this transition smoothly, ensuring they continue to thrive.

There is a multitude of herbs that can assist our chickens in these cooler times. Ginger, cinnamon, and many others are warming herbs. These potent plants bring a warmth that can help chickens adjust to the colder temperatures and shorter days that come with autumn and winter.

First, let's talk about ginger. This spicy root has a long history of use in both culinary and medicinal applications. In chickens, it can serve multiple purposes. For one, ginger is known for its warming properties. It helps to increase circulation, which can aid in maintaining body temperature as the weather gets colder. It's also excellent for digestion and can assist in absorbing the extra nutrients your chickens need during this time. Its anti-inflammatory properties also come into play, promoting general wellness in your flock.

To incorporate ginger into your chickens' diet, you can add fresh, grated ginger to their feed, or brew a strong tea to mix with their water. It can be used regularly throughout the autumn and winter months, but remember, like any supplement, it shouldn't make up more than 1-2% of their diet.

Next, let's consider cinnamon. Besides being a familiar flavor in our kitchens, cinnamon is a valuable ally for our feathered friends. Like ginger, cinnamon is warming and supports circulation. Additionally, it has antimicrobial properties that can help keep your chickens healthy during a time when they may be more susceptible to illness. Sprinkle a bit of cinnamon into your chickens' feed or add a stick of cinnamon to their water container for a warming touch.

Echinacea, though not a warming herb in the traditional sense, also deserves a mention. It's often used to support the immune system, which is particularly beneficial during the transition into colder weather. Echinacea can be grown in your garden and its leaves, flowers, and roots can all be used.

There are also several herbs like fenugreek and fennel seeds that can offer warmth. Fenugreek seeds can be sprouted to provide a highly nutritious and warming feed supplement. Fennel seeds can be sprinkled directly into their feed, providing a warm and aromatic treat that supports both digestive and reproductive health.

After uncovering the benefits of warming herbs such as ginger, cinnamon, fenugreek, and fennel, let's now shift our attention to constructing an autumnal diet for our flock, using these herbs and other nutritionally rich ingredients to give them a strong foundation for the coming winter.

Chickens are intuitive eaters. As the days grow shorter and the temperatures drop, they naturally start to crave foods that are denser and higher in energy to prepare them for the winter ahead. Their body knows it needs to layer up fat and energy stores to comfortably get through the cold months. As chicken keepers, we can help facilitate this process by adjusting their feed accordingly.

Starting with grains, the heart of any chicken diet, increase the quantity of whole grains during the autumn months. Whole grains, such as corn, wheat, barley, and oats, are a great source of energy for your chickens. The process of breaking down these whole grains also generates body heat, helping them stay warm. These grains can be scattered on the ground to encourage natural foraging behaviors, or mixed in with their daily feed.

Next, we add in the warming herbs. We've learned how ginger and cinnamon can be beneficial, along with fenugreek and fennel seeds. These can be added directly to their feed or given as separate treats. A word of caution: it's important not to overload your chickens' diet with these herbs. While beneficial, they should only make up a small percentage of the overall diet.

Protein is another critical element to consider. As chickens prepare for winter, their molting process usually occurs. This is when they shed old feathers and grow new ones, and it requires a good deal of protein. Thus, upping the protein content in their diet can be beneficial. This can come from high-protein grains like quinoa or buckwheat, or from mealworms or other insect treats.

Adding more greens might seem counterintuitive in a season where everything is turning brown, but dark leafy greens are packed full of vitamins and nutrients that can help boost your chickens' immune system during the colder months. Kale, spinach, or beet greens can be hung in the coop for chickens to peck at throughout the day.

Supplementing their diet with additional fats is another way to support your flock in the fall. Flaxseeds are a great option because they provide not only fats but also valuable Omega-3 fatty acids. These fats provide an extra energy source that chickens can tap into during the colder winter months.

As we embrace the charm of autumn and its promise of a cozy winter, let's delve deeper into the topic of winter preparations for your flock. After addressing their nutritional needs, it's time to turn our focus towards our feathered friends' overall environment. This includes their coop, the outdoor enclosure, and any other space your chickens use on a regular basis.

When it comes to winter preparation, the coop is the heart of the matter. This is where your chickens will spend most of their time during the cold months, and ensuring it provides adequate warmth and protection is paramount. There are several key aspects to consider when evaluating and winterizing your coop.

First and foremost, the coop should provide protection from the elements. Wind, snow, and ice can be extremely uncomfortable, if not downright dangerous, for your chickens. A good coop will have solid walls to block out the wind and a watertight roof to keep everything dry. If your coop is lacking in either of these areas, autumn is the perfect time to make improvements.

Insulation is another critical factor in coop comfort. It's important to remember that chickens are pretty hardy creatures, and they have their own built-in layer of insulation: feathers. However, a well-insulated coop can make their winter experience more pleasant. Straw bales stacked around the coop can add a layer of insulation and can also be a fun place for chickens to peck and scratch.

Ventilation is a factor that's often overlooked, but it plays a crucial role in maintaining a healthy environment inside the coop. During winter, the coop doors and windows will often be closed to keep out the cold, but this can lead to a build-up of moisture from the chickens' breath and droppings. Too much moisture can lead to respiratory issues and frostbite. So, make sure your coop has adequate ventilation, allowing fresh air in and moist air out.

The coop's interior layout might also need some adjustments. Roosting bars are where your chickens will sleep and spend much of their time. They should be positioned away from drafts, but still have good air circulation. Lowering the roosting bars can help prevent injuries if a chicken slips due to frost or ice.

Now, let's step outside the coop and examine the run or any other outdoor space your chickens have access to. It's a good idea to have a covered area where your chickens can escape from falling snow or sleet. This can be as simple as a tarp strung up over part of the run or a lean-to built off the side of the coop. You may want to consider wrapping your run so your chickens aren't exposed to freezing temperatures. There are many options for materials to wrap your run with, from tarps to 6ml painter's plastic. Providing an outdoor space where your chickens can get fresh air, even in bad weather, can help prevent cabin fever.

Water access is another vital consideration during the winter months. Chickens need access to fresh, unfrozen water every day. Heated waterers can be a worthwhile investment, especially in areas with harsh winters.

Keeping these points in mind and preparing accordingly during autumn will provide a safe, comfortable winter habitat for your chickens. As you make these changes, remember to observe your chickens. They're the best indicator of whether or not the environment meets their needs.

Part IV: Winter Warm-ups: Herbal Tonics for the Cold Months

Let's shift our focus now to the heart of winter, a season often synonymous with chills, frosty mornings, and snowy landscapes. While there's a stark beauty to the season, for our feathered friends, winter presents a unique set of challenges and demands special care, particularly in terms of providing warmth and supporting their overall health.

When the mercury drops, chickens, much like us, experience a series of physiological changes. They fluff up their feathers to trap warm air close to their bodies and spend more time in the coop to escape the cold. They might huddle together on the roost at night to share body heat.

Chickens are fairly resilient to the cold thanks to their feather insulation and high metabolism, but that doesn't mean we can't help improve their comfort and well-being during this frosty season.

Just as you swap your salads for soups during winter, chickens also need an adjusted diet. They require more energy to maintain their body temperature, which means their food intake increases. Their nutritional needs shift towards energy-dense foods that help them generate more heat. We'll delve deeper into winter nutrition in a bit, but for now, let's focus on understanding why these changes are necessary.

As we touched on earlier, winter comes with shorter days and longer nights. This reduction in sunlight impacts the laying habits of chickens. Most hens reduce or even cease laying during winter, reserving their energy for warmth instead of egg production. This natural pause gives their reproductive system a much-needed break. As caregivers, it's our responsibility to respect and support this natural cycle rather than fight it.

Another crucial aspect of winter care is to be on the lookout for signs of frostbite, a common issue in the winter months. Chicken combs, wattles, and feet are most susceptible to frostbite, as they are unfeathered and have more direct exposure to the cold. Regular checks and immediate treatment, if any signs of frostbite are noticed, can save your chickens a lot of discomfort.

The importance of providing warmth to your chickens during winter extends beyond just physical well-being. Chickens, like many animals, can get moody or stressed due to uncomfortable weather conditions. Long-term stress can lower their immunity, making them more prone to diseases. A stressed chicken is an unhappy chicken, and we all want our flocks to be as happy as they can be, don't we?

So, what can you do to ensure your chickens stay warm and comfortable in winter? One effective strategy involves using warming herbs and tonics, both as a preventive measure and a treatment method. These herbs work by boosting your chickens' natural defenses, supporting their immunity, and providing them with extra nutrients to manage the cold better. Winter care for your chickens isn't just about providing heat; it's about understanding and catering to their changing needs. It's about being proactive so small issues don't turn into larger problems. Most importantly, it's about nurturing a space where your chickens can thrive, not just survive, during the cold months.

A wonderful place to start when thinking about winter warmers is to consider incorporating garlic and thyme into your chickens' care regimen. Both of these herbs have a long-standing reputation in both the culinary world and traditional medicine for their powerful properties. Let's dig deeper into why they deserve a place in your winter chicken care toolkit.

Garlic, the fragrant bulb that's a staple in kitchens worldwide, is nothing short of a superfood for your chickens. Bursting with compounds like allicin and sulfur, it's a potent natural antibiotic. It's antifungal, antiviral, and has antioxidant properties, making it a brilliant ally in boosting your chickens' immunity.

An added benefit of garlic is that it's a natural wormer. Parasites can be a problem any time of the year, but why not give your chickens that extra bit of protection during winter? Including crushed or minced garlic in your flock's water can help rid them of internal parasites and promote overall gut health. Remember, a healthy gut contributes to a healthy immune system.

Not to forget, chickens seem to enjoy the taste of garlic. Introducing this powerful bulb into their diet can also stimulate their appetite, encouraging them to eat more and thus helping them maintain their body temperature.

Now, let's turn the spotlight on thyme. This aromatic herb is a source of vitamins A and C and contains essential minerals like iron, magnesium, and potassium. Vitamin C is particularly important during winter, as it can help support your chickens' immune system, allowing them to better ward off potential infections.

Thyme also possesses potent antiseptic properties, which can come in handy if any of your chickens get small cuts or wounds. The essential oils present in thyme, such as thymol, have shown to be effective in controlling and eliminating certain harmful organisms. And if you thought that was impressive, wait until you hear that thyme is also a natural decongestant. It can help alleviate respiratory issues, a common concern in the cold winter months when chickens spend more time huddled up inside the coop.

There are multiple ways to incorporate garlic and thyme into your chickens' winter regimen. A simple method is to add crushed garlic cloves and dried thyme to their water or sprinkle it over their feed. You could even make an herbal tonic by steeping these herbs in hot water, allowing it to cool, and then offering it to your chickens. Remember, though, that moderation is key. Too much of any herb can be overwhelming and even detrimental to your chickens.

Let's be clear: garlic and thyme are not magic bullets. They won't single-handedly keep your chickens warm and healthy throughout winter. What they offer, instead, are additional layers of support, enabling your chickens to better manage the cold season. They are valuable tools in your winter care kit, complementing other essential care practices like providing adequate shelter, fresh food, and clean water.

Garlic and thyme are just two of the many herbal stars that can shine bright in your chickens' winter care routine. They are fantastic, but they work best in combination with other warming herbs and thoughtful practices. So, let's delve into some remedies and ideas for winter wellness that can elevate your flock's health during those chilly months.

1. Winter Wellness Tonic

Ingredients:

- 4 cloves of garlic, crushed
- 2 tablespoons of fresh thyme leaves
- 2 tablespoons of dried oregano
- 1 tablespoon of crushed ginger root
- Apple cider vinegar

Instructions:

a. Mix garlic, thyme, oregano, and ginger root in a glass jar.
b. Cover with apple cider vinegar, ensuring all ingredients are submerged.
c. Seal the jar and let it steep in a cool, dark place for 2-4 weeks.
d. Strain and add a tablespoon per gallon of water of this tonic to your chickens' waterer.

This tonic brings together the antiviral, antibacterial properties of garlic, the respiratory support of thyme, the immune-boosting oregano, and ginger's warmth. It's a powerhouse of protection for winter.

2. Spiced Warming Feed Mix

Ingredients:

- 4 cups of regular chicken feed
- 2 tablespoons of crushed fenugreek seeds
- 1 tablespoon of ground cinnamon
- 1 tablespoon of dried, crushed rosemary

Instructions:

a. Mix the regular chicken feed with the fenugreek seeds, cinnamon, and rosemary.
b. Serve as usual. You can use this mix daily.

Fenugreek can provide warmth, cinnamon offers a sweet-spicy touch chickens enjoy, and rosemary is renowned for its digestion support. This is a comforting, warm meal for those cold days.

3. Respiratory Relief Steam

Ingredients:

- Fresh eucalyptus leaves
- Fresh mint leaves
- Boiling water

Instructions:

a. Place eucalyptus and mint leaves in a large heat-resistant bowl.
b. Pour boiling water over the leaves and place the bowl in your chicken coop.
c. Allow the steam to fill the area, providing respiratory relief for any congested chickens.

Eucalyptus and mint are fantastic natural decongestants, and this steam treatment can be a soothing experience for your chickens on those damp, cold days.

4. Herbal Immunity Mash

Ingredients:

- Your chicken feed
- 1 tablespoon of turmeric powder
- 1 tablespoon of dried nettle leaves
- A handful of crushed elderberries

Note: If you would like to serve this to them warm, you could always allow the chicken feed to soak in some hot water for 10 to 15 minutes. Test the mixture on the inside of your wrist before you serve this to your chickens to be sure you will not scald their mouth.

Instructions:

a. Mix cooked oats or barley with turmeric, dried nettle leaves, and elderberries.
b. Serve warm as a treat.

Here, turmeric acts as a natural anti-inflammatory, nettle is packed with vital nutrients, and elderberries offer immune support. It's a nourishing dish that can be served as a special treat.

These remedies are more than just food; they are a means of connection, care, and support for your chickens during a challenging season. They combine the wisdom of traditional herbal practices with practical poultry care.

You may tailor these remedies according to your flock's specific needs or preferences. The key is to observe, understand, and be willing to adapt. Each ingredient, each mix, and every practice should align with the unique needs of your chickens.

Observing and adapting to the unique needs of your chickens will lead you to ensure your chickens' comfort and health through the coldest months. While the earlier remedies are tools to help you along the way, they are part of a broader, more holistic approach that calls for a complete understanding of what your chickens need during winter. Let's dive into these areas of focus that can help you create a comforting and healthy environment for your flock.

During winter, the importance of shelter cannot be overstated. Chickens need a dry, draft-free, yet well-ventilated space to roost. Insulating the coop without sealing it entirely helps maintain an even temperature, and using deep bedding, like straw, can create a warm floor. Regular checks for any leaks or drafts and fixing them promptly can keep your chickens warm and protected.

Water access can be a challenge in freezing temperatures. Ensuring a constant supply of fresh, unfrozen water is vital. Heated waterers or simple solutions like placing a small, safe heater near the water source can make a significant difference. Staying vigilant for icy conditions and being ready to replace the water if it does freeze is a daily task that pays off in healthy, hydrated chickens.

Beyond the warming herbs and spices, your chickens may need more calories during the cold season to maintain body temperature. Including more grains like corn in their diet or increasing the regular feed just slightly can meet this need. Balancing these additional calories with sufficient protein and other nutrients ensures a well-rounded winter diet.

Though snow and cold can restrict some outdoor activities, creating opportunities for exploration is crucial. Covered runs, windbreaks using hay bales or wooden planks, and even temporary structures to protect against snow can make outside areas more accessible. Placing perches, treat baskets, or other engagement tools in these protected spaces gives your chickens the incentive to explore, exercise, and stay mentally stimulated.

Winter can be hard on chickens, especially the young and old. Regular health checks for signs of frostbite, respiratory issues, or general distress can catch problems early. Having a first-aid kit ready, with essentials like petroleum jelly for combs and wattles, herbal salves for minor cuts or frostbites, and some essential oils like lavender for calming stressed birds, can be a lifesaver.

The shorter days of winter can affect laying patterns. While some keepers use artificial lighting to maintain egg production, it's a choice that requires careful consideration. If you decide to add light, do so gradually, and monitor your chickens for any signs of stress or fatigue. Winter is the time of year when hens get a well-deserved break from their laying cycle. We should learn to allow them to have this time to focus on using their energy to get through the winter. Respecting their natural rhythms means accepting reduced laying and focusing on their overall well-being.

Winter cleaning is different but no less critical. A damp coop can become a breeding ground for disease. Regular cleaning, making sure bedding is dry, and maintaining good ventilation without drafts can keep the coop healthy. Integrating herbs like mint, lavender, or pine shavings can add a fresh scent, and some added antibacterial benefits.

Your presence, your touch, your voice - these connections with your flock are more important in winter when life can become a bit more isolated for your chickens. Regular interactions, talking to them, handling them gently, and observing their behaviors closely can make winter a time of deepening bonds. We want to create a winter world where your chickens feel safe, warm, nourished, engaged, and loved. It's about balancing their physical needs with their emotional ones and being present and attentive to their unique personalities and preferences.

Winter care for chickens is not just a series of tasks; it's a philosophy of life. It's about embracing the season, understanding its challenges and beauty, and navigating it with grace and compassion.

Just remember that all of these remedies mentioned throughout the book are designed as a supplement to, not a replacement for, a balanced chicken diet. Your chickens still need their regular feed to get the full spectrum of nutrients necessary for their health and productivity. Over-supplementing one nutrient while forgetting about others can lead to a diet that doesn't fully support the broad spectrum of your chickens' needs. Equally, it's important to remember that chickens are individuals. Some might gobble up ginger and cinnamon with glee, while others might prefer fenugreek or fennel seeds. Observing your flock's reactions and preferences can guide adjustments and modifications to their diet. Your understanding of your chickens' behaviors, preferences, and needs will be instrumental in applying these concepts effectively.

The Cooked Oatmeal Mistake: Why This Common Treat is a No-No for Chickens

Winter has a way of inspiring compassionate chicken keepers to serve their backyard chickens a steaming bowl of oatmeal. These images, filled with warmth and affection, seem perfect for the season. But is this popular and seemingly innocent treat truly suitable for your feathered friends? Let's explore the truth behind oatmeal for chickens.

The controversy surrounding oatmeal as a treat for chickens is rooted in good reason. While it's a staple breakfast for humans, filled with health benefits, chickens are not little people with feathers. They have unique dietary needs, and oatmeal, unfortunately, is detrimental to their health.

The key issue lies in oats' content of beta-glucan. This compound is poorly digested by chickens and can form a thick gel-like substance in their intestines. The consequences of this can be severe, leading to conditions like necrotic enteritis and preventing the absorption of vital nutrients. A chicken's resilience during winter hinges on a nutritionally sound diet, and oatmeal can dilute their diet, making them less capable of absorbing essential nutrients from their regular feed.

It might seem like a small act of kindness, offering a warm bowl of oatmeal, but it's essential to understand the underlying risks. You invest in high-quality, complete feeds, and it's counterproductive to undermine that investment with foods that not only offer no benefit but might actually harm your flock.

So, what can you do if you're tempted to offer a warm treat during the cold months? The solution is delightfully simple and nutritious. Replace the oatmeal with their everyday LAYER FEED. Just add warm water to pellets or crumbles and serve it in their designated feed bowl or tray. If you wish to elevate this treat, a sprinkle of cinnamon or a thoughtful addition of seeds, fruits, veggies, mealworms, or other favorite treats can create a "gourmet" version. Just remember to exercise restraint with these extras.

In the end, understanding the difference between human and chicken dietary needs helps avoid well-intentioned mistakes. By embracing alternatives, you can still offer warmth and love without compromising your flock's health. The winter months can be a time of nourishment, comfort, and joy without risking the well-being of your cherished chickens. It all comes down to informed choices and thoughtful care.

Epilogue: A Journey Beyond the Coop

The journey you've embarked upon in these pages goes far beyond the confines of a chicken coop or the boundaries of a backyard. It's a journey into a world where simplicity meets complexity, where tradition dances with innovation, and where understanding blossoms into empathy.

From the first crow of a rooster to the last settling cackle at dusk, you've explored the multifaceted universe that exists in the company of chickens. You've discovered the magic that resides in the everyday, in the clucking of a hen or the intricate design of a feather. You've uncovered secrets that turn mundane tasks into mindful rituals.

The wisdom gathered here is not meant to be a definitive guide but a trusted companion, a friend that accompanies you on your own unique path. Each flock is different; each chicken keeper's experience is distinct. Embrace that uniqueness. Celebrate it. Allow it to guide you to new understandings and deeper connections.

As you close this book, know that the journey is far from over. In the appendices that follow, you'll find valuable information, resources, and remedies. Consider it a treasure trove filled with the practical magic of herbs.

But more than that, let this book be a reminder that life's most profound lessons often come dressed in feathers and clucking softly from a nest. Let it inspire you to pause, listen, observe, and appreciate your feathered friends.

Chickens, in their humble and profound way, have the ability to transform a backyard into a sanctuary, a daily routine into a dance, and a simple egg into a symbol of life's extraordinary beauty.

May your journey with chickens be filled with discovery, joy, and the deep satisfaction that comes from a connection well-nurtured.

See you in the coop, dear friends. The adventure has only just begun.

With gratitude,

Miss Mary and her HAPPY Chickens

P.S.: Don't forget to explore the appendices. They're packed with gems waiting to spark your curiosity and ignite your creativity. From herbal concoctions to delightful remedies for your flock, it's a garden of delights that continues the conversation we've started here.

Appendix 1

Cluckin' Good Greens: Safe Herbs for Your Feathered Friends

Herbs, spices, and plants have long played an essential role in human and animal nutrition. When it comes to chickens, these plants can provide numerous benefits, from enhancing flavor in eggs to promoting overall health and well-being. Here's a guide about the different herbs and spices that are safe and beneficial for your feathered friends:

A List of Safe Herbs, Spices, and Plants for Your Chickens, Including Their Beneficial Properties for Your Flock

- Aloe Vera: Supports digestive health and can be applied topically for skin issues.
- Anise Seed: Stimulates laying and aids in digestion.
- Arnica: Topical use in wound healing.
- Basil: Enhances the respiratory health of chickens and acts as an antibacterial agent.
- Black Pepper: Can be used in small amounts to aid digestion
- Borage: Stimulates laying and has a positive impact on respiratory health.
- Calendula: Enhances yolk color and has anti-inflammatory properties.
- Caraway Seeds: Supports digestive function.
- Cardamom: Rich in nutrients and supports respiratory health
- Catnip: Acts as a natural insect repellent.
- Chamomile: Calming and relaxing, this herb is also an anti-inflammatory.
- Cayenne Pepper: Improves blood circulation and can be a metabolic stimulant.
- Chervil: High in vitamins and minerals, supports overall health.
- Chicory: Aids in parasite prevention and digestion.
- Cilantro: Aids in digestion.
- Cinnamon: Supports digestive wellness and has natural antibacterial qualities.
- Comfrey: Known for skin healing properties, supports bone health and respiratory health.
- Coriander Seeds: Boosts digestive function..
- Cumin: Aids in digestion.
- Dandelion: A great source of vitamins and minerals, aids in digestion.
- Dill: Supports both digestion and respiratory function.
- Echinacea: Known for boosting the immune system and promoting overall well-being.
- Elderberry (only the berries of the plant): Known for boosting the immune system and provides respiratory support.
- Fennel: Stimulates egg laying and supports overall reproductive health.
- Fenugreek: Supports digestive health.
- Feverfew: Natural insect repellent.
- Garlic: Boosts immunity and acts as a natural wormer.
- Ginger: Stimulates digestion and is helpful during molting
- Hops: Calming effect may help with anxious chickens.
- Horsetail: Supports feather growth and bone health.
- Kale: High in nutrients and antioxidants, great for general health.
- Lavender: Has a calming effect and can be used to reduce stress and promote relaxation.
- Lemon Balm: Acts as a calming herb and is a nice treat for chickens.
- Lemongrass: Aromatic, acts as an insect repellent.

- Marjoram: Known to be a laying stimulant for hens.
- Mint: Aids in digestion, and its strong aroma helps in pest control around the coop.
- Mugwort: Parasite control and digestive aid.
- Mustard Greens: Stimulates egg laying.
- Nettle: High in nutrients, nettle supports blood health and vitality. Great for egg production.
- Nutmeg: Contains antibacterial properties. Use in small amounts.
- Oregano: Known for its antibiotic properties, oregano can boost the immune system.
- Papaya Leaf: Aids in digestion, especially proteins.
- Paprika: Enhances yolk color and is a rich source of vitamins.
- Parsley: Rich in vitamins, it can boost egg production and is known to help during molting.
- Red Clover: Supports respiratory health and laying.
- Rosemary: Supports respiratory health and provides overall well-being.
- Sage: Contains antioxidant properties and supports general wellness.
- Sorrel: Rich in Vitamin C and supports digestive health.
- Tarragon: An aromatic herb that chickens love and supports appetite
- Thyme: Supports respiratory health and contains antibacterial properties.
- Turmeric: Contains anti-inflammatory properties and promotes vibrant plumage.
- Valerian: Calming effect, good for stressed or nervous birds.
- Watercress: High in vitamins and promotes overall wellness.
- Wheatgrass: Nutrient-dense and provides support for overall vitality.
- White Pepper: Similar to black pepper, aids digestion. Use in small amounts.
- Wood Betony: Calms nerves and supports digestion.
- Yarrow: Acts as a natural astringent and supports wound healing.
- Zinnia Flowers: Add color and can have calming effects.

Notes:
- Quality Matters: Always source herbs from a reputable provider or grow them yourself to ensure they are free from pesticides and other harmful chemicals.
- Moderation is Key: Herbs should be used as a supplemental addition to a balanced chicken diet, not as a replacement for proper nutrition.
- Research Each Herb: Understanding each herb's unique properties helps you use them effectively.
- Fresh vs. Dried: Both fresh and dried herbs can be used, but remember that drying concentrates the properties.
- Experiment and Observe: Different chickens may have different preferences, so feel free to experiment with various herbs and observe which ones your chickens seem to favor.
- Drying and Storing: If you have an abundance of fresh herbs, consider drying them for later use. Drying retains the essential oils and flavors, and dried herbs can be stored for months, ensuring a steady supply for your flock.
- Creative Serving Ideas: You can serve herbs fresh, dried, or even brewed as a tea. Mix them into the feed, scatter them around the coop, or add them to nesting boxes to create a stimulating and enriching environment for your chickens.
- Home-Grown Advantage: Growing these herbs at home not only ensures quality but also provides a fun project that connects your gardening with the care of your chickens.

Exploring the world of herbs and spices with your chickens can be a rewarding experience, not only in terms of their health benefits but also in engaging your chickens' senses. It's a way to enrich their environment and diet while knowing you are providing natural and wholesome additions that contribute to their well-being. Feel free to mix and match, and let your flock enjoy the flavors of these herbs and spices!

Fowl Foliage: Herbs to Avoid in Your Chicken Coop

While many herbs and spices are beneficial for your flock, some can be quite harmful or even deadly. It's vital to understand which plants to keep away from your coop and your chickens' foraging areas. Let's delve into a list of herbs, plants, and spices that are toxic to chickens and why they should be avoided.

A List of Toxic Herbs, Plants and Spices

- Aconite (Monkshood): Highly poisonous, affects the heart, and can lead to death.
- Autumn Crocus: Contains colchicine, causing gastrointestinal problems.
- Azalea: Contains toxins that can cause gastrointestinal irritation, drooling, and diarrhea.
- Belladonna (Deadly Nightshade): Highly toxic due to the presence of atropine and scopolamine.
- Bleeding Heart: May lead to convulsions and heart issues.
- Bloodroot: Contains sanguinarine, which is harmful to the digestive system.
- Boxwood: May cause vomiting, diarrhea, and respiratory failure.
- Bracken Fern: Known to cause bracken poisoning, leading to blood clotting disorders.
- Buttercup: Irritates the digestive tract and may lead to mouth sores.
- Caladium: Can lead to oral irritation, drooling, and difficulty swallowing.
- Calla Lily: Contains oxalates, leading to oral pain and digestive problems.
- Cassia (a type of cinnamon): Contains coumarin, which may cause liver damage.
- Castor Bean Plant: Contains ricin, one of the most toxic substances known, leading to severe abdominal pain, drooling, and convulsions.
- Cherry Trees: Wilted cherry leaves produce cyanide, a deadly toxin.
- Chrysanthemum: Contains pyrethrins that may affect the nervous system.
- Daffodil: The bulb is the most toxic part, causing severe gastrointestinal issues.
- Datura (Jimson Weed): Highly toxic; causes hallucinations and seizures.
- Elderberry (leaves and stems): While the berries are very beneficial to your flock the leaves and stems contain cyanogenic glycosides that can lead to cyanide poisoning.
- Foxglove: Contains digitalis, known for heart disturbances.
- Golden Chain Tree: Contains alkaloids that affect the nervous system.
- Hellebore: Toxic to the heart, leads to drooling, abdominal pain, and collapse.
- Hemlock: All parts are toxic, which leads to nervous system disorders.
- Horse Chestnut: May cause vomiting and abdominal pain.
- Hydrangea: Contains cyanogenic glycosides, which can be lethal.
- Iris: Causes severe digestive disturbances.
- Ivy: Causes gastrointestinal problems and labored breathing.
- Jack-in-the-Pulpit: Leads to irritation of the mouth and throat.
- Jerusalem Cherry: Contains solanocapsine, affecting the gastrointestinal system.
- Lantana: Damages the liver, leading to jaundice and weakness.
- Larkspur: May cause neuromuscular paralysis.
- Lily of the Valley: Contains cardiac glycosides, affecting the heart.
- Lupine: Certain species may cause nervousness and difficulty breathing.
- Mayapple: Toxic except for the ripe fruit, causing digestive problems.
- Mistletoe: Known to cause gastrointestinal problems and difficulty breathing.
- Morning Glory: Seeds may cause hallucinations and diarrhea.

- Mountain Laurel: Affects the digestive and nervous systems.
- Oleander: All parts are toxic, affects the heart, and can be fatal.
- Pokeweed: Affects the digestive system, leading to drooling, convulsions, and difficulty breathing.
- Poinsettia: Causes mouth irritation and stomach upset.
- Privet: Leads to gastrointestinal and heart issues.
- Rhubarb: Leaves contain oxalic acid, leading to kidney problems.
- Sago Palm: Highly toxic, leads to liver failure.
- Sweet Pea: Contains amino acids that can cause nervous symptoms.
- Tansy: May cause vomiting, seizures, and miscarriages in hens.
- Tobacco: All parts are toxic, leading to hyperexcitability and convulsions.
- Yellow Jasmine: All parts are toxic, affecting the heart and nervous system.
- Yew: Highly toxic, affects the central nervous system, and can lead to death.
- Nutmeg (in high quantities): Can cause hallucinations and seizures.
- Salt: Though not a spice, excessive salt can lead to salt poisoning.

This list covers a wide range of plants that could be found in gardens or wild landscapes and highlights the importance of being cautious with the environment your chickens inhabit. The information about these herbs, plants, and spices should serve as a guide to ensure the safety of your flock and help you recognize any unusual behavior that could be a sign of poisoning.

Always remember to balance the diet of your chickens with safe and nutritious foods and avoid the temptation to feed them leftovers or scraps that might contain these harmful substances. It's all about creating a nurturing and secure environment for your feathered friends to thrive.

Notes:
- It's not only the knowledge of what plants to avoid that's essential but understanding why they should be avoided can assist in making educated choices about planting around the coop or feeding scraps.
- Sensitivity Varies: Some chickens may be more sensitive to certain plants, and reactions can vary.
- Unpredictable Reactions: Even if a plant is only mildly toxic to chickens, the reaction can be unpredictable.
- Secure the Coop Area: Make sure that toxic plants are not accessible within the chicken's reach.
- Being aware of these potentially harmful herbs, spices, and plants helps ensure a safe environment for your flock. It's a crucial part of responsible chicken care and can prevent unnecessary suffering or even the tragic loss of a feathered friend. Always double-check the safety of any plant you intend to introduce to your chickens, and when in doubt, err on the side of caution.

✳This list is by no means exhaustive; it is provided to educate you and spark your curiosity to investigate more herbs. Whether an herb is considered safe or should be avoided, it's always wise to research each one individually. Doing so will not only enhance your understanding but also help you grasp the specific effects that the herb may have on your flock.

Herbal Suppliers and Resources for Purchasing Quality Herbs

When it comes to using herbs for your chickens, quality is paramount. Fresh, organic, and sustainably sourced herbs ensure the health and well-being of your flock. Here's a list of suppliers and resources that can be your go-to places for quality herbal products. I am not affiliated with any of the suppliers mentioned below.

Reputable Herbal Suppliers

1. Mountain Rose Herbs: Specializing in certified organic herbs and essential oils. Perfect for those looking to support sustainable farming.
2. Starwest Botanicals: Offers a broad range of bulk herbs and spices. They also carry certified organic products.
3. Frontier Co-op: With a focus on natural and organic products, Frontier is committed to ethical sourcing.
4. Bulk Herb Store: A family-owned business providing quality herbs and educational resources.
5. Penn Herb Company: Established in 1924, Penn offers quality herbs and natural remedies.
6. Herb Pharm: If tinctures and herbal extracts are what you need, Herb Pharm has a wide selection.
7. Pacific Botanicals: Committed to organic and wildcrafted herbs, they focus on purity and quality.
8. Dandelion Botanical Company: Known for their handcrafted products and commitment to the environment.
9. Blessed Herbs: Offers a variety of cleansing products and herbal blends.
10. Banyan Botanicals: They provide Ayurvedic herbs and products, focusing on sustainable sourcing.
11. Jean's Greens Herbal Tea Works & Herbal Essentials: A reliable source of tea herbs, oils, and natural beauty products.
12. Monterey Bay Spice Company: With a large selection of organic and conventional herbs, it's a great option for bulk purchases.
13. Nature's Herbal: Family-operated and specializing in locally sourced and wildcrafted herbs.
14. Earthwise Organics: Offers a variety of herbal products, including special blends for chickens.
15. The Growers Exchange: Ideal for those who want to grow herbs themselves. They offer quality plant starters.
16. Kalyx: With a vast catalog of herbs and natural products, Kalyx provides both bulk and retail options.
17. Herbalist & Alchemist: They offer herbal extracts, compounds, and custom formulations.
18. Bio-Botanica®: Known for its organic, kosher, and halal-certified products, specializing in herbal extracts.
19. Botanic Universe: A one-stop shop for essential oils, herbs, and botanicals.
20. Dragon Herbs: They provide Chinese herbs, herbal products, and supplements.

Notes:

- Selecting a reputable supplier is crucial in ensuring that the herbs are of high quality, ethically sourced, and free from contaminants. It's also wise to consider the freshness of the herbs, as freshly harvested herbs often have higher potency.
- Always look for suppliers that provide details about the origins of the herbs, growing methods, and any certifications like organic, kosher, or halal. Some suppliers even provide lab testing reports, ensuring that the herbs meet specific quality standards.
- Consider subscribing to newsletters or blogs of these suppliers, as they often share valuable insights and knowledge about herbs, their uses, and how to incorporate them into daily life.

Appendix 2
Dosage and Safety Guidelines for Herbal Treatments

Understanding Safe Dosages for Herbal Treatments

Herbal treatments are a wonderful way to enrich the lives of our chickens, providing natural solutions to common health concerns and enhancing their overall well-being. But as with anything in life, balance is key, and understanding the safe dosages for herbal treatments is vital.

When dealing with herbs, it's essential to remember that chickens are not just smaller versions of humans. They have unique digestive systems, metabolic rates, and sensitivities. What may seem like a small amount to us can be a significant dose for them. Therefore, accurate knowledge of the correct dosages becomes not just a matter of efficacy but of safety.

One of the first steps in understanding safe dosages is recognizing the potency of herbs. Different herbs have different levels of potency, and this can be influenced by factors such as the growing conditions, harvest time, and preparation method. A carefully cultivated herb can have a significantly different impact on a chicken's system than the same herb grown under different conditions.

Next, let's look at the individual needs of your chickens. Factors like age, size, breed, and current health can all play a role in how an herb will affect them. Younger birds might be more sensitive, and a bird that's already under the weather might react differently to a particular herb. Being mindful of these factors allows for a more tailored approach to herbal treatments, ensuring that the benefits are maximized without risking harm.

Dosages should be carefully measured and consistently applied. Using standardized measurements like teaspoons or grams can help with this. Avoid eyeballing or estimating, as small variations can make a big difference. It's a good idea to start with a smaller dose and observe how your flock reacts. If all seems well, the dosage can be gradually increased to the recommended level. Remember, each flock is different, and what works for one may not be suitable for another.

Also, the form in which the herb is administered can affect the dosage. Fresh herbs, dried herbs, tinctures, and oils all require different measurements. For example, dried herbs are typically more concentrated than fresh ones, so a smaller amount will often suffice. Understanding these distinctions and adjusting dosages accordingly is an essential part of safe herbal treatment.

It's equally important to be aware of potential interactions between herbs and other supplements or medications your chickens might be receiving. While herbs offer many benefits, they are not always compatible with other substances. Researching and consulting with knowledgeable experts can prevent unintended side effects or reduced efficacy of the treatment.

Please keep in mind that not all herbs are suitable for all chickens, and some might even be toxic in certain situations. Knowledge of what to avoid is as vital as knowing what to use. The same herb that might soothe one condition could exacerbate another. This emphasizes the importance of a holistic understanding of your flock's needs and the specific properties of the herbs you're using.

Here are some guidelines for safe dosages of common herbs used for chickens. It's essential to note that these are general recommendations and might need to be adjusted based on your flock's specific needs, size, and breed.

Garlic
- Mixed into Feed: 1-2 crushed cloves per chicken, mixed into daily feed.
- Water: 1 clove per gallon of water, minced or crushed.
- Given Directly: A small minced clove can be offered directly.

Oregano
- Mixed into Feed: 1-2 teaspoons of dried oregano per chicken per week.
- Water: A pinch of dried oregano per gallon of water.
- Tincture: If using an oregano tincture, 1-2 drops per chicken diluted in water.

Thyme
- Mixed into Feed: 1 teaspoon of dried thyme per chicken per week.
- Water: 1 teaspoon per gallon of water.
- Given Directly: Fresh thyme leaves can be offered directly as a treat.

Lavender
- Mixed into Feed: 1 teaspoon of dried lavender per chicken per week.
- Water: 2 teaspoons per gallon of water for a calming effect.
- Tincture: Use sparingly 1-2 drops of lavender tincture per chicken.

Mint
- Mixed into Feed: 1-2 teaspoons dried mint per chicken per week.
- Water: 1-2 sprigs of fresh mint per gallon of water.
- Given Directly: Fresh mint leaves can be offered directly.

Chamomile
- Mixed into Feed: 1 teaspoon dried chamomile per chicken per week.
- Water: 1-2 teaspoons of dried chamomile per gallon of water.
- Tincture: 1-2 drops of chamomile tincture per chicken, diluted.

Nettle
- Mixed into Feed: 1 teaspoon dried nettle per chicken per week.
- Water: A pinch of dried nettle per gallon of water.
- Given Directly: Fresh nettle (wilted to remove sting) can be offered directly.

Basil
- Mixed into Feed: 1 teaspoon dried or fresh basil per chicken per week.
- Water: 1 teaspoon of fresh basil per gallon of water.
- Given Directly: Fresh basil leaves can be offered directly.

Sage

- Mixed into Feed: 1 teaspoon dried sage per chicken per week.
- Water: A small pinch of dried sage per gallon of water.
- Tincture: 1 drop of sage tincture per chicken, diluted.

Parsley
- Mixed into Feed: 1 tablespoon of fresh parsley per chicken per week.
- Water: 1 teaspoon of fresh parsley per gallon of water.
- Given Directly: Fresh parsley sprigs can be offered directly.

Dandelion
- Mixed into Feed: Fresh or dried dandelion leaves can be mixed at a ratio of 1 teaspoon per chicken per week.
- Water: A small handful of fresh dandelion leaves per gallon of water.
- Given Directly: Fresh dandelion leaves and flowers can be offered directly.

Rosemary
- Mixed into Feed: 1 teaspoon dried rosemary per chicken per week.
- Water: 1 sprig of fresh rosemary per gallon of water.
- Tincture: 1-2 drops of rosemary tincture per chicken, diluted.

Marjoram
- Mixed into Feed: 1 teaspoon dried marjoram per chicken per week.
- Water: A small pinch of dried marjoram per gallon of water.
- Given Directly: Fresh marjoram leaves can be offered directly.

Fennel Seeds
- Mixed into Feed: 1 teaspoon of fennel seeds per chicken per week.
- Water: 1/2 teaspoon of fennel seeds per gallon of water.
- Given Directly: A small pinch of fennel seeds can be offered directly.

Cilantro
- Mixed into Feed: 1 tablespoon of fresh cilantro per chicken per week.
- Water: 1 sprig of fresh cilantro per gallon of water.
- Given Directly: Fresh cilantro leaves can be offered directly.

Turmeric
- Mixed into Feed: 1/4 teaspoon turmeric powder per chicken per week.
- Water: A pinch of turmeric powder per gallon of water.
- Tincture: 1 drop of turmeric tincture per chicken, diluted.

These dosages are a starting point. As with previous guidelines, it's essential to use these herbs in combination with proper care, as discussed in previous chapters. The freshness, quality, and type (dried or fresh) of the herb also play a vital role in determining the proper dosage. Always make sure the herbs are free from pesticides or other chemicals that might be harmful to your flock. Observation and adaptation will be key in ensuring the optimal health and happiness of your chickens. Herbs complement, rather than replace, good husbandry practices such as proper feeding, clean water, and suitable shelter. The key to success with herbal treatments lies in understanding your flock's unique needs and being willing to learn, adapt, and grow along with them.

The Impact of Herb Quality on Safety

Herb quality is a critical factor that directly affects the safety and effectiveness of herbal treatments, not only for humans but also for our feathered friends, such as chickens. Understanding the importance of herb quality in chicken care requires a deeper look into various elements, including the source, freshness, preparation, storage, and potential contamination of herbs.

1. Source of Herbs

- Wild vs. Cultivated: Wild herbs may contain higher levels of active compounds but can also be at risk for contamination with pesticides or pollutants. Cultivated herbs, particularly those grown organically, offer more control over growing conditions.
- Soil Quality: The soil in which the herbs are grown can affect their nutrient content. Nutrient-rich soil typically yields healthier, more potent herbs.
- Location and Climate: The geographical location and the climate where the herbs are grown can also affect their quality. Different regions may have unique soil compositions and weather conditions that influence the herb's growth and chemical composition.

2. Freshness of Herbs

- Dried vs. Fresh: While dried herbs are convenient, they may lose potency over time. Fresh herbs often contain more active compounds but must be used quickly to avoid spoilage.
- Harvest Time: The time of harvest can influence the herb's quality. For example, some herbs are best harvested in the morning when their oil content is highest.

3. Preparation of Herbs

- Processing: How an herb is processed can impact its quality. Over-processing or harsh processing methods can degrade valuable compounds.
- Form: Whether the herb is used as a whole, crushed, or ground can affect how quickly it releases its compounds. This needs to be considered in dosing and safety.

4. Storage of Herbs

- Shelf Life: Herbs, especially dried ones, have a shelf life. Using them past their prime can lead to reduced effectiveness and even potential health risks.
- Storage Conditions: Proper storage conditions (cool, dark, and dry places) can preserve the herb's quality. Improper storage can lead to mold growth or degradation.

5. Potential Contamination

- Pesticides and Chemicals: If not grown organically, herbs might be exposed to various chemicals and pesticides that could remain as residues. This could pose a threat to the health of the chickens.
- Heavy Metals: Contamination with heavy metals like lead or mercury is a concern, especially in wild-collected herbs. These contaminants can lead to serious health problems in chickens.
- Microbial Contamination: Improper handling and storage can lead to contamination with harmful microbes, causing illnesses.

6. Considerations for Specific Treatments

- Tinctures: The quality of the alcohol or apple cider vinegar used in tinctures can affect safety. Using food-grade alcohol is essential. If you opt for apple cider vinegar, the variety with the mother is best.
- Teas and Infusions: Water quality, steeping time, and temperature all play a role in creating a safe and effective herbal tea or infusion.

7. Ethical Considerations

Sustainable Harvesting: Choosing sustainably harvested herbs ensures that wild populations are not depleted and that ecosystems are not harmed.

The quality of herbs plays an invaluable role in the safety and effectiveness of herbal treatments for chickens. By paying attention to the source, freshness, preparation, storage, and potential contamination of herbs, chicken keepers can ensure that their flock benefits from the therapeutic properties of these natural remedies. Awareness and vigilance are essential in selecting and using herbs in a manner that supports the health and well-being of your chickens.

The Importance of Gradual Introduction of New Herbs

Embarking on a journey of incorporating herbal treatments into the care of chickens can be an enlightening and fulfilling experience. Just as in human nutrition and wellness, the potential benefits of herbs for chickens are vast. However, what's vital to recognize is the importance of gradually introducing new herbs to your flock's diet and care routine. The process is not about tossing a blend of herbs into the feed and hoping for the best; it involves mindfulness, observation, and a step-by-step approach. Let's explore why this is so essential and how to do it effectively.

1. Recognizing Individual Needs and Preferences

Chickens, like people, have individual tastes and needs. What may be appealing and beneficial to one chicken may not be the same for another. A gradual introduction allows you to observe how each chicken responds, whether it's a positive reaction, indifference, or even a dislike. This observation helps in tailoring the right blend for your flock.

2. Minimizing the Risk of Adverse Reactions

While herbs generally offer gentle care, the possibility of an adverse reaction cannot be completely ruled out. Introducing herbs gradually minimizes the risk, allowing you to identify any unusual behavior or signs of distress early on. If a negative reaction is observed, the specific herb can be identified and removed or reduced in quantity.

3. Understanding the Digestive Adaptation

Chickens have unique digestive systems, and introducing a new herb can be a new experience for them. A gradual introduction helps the digestive system adapt to the new ingredient, minimizing potential digestive discomfort or upset.

4. Preventing Overwhelm and Confusion

Introducing too many herbs at once can be overwhelming, both for the chickens and for the caregiver. You might find it challenging to discern what's working and what's not. By adding one herb at a time, you create a clear pathway to understanding the effects and benefits of each herb.

5. Ensuring Proper Dosage and Application

The gradual introduction allows you to experiment with different dosages and applications, be it in feed, water, or direct application. It's about finding the 'sweet spot' where the herb is effective but not overpowering or detrimental.

6. Building Trust and Acceptance

Introducing something new to chickens may be met with suspicion or reluctance. Gradually adding herbs can help in building trust, allowing chickens to get used to the new taste or smell. It fosters a sense of acceptance and eases them into the change.

7. Incorporating Herbs into Different Seasons

Not all herbs are suitable for every season. Introducing herbs gradually also means aligning with the seasons and the specific needs of the chickens during that time. This alignment ensures that the herbs are not only accepted but are seasonally appropriate.

8. Appreciating the Role of Each Herb

Each herb has a unique role. By adding them one by one, you develop a deeper understanding and appreciation for what each herb brings to the flock's wellness. It also enables more precise adjustments in the future.

9. Steps for Gradual Introduction

Here's a simple approach to gradually introducing herbs:

- Start Small: Begin with a small amount and watch for reactions.
- One Herb at a Time: Focus on one herb for a week or so before introducing another.

- Observe and Adjust: Pay attention to the flock's reaction and adjust accordingly.
- Keep Records: Documenting the process helps in understanding what works best.

The gradual introduction of herbs into the care of chickens is not just a safety measure; it's an art and science. It's about creating a harmony where each herb finds its place in the symphony of your flock's health and well-being. It's about being present, patient, and perceptive. The path to herbal care for chickens isn't a race but a graceful dance, one step at a time, leading to a more natural, wholesome, and vibrant life for your cherished flock.

Addressing Potential Allergic Reactions in Chickens

When we think of allergies, we often consider human reactions to various substances, ranging from food to pollen. However, it's crucial to understand that chickens, like other animals, can also have sensitivities and even allergic reactions to certain substances, including herbs. The exploration of herbs as a means to enhance the health and well-being of chickens must include a firm understanding of potential allergic reactions. While rare, these reactions can occur, and knowing how to identify and respond to them is a vital part of responsible chicken care.

1. Identifying Potential Allergens

Not all herbs are created equal, and some may have the potential to cause an allergic reaction in certain chickens. Common allergens in humans don't necessarily translate to chickens, so it requires careful observation and understanding.

2. Signs of an Allergic Reaction

Unlike humans, chickens cannot verbally communicate discomfort or distress. Recognizing an allergic reaction in a chicken involves watching for physical signs. Some common indicators might include:

- Skin Irritation: Redness, swelling, or itching, particularly around the face and wattles.
- Respiratory Issues: Difficulty breathing, coughing, or wheezing.
- Digestive Problems: Diarrhea, vomiting, or refusal to eat.
- Behavioral Changes: Increased aggression or withdrawal from the flock.

3. Prevention through Gradual Introduction

As discussed in the previous section, the gradual introduction of new herbs into a chicken's diet or care routine can help in identifying potential allergic reactions. Introducing one herb at a time and observing any changes allows for immediate identification and removal of the offending herb.

4. Immediate Response

If an allergic reaction is suspected, immediate removal of the suspected herb is essential. Monitoring the chicken and providing fresh water and comfort is often the first step in care.

Depending on the severity of the reaction, consultation with a veterinarian or poultry specialist might be necessary.

5. Understanding Cross-Reactivity

In some cases, an allergic reaction to one herb may indicate a sensitivity to others in the same family. Being aware of these relationships can prevent further allergic reactions.

6. Long-term Care and Monitoring

Once an allergic reaction has been identified, long-term care includes the permanent removal of the offending herb from the chicken's diet or care routine. Keeping a record of the reaction can help in future care and the sharing of information with other poultry keepers or professionals.

7. Consideration of Environmental Factors

Sometimes, what appears to be an allergic reaction may be a response to an environmental factor, such as a change in bedding or the introduction of a new cleaning product. Being aware of all changes in a chicken's environment is crucial in accurately identifying and addressing potential allergic reactions.

8. Professional Consultation

In some cases, the guidance of a veterinarian or poultry specialist may be necessary. Building a relationship with a professional who understands both traditional poultry care and herbal treatments can be invaluable in addressing potential allergic reactions.

9. Educating Yourself

Understanding potential allergens and how they may affect chickens requires research and education. Various resources, ranging from books to workshops, can provide essential knowledge in this area.

10. Community Engagement

Connecting with other poultry keepers who utilize herbal treatments can offer support, insights, and shared experiences. Learning from others' successes and challenges can be enlightening.

Addressing potential allergic reactions in chickens is a multifaceted responsibility that requires awareness, observation, and action. While the incidence of allergic reactions in chickens due to herbs may be rare, the possibility cannot be ignored. Creating a safe and nurturing environment for chickens involves understanding their unique needs and responses. The joy of raising chickens and enhancing their lives with herbal treatments comes with the responsibility of recognizing and addressing their individual needs, including the rare but significant occurrence of allergic reactions. In doing so, we foster a more profound connection with our feathered friends and ensure their health, happiness, and well-being.

Understanding the Role of Age, Breed, and Size in Herb Safety

When it comes to administering herbal remedies to chickens, one size certainly does not fit all. The factors of age, breed, and size play a vital role in determining the right approach to herb safety. Each of these factors brings unique considerations that must be taken into account to ensure that herbal treatments are safe and effective.

1. Age Considerations

- Chicks: The young chicks are more sensitive to herbs. Their digestive systems are still developing, and their immunity is not fully formed. Therefore, caution must be exercised when introducing herbs to young birds.
- Laying Hens: Mature hens may have specific nutritional and health needs, especially during laying periods. Certain herbs can support or disrupt laying, depending on their properties.
- Older Birds: Older chickens might have different health issues that can be either alleviated or exacerbated by certain herbs. Their metabolism might also differ from younger birds.

2. Breed Specifics

- Commercial vs. Heritage Breeds: Different breeds of chickens can react differently to herbal treatments. Commercial breeds often grow faster and might have specific health concerns that need attention. Heritage or rare breeds might have unique characteristics that need to be considered.
- Size of the Breed: Larger breeds might require different dosages than smaller breeds. Understanding the average size and weight of specific breeds can guide dosage decisions.
- Known Sensitivities: Some breeds might have known sensitivities or intolerances to certain herbs. Knowledge of these specificities can prevent unnecessary health issues.

3. Size and Weight Factors

- General Guidelines: The size and weight of the chicken must guide the dosage of any herbal treatment. Larger birds generally require larger doses, while smaller birds require smaller doses.
- Adjusting for Growth: As chickens grow, their size and weight change, and so should the dosage of the herbal treatments.
- Avoiding Overdosing: Understanding the correct dosage for a bird's size is crucial to avoid overdosing, which can lead to toxic effects or other health issues.

4. Interactions with Other Factors

- Health Conditions: A bird's current health condition, whether related to age, breed, or size, can influence how it reacts to an herb. Pre-existing health conditions must be considered when choosing and dosing herbs.
- Diet: The diet of a chicken, including what it forages, can affect how it metabolizes herbs. Chickens with a varied diet might react differently to certain herbs than those on a more controlled diet.

5. Practical Tips for Considering Age, Breed, and Size

- Consult Experts: If unsure about the specific needs of a bird related to age, breed, or size, it can be beneficial to consult a veterinarian or an experienced chicken keeper.
- Start Slow: When introducing a new herb, start with a smaller dosage and observe how the bird reacts. This approach allows for adjustments based on the bird's unique characteristics.
- Keep Records: Maintaining records of what herbs have been given, in what dosages, and how the birds reacted can provide valuable insights for future care.

6. Potential Pitfalls to Avoid

- Assuming Uniformity: Not all chickens are the same. Assuming that all birds will react the same way to an herb can lead to problems.
- Ignoring Individual Needs: Each bird might have individual needs and characteristics that need to be considered. Ignoring these can lead to ineffectiveness or harm.

Age, breed, and size are essential factors that must be understood and respected when using herbal treatments in chicken care. These factors influence not only the choice of herbs but also the dosage and method of administration. By taking these aspects into account, chicken keepers can provide herbal treatments that are not only safe but also tailored to the specific needs and characteristics of their flock. It's a nuanced approach that requires careful observation, knowledge, and flexibility, but it's one that can significantly enhance the well-being of the chickens.

Finally, always keep a keen eye on your flock after administering any herbal treatments. Look for changes in behavior, appetite, or physical appearance. Any unexpected changes might be a sign that the dosage needs adjusting or that the herb is not suitable for your particular flock.

In conclusion, understanding safe dosages for herbal treatments is a complex but rewarding endeavor. It requires careful attention to detail, a willingness to learn and adapt, and a deep respect for the unique needs of your chickens. By embracing these principles, you can provide your flock with the enriching benefits of herbal treatments, confident that you're doing so in a way that is not just effective but safe and compassionate as well. The relationship between a chicken keeper and their flock is one of trust and care, and a thoughtful approach to herbal treatments reflects and strengthens that bond.

Appendix 3

Reference Guide for Common Chicken Ailments and Recommended Herbal Remedies

In this appendix, we delve into the world of common chicken ailments and explore the natural remedies that can alleviate or cure these conditions. From respiratory issues to digestive problems, we've carefully curated a selection of herbal solutions that are not only effective but also gentle on your feathered friends. Whether you're a seasoned expert or just beginning your journey into chicken care, this guide will provide you with the knowledge and confidence to address various health challenges using the healing power of plants.

1. Respiratory Issues

Respiratory issues in chickens are common and can manifest in various ways, such as wheezing, coughing, nasal discharge, and labored breathing. These symptoms may be indicative of underlying problems like infections, environmental irritants, or nutritional deficiencies. The causes can range from viral and bacterial infections to exposure to dust, ammonia, or poor ventilation in the coop. Understanding the specific signs and identifying potential triggers are essential in managing and alleviating these respiratory ailments. Herbal remedies, proper care, and attention to the living conditions of the chickens can often provide relief and support their overall well-being.

Breathe Easy Tonic

The Breathe Easy Tonic is a gentle yet effective herbal remedy designed to alleviate respiratory issues in chickens. By combining the soothing properties of Eucalyptus, Thyme, and Peppermint, this tonic helps ease symptoms like wheezing, coughing, and nasal discharge, promoting clearer breathing and overall comfort.

Ingredients:
• 2 tablespoons of Eucalyptus leaves
• 1 tablespoon of Thyme
• 1 teaspoon of Peppermint leaves
• 2 cups of distilled water

Directions:
• Combine all the herbs in a small pot with 2 cups of distilled water.
• Bring the mixture to a gentle boil and then simmer for 15-20 minutes.
• Strain the herbs, allowing the liquid to cool to room temperature.
• Administer the tonic by adding a 1/4 cup of the tonic to 1 gallon of the chicken's drinking water or 5 drops directly into the beak using a dropper.

The Breathe Easy Tonic serves as a natural support for chickens experiencing respiratory discomfort. Eucalyptus acts as an expectorant, helping to clear mucus, while Thyme has antibacterial properties that can combat underlying infections. Peppermint adds a soothing effect, calming irritation in the respiratory tract.

Notes:
- Eucalyptus: Known for its strong aromatic properties, Eucalyptus helps in opening up the airways and clearing mucus.
- Thyme: Thyme's antibacterial qualities can aid in fighting infections that may be causing respiratory issues.
- Peppermint: Peppermint provides a cooling sensation, easing any discomfort in the throat or respiratory system.
- Quality matters, so select fresh or dried herbs from reputable sources.
- Consistent treatment with this tonic is key to seeing improvements.
- Storage: Store the tonic in a cool, dark place, and use it within one week for optimal freshness.
- Dosage and Administration: 1/4 cup of the tonic can be added to 1 gallon of the chicken's drinking water or administer 5 drops directly once or twice a day. Observe your chicken for signs of improvement.
- Treatment Duration: Continue the treatment for 7-10 days or until symptoms subside. Regular monitoring and patience are essential in natural healing.
- IMPORTANT: Ensure the correct dosage, as too much can be overpowering.

This remedy offers a thoughtful blend of herbs that work in harmony to support your chicken's respiratory health. By understanding the purpose and properties of each ingredient, you can confidently administer this tonic, knowing that quality, consistency, and correct dosage are integral to its success.

Respiratory Reviver

Respiratory Reviver Tonic is a specialized blend crafted to support chickens experiencing respiratory challenges, such as infectious bronchitis. Utilizing the potent properties of Thyme, Eucalyptus Leaves, Crushed Garlic, and Oregano, this tonic can be added to water or administered directly to provide immediate relief and ongoing support.

Ingredients:
- 2 tablespoons of Thyme
- 1 tablespoon of Eucalyptus Leaves
- 3 cloves of Garlic (crushed)
- 1 teaspoon of Oregano
- 1 quart of Water

Directions:
- Combine the Thyme, Eucalyptus Leaves, Crushed Garlic, and Oregano in a medium saucepan with the water.
- Bring the mixture to a gentle boil, then reduce the heat and simmer for 20 minutes.
- Remove from heat and allow to cool.
- Strain the herbs, retaining the liquid.
- Store the tonic in a clean, airtight container in the refrigerator.

- Administer the tonic by adding 1 cup of the tonic to 1 gallon of the chicken's drinking water or 5-10 drops directly into the beak using a dropper.

The Respiratory Reviver Tonic combines herbs known for their respiratory support and antimicrobial properties. Thyme acts as a natural expectorant, helping to clear mucus, while Eucalyptus Leaves provide a cooling and soothing effect. Crushed Garlic offers potent antimicrobial benefits, and Oregano's antiviral properties further enhance the remedy's effectiveness. Together, they create a balanced approach to respiratory health, making it an ideal choice for chickens with respiratory challenges.

Notes:
- Thyme: Rich in antioxidants; using fresh or high-quality dried Thyme ensures optimal respiratory support.
- Eucalyptus Leaves: Ensure the use of fresh or quality dried leaves for the best cooling effects.
- Crushed Garlic: Fresh garlic offers potent antimicrobial benefits; consistency in usage will provide the best results.
- Oregano: Its antiviral effects are maximized when combined with other herbs in this blend.
- Storage: Keep the tonic refrigerated, and use it within two weeks for best results.
- Dosage: Administer the tonic by adding 1 cup of the tonic to 1 gallon of the chicken's drinking water or 5-10 drops directly into the beak using a dropper. Observe your chicken's response and adjust the dosage if needed, considering the size and symptoms.

The Respiratory Reviver Tonic offers a multifaceted approach to managing respiratory challenges in chickens. By understanding the unique properties of each ingredient, you can create a supportive environment for your chickens, promoting respiratory ease and overall well-being.

Bronchial Booster Feed Mix

Bronchial Booster Feed Mix is a specially formulated herbal blend designed to support the bronchial health of chickens. By incorporating the healing properties of Fennel, Mullein, and Echinacea, this feed mix aids in soothing respiratory discomfort, reducing inflammation, and enhancing the immune response.

Ingredients:
- 2 tablespoons of Fennel
- 2 tablespoons of Mullein
- 1 tablespoon of Echinacea
- 5 pounds of Chicken Feed

Directions:
- Grind the Fennel, Mullein, and Echinacea into a fine powder.
- Mix the ground herbs thoroughly with the chicken feed, ensuring even distribution.
- Store the feed mix in an airtight container away from direct sunlight.
- Replace your chicken's regular feed with this blend as needed, observing for positive changes in respiratory health.

Bronchial Booster Feed Mix offers a targeted approach to respiratory health in chickens. Fennel is known for its anti-inflammatory and digestive support, while Mullein acts as a gentle expectorant, aiding in the clearance of mucus. Echinacea enhances the overall blend with its immune-boosting properties. Together, these herbs create a synergistic effect, supporting the bronchial system and overall well-being of your chickens.

Notes:
- Fennel: Its anti-inflammatory benefits are best harnessed using fresh or high-quality dried seeds.
- Mullein: Known for its gentle action on the respiratory system, ensure the use of clean, pesticide-free Mullein.
- Echinacea: Quality matters; using fresh or high-quality dried Echinacea ensures optimal immune support.
- Storage: Store the feed mix in a cool, dry place, and use it within one month for the best results.
- Dosage: Observe your chicken's response and adjust the feeding amount based on size and needs.

Bronchial Booster Feed Mix is a thoughtful blend that goes beyond mere symptom relief, addressing the underlying needs of chickens dealing with bronchial challenges. By understanding the unique characteristics of each ingredient, you can provide a nurturing and supportive environment that promotes your chicken's return to health and vitality.

Feathered Friend's Respiratory Salve

Feathered Friend's Respiratory Salve is a soothing blend crafted to ease respiratory discomfort in chickens. Infused with calming herbs like Lavender, Chamomile, Peppermint, and Eucalyptus, this salve can be applied externally to provide relief from symptoms such as wheezing and nasal congestion.

Ingredients:
- 1 tablespoon of Lavender flowers
- 1 tablespoon of Chamomile flowers
- 1 teaspoon of Peppermint leaves
- 1 teaspoon of Eucalyptus leaves
- 1/2 cup of Coconut or Olive Oil
- 2 tablespoons of Beeswax

Directions:
- Combine the herbs with the oil in a double boiler and gently heat for 1-2 hours, allowing the herbs to infuse into the oil.
- Strain the herbs, returning the infused oil to the double boiler.
- Add the beeswax, stirring until melted and fully combined.
- Pour the mixture into small jars or tins and allow it to cool and solidify.

Feathered Friend's Respiratory Salve acts as a comforting balm for chickens experiencing respiratory distress. The combination of Lavender and Chamomile offers calming effects, while

Peppermint and Eucalyptus provide a refreshing sensation that can open airways. The salve's gentle formulation allows for easy application to the chicken's beak and nostrils, where it can provide immediate relief.

Notes:
- Lavender & Chamomile: These herbs are known for their calming properties, helping to soothe irritation.
- Peppermint & Eucalyptus: Both herbs offer a cooling effect and can help clear congestion.
- Coconut or Olive Oil: These oils serve as the base, allowing for smooth application. Choose cold-pressed and unrefined options for the best quality.
- Beeswax: Adds a firm texture to the salve, making it easy to handle. Ensure it's pure and free from additives.
- Quality selection is vital, so choose organic or well-sourced herbs.
- Consistency in the application will enhance the benefits
- Storage: Store the salve in a cool, dark place. It should remain effective for up to a year.
- Dosage and Administration: Apply a small amount to the chicken's beak and nostrils once or twice a day, as needed.
- Treatment Duration: Continue treatment until symptoms subside, typically within a week or two.

Feathered Friend's Respiratory Salve is a thoughtful blend of natural ingredients, each serving a specific purpose in supporting respiratory health. By understanding the role of each component and adhering to guidelines on quality, consistency, storage, and administration, you can offer this gentle remedy to your chickens with confidence and care.

Bronchial Soothing Tonic

The Bronchial Soothing Tonic is a gentle yet effective herbal blend designed to alleviate respiratory infections in chickens. By combining the healing properties of Echinacea, Thyme, Mullein, and Licorice Root, this tonic helps soothe the respiratory tract, reduce inflammation, and boost the immune system.

Ingredients:
- 2 tablespoons of Echinacea
- 1 tablespoon of Thyme
- 1 tablespoon of Mullein
- 1 teaspoon of Licorice Root
- 1 quart of distilled water

Directions:
- Combine the herbs in a medium saucepan with the water.
- Bring the mixture to a gentle boil, then reduce the heat and simmer for 20 minutes.
- Remove from heat and allow to cool.
- Strain the herbs.
- Store the tonic in a clean, airtight container in the refrigerator.
- Directly administer 5 to 10 drops of the tonic to your chicken daily or mix 1 cup of the tonic with 1 gallon of their fresh drinking water per day.

The herbs in the Bronchial Soothing Tonic were carefully selected for their synergistic effects on respiratory health. Echinacea is known for its immune-boosting properties, while Thyme and Mullein act as natural expectorants, helping to clear mucus from the respiratory tract. Licorice Root adds a soothing touch, reducing inflammation and irritation. Together, these herbs create a holistic approach to managing infectious bronchitis in chickens.

Notes:
- Echinacea: Quality matters; using fresh or high-quality dried Echinacea ensures optimal immune support.
- Thyme: Rich in antioxidants, Thyme contributes to overall health. Consistency in using the remedy will yield the best results.
- Mullein: Known for its gentle action on the respiratory system, Mullein should be free from contaminants.
- Licorice Root: Its anti-inflammatory properties are enhanced when used in conjunction with other herbs.
- Storage: Keep the tonic refrigerated, and use it within two weeks for best results.
- Dosage: Directly administer 5 to 10 drops of the tonic to your chicken daily or mix 1 cup of the tonic with 1 gallon of their fresh drinking water per day. Adjusting the dosage based on the chicken's size and symptoms may be necessary; observe the chicken's response and adjust as needed.

This remedy offers a natural approach to managing infectious bronchitis, focusing on both symptom relief and overall wellness. By understanding the individual properties of each ingredient, you can confidently administer this tonic to support your chicken's health.

Respiratory Relief Water Additive

The Respiratory Relief Water Additive is a specialized herbal concoction designed to ease respiratory distress. Infused with Peppermint, Elderberry, Garlic, and Oregano, this additive not only clears the respiratory passages but also fortifies the immune system.

Ingredients:
- 2 tablespoons of Peppermint
- 1 tablespoon of Elderberry
- 1 clove of Garlic (crushed)
- 1 teaspoon of Oregano
- 1 gallon of distilled water Water

Directions:
- Place the herbs and garlic in a large pot and add the water.
- Bring to a gentle boil, then reduce heat and simmer for 30 minutes.
- Allow the mixture to cool, then strain to remove the solids.
- Add the additive to your chicken's drinking water, using 1 cup per gallon of fresh water.
- Refresh daily to ensure potency and freshness.

This water additive combines herbs known for their respiratory and immune-boosting properties. Peppermint provides a cooling effect, easing respiratory discomfort, while Elderberry supports immune function. Garlic adds a layer of natural antimicrobial action, and Oregano's antiviral properties further enhance the remedy's effectiveness. Together, they create a balanced approach to respiratory health, making it an ideal choice for chickens with infectious bronchitis.

Notes:
- Peppermint: Its cooling properties are most effective when using fresh or high-quality dried leaves.
- Elderberry: Ensure the use of ripe berries or quality extracts for optimal immune support.
- Garlic: Fresh garlic offers potent antimicrobial benefits; consistency in usage will provide the best results.
- Oregano: Its antiviral effects are maximized when combined with other herbs in this blend.
- Storage: Store any unused portion in the refrigerator and use it within one week.
- Dosage: Observe your chicken's response and adjust the dosage if needed, considering the size and symptoms.

The Respiratory Relief Water Additive offers a multifaceted approach to managing infectious bronchitis in chickens. By understanding the unique properties of each ingredient, you can create a supportive environment for your chickens, promoting respiratory ease and overall well-being.

Cluckers' Comfort Feed Additive

Cluckers' Comfort Feed Additive is a nourishing blend designed to support chickens during recovery from respiratory infections. Combining the healing properties of Fenugreek, Anise, Rosemary, Turmeric, and Flax Seed, this additive enhances digestion, boosts immunity, and promotes overall well-being.

Ingredients:
- 2 tablespoons Fenugreek
- 1 tablespoon Anise
- 1 tablespoon Rosemary
- 1 teaspoon Turmeric
- 2 tablespoons Flax Seed (freshly ground)
- 5 pounds of Chicken Feed

Directions:
- Grind the Fenugreek, Anise, Rosemary, Turmeric, and Flax Seed into a fine powder.
- Combine the herbal mixture with the chicken feed, ensuring even distribution.
- Store the feed in an airtight container away from direct sunlight.
- Replace your chicken's regular feed with this blend as needed, observing for positive changes in health and vitality.

Cluckers' Comfort Feed Additive offers a multifaceted approach to recovery. Fenugreek and Anise support digestion, while Rosemary's antioxidant properties aid in overall health.

Turmeric's anti-inflammatory effects provide additional comfort, and Flax Seed's Omega-3 fatty acids promote healthy feathers and skin. Together this blend supports your chicken's return to health following respiratory infections.

Notes:
- Fenugreek: Known for digestive support; quality matters, so choose fresh or high-quality dried seeds.
- Anise: Enhances flavor and supports digestion; consistency in feeding will provide the best results.
- Rosemary: Rich in antioxidants; ensure the use of fresh or quality dried leaves.
- Turmeric: Its anti-inflammatory benefits are maximized when combined with other herbs.
- Flax Seed: Provides Omega-3 fatty acids; grind fresh for optimal nutritional value.
- Storage: Store the feed in a cool, dry place, and use it within one month for the best results.
- Dosage: Observe your chicken's response and adjust the feeding amount based on size and needs.

Cluckers' Comfort Feed Additive is a thoughtful blend that goes beyond mere symptom relief, addressing the underlying needs of chickens recovering from a respiratory infection. By understanding the unique characteristics of each ingredient, you can provide a nurturing and supportive environment that promotes your chicken's return to health and happiness.

Cluck Clear Water Additive

Cluck Clear Water Additive is an herbal infusion designed to support respiratory health in chickens. By blending Lemon Balm, Oregano, and Rosemary, this water additive provides a natural way to ease symptoms such as coughing, sneezing, and nasal congestion, making it a convenient addition to your chickens' daily care routine.

Ingredients:
- 2 tablespoons of Lemon Balm leaves
- 1 tablespoon of Oregano leaves
- 1 tablespoon of Rosemary leaves
- 4 cups of distilled water

Directions:
- Combine the herbs in a pot with 4 cups of water.
- Bring the mixture to a boil and then reduce to a simmer for 15-20 minutes.
- Strain the herbs, allowing the liquid to cool to room temperature.
- Allow the infusion to cool completely
- Administer 5 to 10 drops directly to affected chickens or 1/4 cup of the infusion directly to 1 gallon of the chicken's drinking water

Cluck Clear Water Additive serves as a gentle support for chickens experiencing respiratory discomfort. Lemon Balm is known for its calming effects, Oregano possesses antibacterial properties, and Rosemary aids in opening the airways. Together, these herbs create a balanced blend that can be easily added to the drinking water, offering daily support for respiratory well-being.

Notes:
- Lemon Balm: This herb offers calming properties and can help soothe the respiratory tract.
- Oregano: Known for its antibacterial qualities, Oregano can assist in combating underlying infections.
- Rosemary: Rosemary helps in opening up the airways and clearing congestion..
- Select fresh or dried leaves from reputable sources for the best quality.
- Consistency in treating with this infusion is essential for optimal results.
- Storage: Store any unused portion of the infusion in the refrigerator for up to one week.
- Dosage and Administration: Add approximately 1/4 cup of the infusion to 1 gallon of the chickens' drinking water daily.
- Treatment Duration: Continue the treatment for 7-10 days or until symptoms subside. Regular monitoring will help you gauge the effectiveness.
- IMPORTANT: Ensure the correct dosage to maintain a pleasant flavor in the water

Cluck Clear Water Additive offers a simple yet effective way to incorporate herbal support into your chickens' daily routine. By understanding the unique properties of each herb and adhering to guidelines on quality, consistency, storage, and administration, you can provide this remedy with confidence. It's a thoughtful approach to natural care that aligns with the overall well-being of your feathered friends.

Henhouse Healing Tincture

Henhouse Healing Tincture is an herbal remedy specifically formulated to support respiratory health in chickens. Combining the potent benefits of Elderberry, Sage, and Fennel, this tincture provides a natural approach to easing respiratory symptoms and enhancing overall well-being.

Ingredients:
- 1/4 cup of Elderberry
- 1/4 cup of Sage leaves
- 1/4 cup of Fennel seeds
- 1 cup of Distilled Water
- 1 cup of Alcohol (like vodka or brandy) or Apple Cider Vinegar (organic with the mother)

Directions:
- Combine the Elderberry, Sage, and Fennel in a glass jar.
- Add the Distilled Water and Alcohol or Apple Cider Vinegar, ensuring the herbs are fully submerged.
- Seal the jar and allow it to steep in a cool, dark place for 4-6 weeks, shaking occasionally.
- Strain the herbs, transferring the liquid to a clean bottle with a dropper.
- Administer 5 to 10 drops directly into the beak.

Henhouse Healing Tincture offers a blend of herbs known for their respiratory and immune-boosting properties. Elderberry is rich in antioxidants, Sage provides anti-inflammatory benefits, and Fennel aids in digestion. Together, they create a balanced remedy to support respiratory health.

Notes:
- Elderberry: Renowned for its immune-boosting properties, Elderberry can be a key ingredient.
- Sage: Sage's anti-inflammatory effects can help soothe the respiratory tract..
- Fennel: Fennel not only supports respiratory health but also aids in digestion, enhancing overall well-being.
- Alcohol or Apple Cider Vinegar: These act as preservatives and extraction agents. Choose a clean, high-proof alcohol or organic Apple Cider Vinegar with the mother for optimal benefits.
- Quality matters, so choose organic or wild-harvested herbs.
- Consistency in using this tincture is essential for the best results
- Storage: Store the tincture in a cool, dark place. It should remain potent for up to a year.
- Dosage and Administration: 5 to 10 drops administered directly to the chicken once or twice a day.
- Treatment Duration: Continue the treatment for 7-10 days or until symptoms subside, keeping a close eye on progress.

Henhouse Healing Tincture is a carefully crafted remedy that brings together herbs with complementary properties. Understanding the role of each ingredient and adhering to guidelines on quality, consistency, and correct administration ensures that this tincture can be a valuable part of your natural care routine for chickens.

Nest Soothe Herbal Infusion

Nest Soothe Nesting Herbs is a unique blend of herbs designed to create a calming and therapeutic environment within the chicken's nest. Infused with Lavender, Spearmint, Hyssop, Basil, Eucalyptus, Plantain, Oregano, Turmeric, Parsley, and Thyme, these nesting herbs not only provide a pleasant aroma but also offer respiratory support, helping to ease symptoms like congestion and irritation.

Ingredients:
- 1 cup of Lavender flowers
- 1 cup of Spearmint leaves
- 1/2 cup of Hyssop
- 1 cup of Basil leaves
- 1/4 cup of Eucalyptus leaves
- 1/2 cup of Plantain leaves
- 1/4 cup of Oregano leaves
- 1 tablespoon of Turmeric powder
- 1/2 cup of Parsley leaves
- 1/4 cup of Thyme leaves

Directions:
- Mix all the herbs together in a bowl, ensuring an even blend.

- Sprinkle the mixture generously in the nesting areas where the chickens rest.
- Refresh the herbs every few days or as needed to maintain their potency and aroma.

Nest Soothe Nesting Herbs serves as a gentle and natural way to enhance the nesting environment for chickens. The blend of herbs offers various benefits, from Lavender's calming effect to Eucalyptus's ability to clear the airways. The combination creates a soothing ambiance that supports respiratory health and overall well-being, making the nest a place of comfort and healing.

Notes:
- Lavender: Known for its calming properties, Lavender adds a relaxing scent to the nest.
- Spearmint & Hyssop: These herbs offer a refreshing aroma and can help with breathing.
- Basil & Eucalyptus: Both herbs support clear airways and add a pleasant fragrance.
- Plantain & Oregano: Known for their healing properties, they contribute to overall health.
- Turmeric: Adds a warm color and has anti-inflammatory benefits.
- Parsley & Thyme: Provide a fresh scent and have antibacterial qualities.
- Quality matters, so choose organic or wild-harvested herbs.
- Storage: Store any unused portion in a cool, dark place, and it should remain effective for up to 6 months.
- Administration: Sprinkle generously in the nesting areas, refreshing as needed.
- Treatment Duration: Continue to use until you see an improvement in symptoms, or use the herbs as a regular part of the nesting routine.

Nest Soothe Nesting Herbs offers a thoughtful and natural approach to enhancing the nesting environment for chickens. By understanding the unique properties of each herb and adhering to guidelines on quality, consistency, and administration, you can create a nurturing space that aligns with the overall well-being of your feathered friends. It's a simple yet effective way to provide comfort and support, reflecting a deep connection and care for your chickens.

2. Bumblefoot

Bumblefoot, scientifically known as pododermatitis, is a common condition in chickens characterized by inflammation and infection in the foot. It often begins with a small injury or abrasion on the footpad, which allows bacteria to enter and form an abscess or hard kernel. Over time, this can lead to swelling, redness, and discomfort, making it difficult for the chicken to walk. If left untreated, bumblefoot can become chronic and lead to more serious complications. Fortunately, early detection and natural remedies can often alleviate the symptoms and promote healing, making it essential for chicken keepers to regularly inspect their flock's feet and provide proper care.

Foot Soak Bliss

Foot Soak Bliss is a gentle and soothing herbal remedy designed to address bumblefoot in chickens. By combining the healing properties of Calendula, Lavender, and Epsom Salt, this foot soak provides relief from the discomfort and inflammation associated with bumblefoot, promoting healing and relaxation.

Ingredients:
• 2 tablespoons of Calendula flowers
• 2 tablespoons of Lavender flowers
• 1 cup of Epsom Salt
• 1 gallon of warm distilled water

Directions:
• In a large basin, combine the distilled water and Epsom Salt, stirring until dissolved.
• Add the Calendula and Lavender flowers, allowing them to infuse in the water for 10-15 minutes.
• Gently place the chicken's affected foot in the basin, letting it soak for 15-20 minutes.
• Pat the foot dry with a clean towel and allow the chicken to rest.

Foot Soak Bliss serves as a natural and calming treatment for bumblefoot, a common foot infection in chickens. Calendula offers anti-inflammatory benefits, Lavender provides a calming effect, and Epsom Salt helps to draw out impurities and soothe the affected area. Together, these ingredients create a therapeutic soak that can be used regularly to support healing and provide comfort.

Notes:
- Calendula: Known for its healing and anti-inflammatory properties, Calendula helps to reduce swelling and promote healing.
- Lavender: Lavender adds a relaxing scent and has antiseptic qualities that can aid in preventing further infection.
- Epsom Salt: Epsom Salt is known for its ability to draw out toxins and soothe discomfort. Ensure you're using pure Epsom Salt without additives.
- Distilled Water: Using distilled water ensures a clean and pure base for the soak.
- Quality matters, so choose organic or well-sourced dried herbs.
- Storage: A fresh preparation is recommended for each use to maintain potency.

- Dosage and Administration: The soak can be administered once daily or as needed, depending on the severity of the bumblefoot.
- Treatment Duration: Continue treatment until symptoms subside, typically within a week or two, but regular monitoring is essential.

Foot Soak Bliss offers a thoughtful and compassionate approach to treating bumblefoot in chickens. By understanding the unique properties of each ingredient and adhering to guidelines on quality, consistency, and administration, you can provide this gentle remedy with confidence. It's a nurturing and natural way to care for your chickens, reflecting a deep connection and commitment to their well-being.

Bumble Be-Gone Salve

Bumble Be-Gone Salve is a specially formulated herbal remedy designed to target bumblefoot in chickens. By blending coconut oil, shea butter, beeswax, calendula, comfrey, plantain, and tea tree essential oil, this salve offers a natural and effective way to soothe, heal, and protect the affected foot, promoting recovery and comfort.

Ingredients:
• 1/2 cup of coconut oil
• 1/4 cup of shea butter
• 2 tablespoons of beeswax
• 2 tablespoons of calendula flowers
• 2 tablespoons of comfrey leaves
• 2 tablespoons of plantain leaves
• 10 drops of tea tree essential oil

Directions:
• In a double boiler, gently melt the coconut oil, shea butter, and beeswax.
• Add the calendula, comfrey, and plantain, allowing them to infuse in the oil mixture for 1-2 hours.
• Strain the herbs, returning the infused oil to the double boiler.
• Stir in the tea tree essential oil and pour the mixture into small jars or tins.
• Allow the salve to cool and solidify before use.
• Apply a small amount to the affected foot, massaging gently.

Bumble Be-Gone Salve acts as a comprehensive treatment for bumblefoot, a common foot infection in chickens. The combination of coconut oil and shea butter offers a moisturizing base, while calendula, comfrey, and plantain provide healing properties. Beeswax adds a protective layer, and tea tree essential oil offers antiseptic benefits. Together, these ingredients create a balanced salve that can be applied directly to the affected area, offering immediate relief and ongoing support.

Notes:
- Coconut Oil & Shea Butter: These oils provide a moisturizing and nourishing base for the salve. Choose unrefined and cold-pressed options for the best quality.

- Beeswax: Adds a firm texture to the salve, making it easy to handle. Ensure it's pure and free from additives.
- Calendula, Comfrey & Plantain: These herbs are known for their healing properties, helping to soothe irritation and promote recovery.
- Tea Tree Essential Oil: Offers antiseptic qualities, aiding in preventing further infection. Use therapeutic-grade oil for the best results.
- Storage: Store the salve in a cool, dark place. It should remain effective for up to a year.
- Dosage and Administration: Apply a small amount to the affected foot once or twice a day, as needed.
- Treatment Duration: Continue treatment until symptoms subside, typically within a week or two.

Bumble Be-Gone Salve is a thoughtful blend of natural ingredients, each serving a specific purpose in supporting the healing of bumblefoot. By understanding the role of each component and adhering to guidelines on quality, consistency, storage, and administration, you can offer this gentle remedy to your chickens with confidence and care. It's a compassionate approach to natural care that aligns with the overall well-being of your feathered friends.

Cluck Comfort Foot Spray

Cluck Comfort Foot Spray is an invigorating and soothing herbal remedy designed to provide relief for bumblefoot in chickens. Combining the natural benefits of Witch Hazel, Aloe Vera Gel, Peppermint essential oil, and Eucalyptus essential oil, this spray offers a convenient and effective way to cleanse, refresh, and heal the affected foot, promoting comfort and recovery.

Ingredients:
• 1 cup of Witch Hazel
• 1/4 cup of Aloe Vera Gel
• 10 drops of Peppermint essential oil
• 10 drops of Eucalyptus essential oil

Directions:
• In a clean spray bottle, combine the Witch Hazel and Aloe Vera Gel.
• Add the Peppermint and Eucalyptus essential oils, shaking well to blend.
• Spray the affected foot generously, allowing it to air dry or gently pat it dry with a clean towel.
• Repeat as needed, up to twice a day.

Cluck Comfort Foot Spray serves as a gentle yet effective treatment for bumblefoot, a common foot infection in chickens. Witch Hazel acts as a natural astringent, Aloe Vera Gel soothes and moisturizes, while Peppermint and Eucalyptus essential oils provide a refreshing scent and additional antiseptic benefits. Together, these ingredients create a versatile spray that can be used regularly to support healing and provide immediate comfort.

Notes:
- Witch Hazel: Known for its astringent properties, Witch Hazel helps to cleanse and tighten the affected area. Choose alcohol-free Witch Hazel for a gentler effect.

- Aloe Vera Gel: Aloe Vera offers soothing and moisturizing benefits, aiding in healing. Use pure Aloe Vera Gel without additives.
- Peppermint & Eucalyptus Essential Oils: These oils provide a refreshing scent and have antiseptic qualities. Ensure you're using therapeutic-grade oils for the best results.
- Storage: Store the spray in a cool, dark place, and it should remain effective for up to 6 months.
- Dosage and Administration: Spray generously on the affected foot once or twice a day, as needed.
- Treatment Duration: Continue treatment until symptoms subside, typically within a week or two.

Cluck Comfort Foot Spray offers a thoughtful and natural approach to treating bumblefoot in chickens. By understanding the unique properties of each ingredient and adhering to guidelines on quality, consistency, and administration, you can create a nurturing and effective remedy. It's a simple yet powerful way to provide comfort and support, reflecting a deep connection and care for your chickens. Whether used as a standalone treatment or in conjunction with other remedies, Cluck Comfort Foot Spray is a valuable addition to your natural care toolkit.

Foot Fancy Salve

Bumblefoot is a common condition in chickens where a hard, calloused area forms on the foot, often leading to discomfort or even infection. The Foot Fancy salve, made with refreshing mint and soothing calendula, is designed to provide relief and encourage the healing of bumblefoot in your feathered friends.

Ingredients:
• 1 cup fresh mint leaves
• 1 cup fresh calendula petals
• 1 cup coconut oil
• 1 tablespoon beeswax
• A few drops of lavender essential oil (optional)

Directions:
• Place the mint leaves and calendula petals in a double boiler, and cover them with the coconut oil.
• Gently heat the mixture until the coconut oil is melted and the herbs are well-infused about 30 minutes.
• Strain the oil, discard the mint and calendula, and return the infused oil to the double boiler.
• Add the beeswax to the oil, stirring until melted.
• Remove from heat and add a few drops of lavender essential oil if using.
• Pour the mixture into small tins or jars and allow it to cool.
• Apply the salve to the affected foot as needed, massaging gently.

The Foot Fancy salve is a gentle and natural way to help your chickens' feet feel their best. Mint offers a cooling sensation and can alleviate discomfort, while calendula is known for its anti-inflammatory and healing properties. Together, they create a salve that not only soothes but also aids in the healing process of bumblefoot.

Notes:
- Mint Leaves: These provide a cooling and refreshing effect, reducing discomfort associated with bumblefoot.
- Calendula Petals: Known for their healing properties, calendula petals can soothe inflammation and encourage healing.
- Coconut Oil: This acts as a carrier for the herbs and provides additional moisturizing benefits.
- Beeswax: Beeswax gives the salve its consistency and helps form a protective barrier on the skin.
- Lavender Essential Oil (Optional): Lavender adds a pleasant fragrance and has additional calming and antiseptic properties.
- Storage: Store the salve in a cool, dark place. It should remain effective for up to a year.
- Dosage and Administration: Apply a small amount to the affected foot once or twice a day, as needed.
- Treatment Duration: Continue treatment until symptoms subside, typically within a week or two.

The Foot Fancy salve is an example of how simple, natural ingredients can create effective remedies for common ailments. By understanding the properties of these herbs and their beneficial effects, you can create a loving and caring environment for your chickens. This salve is just one way to pamper your feathered friends and keep them clucking happily.

Bumblefoot Balm

Bumblefoot is a common condition in chickens, characterized by swelling, infection, and discomfort in the feet. This Bumblefoot Balm features the natural healing properties of plantain leaf and coconut oil, designed to address the discomfort and inflammation that bumblefoot can cause.

Ingredients:
- 1 cup fresh plantain leaves (finely chopped)
- 1 cup coconut oil
- 1 tablespoon beeswax pellets
- 10 drops lavender essential oil (optional)

Directions:
- Place the chopped plantain leaves and coconut oil in a double boiler or slow cooker.
- Heat gently for several hours to allow the plantain leaves to infuse the oil.
- Strain the oil through a fine-mesh strainer or cheesecloth, discarding the plantain leaves.
- Return the oil to the double boiler and add the beeswax pellets, stirring until melted.
- If using, add the lavender essential oil, mixing thoroughly.
- Pour the mixture into jars or tins and allow to cool and solidify.
- Apply to the affected foot or feet of the chicken once or twice daily until symptoms resolve.

The Bumblefoot Balm is specifically crafted to tackle the inflammation and discomfort that comes with bumblefoot. The soothing coconut oil, coupled with the unique medicinal qualities of plantain leaf, forms a balm that not only helps in reducing pain but also promotes healing.

Notes:
- Plantain Leaf: Plantain leaf is known for its anti-inflammatory, antibacterial, and wound-healing properties. It's an herb that's often used to treat skin irritations and is particularly effective in this remedy.
- Coconut Oil: Coconut oil adds a moisturizing and nourishing touch to the balm. Its antibacterial properties also aid in fighting off any infection.
- Beeswax: This ingredient helps in solidifying the balm, making it easy to apply, and adds a protective layer to the affected area.
- Lavender Essential Oil (Optional): If you choose to add lavender oil, it will further enhance the balm's soothing qualities and adds a pleasant fragrance.
- Storage: Store the balm in a cool, dark place. It should remain effective for up to a year.
- Dosage and Administration: Apply a small amount to the affected foot once or twice a day, as needed.
- Treatment Duration: Continue treatment until symptoms subside, typically within a week or two.

The Bumblefoot Balm provides a gentle, natural alternative to commercial treatments. Its simple and organic ingredients are specifically chosen to offer relief and aid in the healing process for chickens suffering from bumblefoot. By incorporating these beneficial herbs and oils, this remedy can become a go-to solution in your feathered first aid toolkit.

Golden Paste Foot Ointment

Golden Paste Foot Ointment is a rich and nourishing herbal remedy crafted to address bumblefoot in chickens. With a blend of Golden Seal, Plantain, Coconut Oil, and Vitamin E oil, this ointment offers a natural and soothing way to heal, protect, and rejuvenate the affected foot, promoting recovery and overall foot health.

Ingredients:
- 1 tablespoon of Golden Seal powder
- 1 tablespoon of Plantain leaves (finely chopped)
- 1/2 cup of Coconut Oil
- 1 teaspoon of Vitamin E oil

Directions:
- In a small saucepan, gently melt the coconut oil over low heat.
- Add the Golden Seal powder and Plantain leaves, allowing them to infuse in the oil for 10-15 minutes.
- Remove from heat and stir in the Vitamin E oil.
- Pour the mixture into a small jar or tin, allowing it to cool and solidify.
- Apply a small amount to the affected foot, massaging gently once or twice a day.

Golden Paste Foot Ointment serves as a targeted treatment for bumblefoot, a common foot infection in chickens. Golden Seal offers antibacterial and anti-inflammatory benefits, Plantain aids in healing, Coconut Oil provides a moisturizing base, and Vitamin E oil adds nourishment and protection. Together, these ingredients create a luxurious ointment that can be applied directly to the affected area, offering immediate relief and ongoing support for recovery.

Notes:
- Golden Seal: Known for its antibacterial properties, Golden Seal helps to cleanse and heal the affected area. Quality matters, so choose well-sourced Golden Seal powder.
- Plantain: Plantain leaves are known for their healing properties, aiding in soothing irritation and promoting recovery.
- Coconut Oil: Provides a moisturizing and nourishing base for the ointment. Choose unrefined and cold-pressed options for the best quality.
- Vitamin E Oil: Adds nourishment and protection to the skin, aiding in healing. Ensure it's pure Vitamin E oil without additives.
- Storage: Store the ointment in a cool, dark place. It should remain effective for up to a year.
- Dosage and Administration: Apply a small amount to the affected foot once or twice a day, as needed.
- Treatment Duration: Continue treatment until symptoms subside, typically within a week or two.

Golden Paste Foot Ointment is a thoughtful blend of natural ingredients, each serving a specific purpose in supporting the healing of bumblefoot. By understanding the role of each component and adhering to guidelines on quality, consistency, storage, and administration, you can offer this gentle remedy to your chickens with confidence and care. It's a compassionate approach to natural care that aligns with the overall well-being of your feathered friends. Whether used as a standalone treatment or in conjunction with other remedies, Golden Paste Foot Ointment is a valuable addition to your natural care toolkit, reflecting a deep connection and commitment to the health of your chickens.

Tootsie Relief Poultice

Tootsie Relief Poultice is a carefully crafted herbal remedy designed to provide relief and healing for bumblefoot in chickens. By combining Clay, Turmeric, Ginger, Slippery Elm Bark, Marshmallow Root, Chamomile, Flaxseed, and Raw Honey, this poultice offers a natural and soothing way to draw out infection, reduce inflammation, and promote recovery in the affected foot.

Ingredients:
- 2 tablespoons of Clay (Bentonite or Green Clay)
- 1 teaspoon of Turmeric powder
- 1 teaspoon of Ginger powder
- 1 tablespoon of Slippery Elm Bark powder
- 1 tablespoon of Marshmallow Root powder
- 1 tablespoon of Chamomile flowers (finely chopped)
- 2 tablespoons of Flaxseed (ground)
- 1 tablespoon of Raw Honey

Directions:
- In a small bowl, combine the clay, turmeric, ginger, slippery elm bark, marshmallow root, chamomile, and flaxseed.
- Add enough warm water to form a thick paste, stirring well to blend.
- Stir in the raw honey, ensuring a smooth consistency.
- Apply the poultice to the affected foot, covering it with a clean cloth or bandage.
- Leave in place for 20-30 minutes before gently rinsing with warm water.
- Repeat once or twice a day as needed.

Tootsie Relief Poultice serves as a comprehensive treatment for bumblefoot, a common foot infection in chickens. The combination of clay, turmeric, ginger, slippery elm bark, marshmallow root, chamomile, flaxseed, and raw honey creates a potent poultice that draws out infection, reduces swelling, and soothes irritation. Together, these ingredients offer a natural and effective way to support healing and provide comfort to the affected foot.

Notes:
Clay: Known for its drawing properties, clay helps to pull out toxins and impurities. Choose Bentonite or Green Clay for the best results.
Turmeric & Ginger: These spices offer anti-inflammatory benefits, aiding in reducing swelling and discomfort.
Slippery Elm Bark & Marshmallow Root: Provide soothing and healing properties, aiding in recovery.
Chamomile: Chamomile adds a calming effect and supports healing.
Flaxseed: Ground flaxseed adds texture and additional anti-inflammatory benefits to the poultice.
Raw Honey: Offers antibacterial properties and adds a smooth consistency to the poultice.
Storage: Prepare fresh for each use to maintain potency.
Dosage and Administration: Apply to the affected foot once or twice a day, as needed.
Treatment Duration: Continue treatment until symptoms subside, typically within a week or two.

Tootsie Relief Poultice is a thoughtful and natural approach to treating bumblefoot in chickens. By understanding the unique properties of each ingredient and adhering to guidelines on quality, consistency, and administration, you can create a nurturing and effective remedy. It's a hands-on and compassionate way to provide care, reflecting a deep connection and commitment to the well-being of your chickens. Whether used as a standalone treatment or in conjunction with other remedies, Tootsie Relief Poultice is a valuable addition to your natural care toolkit, offering a gentle yet powerful way to address bumblefoot and support overall foot health.

Happy Feet Healing Spray

Happy Feet Healing Spray is a gentle yet potent herbal remedy designed to address bumblefoot in chickens. With a unique blend of Colloidal Silver, Lavender Oil, Frankincense Oil, and Rosemary Oil, this spray offers a convenient and effective way to cleanse, soothe, and heal the affected foot, promoting a swift recovery and overall foot health.

Ingredients:
- 1 cup of Colloidal Silver
- 10 drops of Lavender Oil
- 5 drops of Frankincense Oil
- 5 drops of Rosemary Oil

Directions:
- In a clean spray bottle, combine the Colloidal Silver, Lavender Oil, Frankincense Oil, and Rosemary Oil.
- Shake well to blend the oils with the Colloidal Silver.
- Spray the affected foot generously, allowing it to air dry or gently patting it with a clean towel.
- Repeat as needed, up to twice a day.

Happy Feet Healing Spray serves as a versatile and easy-to-use treatment for bumblefoot, a common foot infection in chickens. Colloidal Silver acts as a natural antimicrobial agent, Lavender Oil soothes and heals, Frankincense Oil promotes skin regeneration, and Rosemary Oil adds a refreshing scent and additional antiseptic benefits. Together, these ingredients create a harmonious spray that can be used regularly to support healing and provide immediate comfort.

Notes:
- Colloidal Silver: Known for its antimicrobial properties, Colloidal Silver helps to cleanse and protect the affected area. Choose a high-quality product with a concentration of 10-20 ppm.
- Lavender Oil: Lavender offers soothing and healing benefits, aiding in recovery. Use therapeutic-grade oil for the best results.
- Frankincense Oil: Promotes skin regeneration and healing. Ensure you're using therapeutic-grade Frankincense oil.
- Rosemary Oil: Adds a refreshing scent and has antiseptic qualities. Choose therapeutic-grade Rosemary oil.
- Storage: Store the spray in a cool, dark place, and it should remain effective for up to 6 months.
- Dosage and Administration: Spray generously on the affected foot once or twice a day, as needed.
- Treatment Duration: Continue treatment until symptoms subside, typically within a week or two.

Happy Feet Healing Spray offers a thoughtful and natural approach to treating bumblefoot in chickens. By understanding the unique properties of each ingredient and adhering to guidelines on quality, consistency, and administration, you can create a nurturing and effective remedy. It's a simple yet powerful way to provide comfort and support, reflecting a deep connection and care for your chickens. Whether used as a standalone treatment or in conjunction with other remedies, Happy Feet Healing Spray is a valuable addition to your natural care toolkit. It's a compassionate and convenient solution that aligns with the overall well-being of your feathered friends, offering a gentle and effective way to address bumblefoot and support overall foot health.

Comfy Foot Balm

Comfy Foot Balm is a luxurious and soothing herbal remedy designed to address bumblefoot in chickens. By combining Shea Butter, Arnica, St. John's Wort, Olive Oil, and Beeswax, this balm offers a nourishing and healing way to treat the affected foot, promoting recovery and overall foot comfort.

Ingredients:
- 1/2 cup of Shea Butter
- 1 tablespoon of Arnica flowers (dried)
- 1 tablespoon of St. John's Wort flowers (dried)
- 1/2 cup of Olive Oil
- 2 tablespocns of Beeswax (grated)

Directions:
- In a double boiler, gently melt the Shea Butter and Beeswax together.
- Add the Olive Oil, Arnica, and St. John's Wort, allowing them to infuse in the oil for 15-20 minutes.
- Strain the herbs, retaining the infused oil.
- Return the oil to the double boiler, and if needed, add more beeswax to reach the desired consistency.
- Pour the mixture into a small jar or tin, allowing it to cool and solidify.
- Apply a small amount to the affected foot, massaging gently once or twice a day.

Comfy Foot Balm serves as a targeted treatment for bumblefoot, a common foot infection in chickens. Shea Butter offers a moisturizing base, Arnica provides anti-inflammatory benefits, St. John's Wort aids in healing, Olive Oil nourishes, and Beeswax adds a protective layer. Together, these ingredients create a rich balm that can be applied directly to the affected area, offering immediate relief and ongoing support for recovery.

Notes:
- Shea Butter: Provides a moisturizing and nourishing base for the balm. Choose unrefined Shea Butter for the best quality.
- Arnica: Known for its anti-inflammatory properties, Arnica helps to reduce swelling and discomfort.
- St. John's Wort: Aids in healing and soothing irritation.
- Olive Oil: Adds nourishment and helps in infusing the herbs. Choose extra virgin Olive Oil for the best quality.
- Beeswax: Adds a protective layer and helps solidify the balm. Choose natural, unbleached Beeswax.
- Storage: Store the balm in a cool, dark place. It should remain effective for up to a year.
- Dosage and Administration: Apply a small amount to the affected foot once or twice a day, as needed.
- Treatment Duration: Continue treatment until symptoms subside, typically within a week or two.

Comfy Foot Balm is a thoughtful blend of natural ingredients, each serving a specific purpose in supporting the healing of bumblefoot. By understanding the role of each component and adhering to guidelines on quality, consistency, storage, and administration, you can offer this gentle remedy to your chickens with confidence and care. It's a compassionate approach to natural care that aligns with the overall well-being of your feathered friends. Whether used as a standalone treatment or in conjunction with other remedies, Comfy Foot Balm is a valuable addition to your natural care toolkit, reflecting a deep connection and commitment to the health of your chickens. It's a nurturing and effective way to address bumblefoot, providing comfort and support when it's needed most.

Kernel Kicker Foot Soak

Kernel Kicker Foot Soak is a specialized herbal remedy designed to address bumblefoot in chickens, particularly when a kernel has developed. By combining Epsom Salt, Baking Soda, Lemon Juice, and Peppermint Oil, this foot soak offers a refreshing and effective way to soften and help remove the kernel, easing discomfort and promoting recovery.

Ingredients:
• 1 cup of Epsom Salt
• 1/2 cup of Baking Soda
• Juice of 1 Lemon
• 5 drops of Peppermint Oil
• 1 gallon of warm water

Directions:
• In a basin large enough for the chicken's foot, dissolve the Epsom Salt and Baking Soda in warm water.
• Add the Lemon Juice and Peppermint Oil, stirring to combine.
• Gently place the affected foot in the soak, allowing it to rest for 15-20 minutes.
• Pat the foot dry with a clean towel, and repeat as needed, up to once a day.

Kernel Kicker Foot Soak serves as a targeted treatment for bumblefoot with a developed kernel, a hardened area that can cause discomfort. Epsom Salt helps to soften the kernel, Baking Soda cleanses, Lemon Juice adds a refreshing touch, and Peppermint Oil provides a soothing sensation. Together, these ingredients create a therapeutic soak that can be used regularly to support the softening and eventual removal of the kernel, offering immediate comfort and ongoing support for recovery.

Notes:
- Epsom Salt: Known for its ability to soften skin and ease discomfort, Epsom Salt is a key ingredient in this soak. Choose a high-quality product.
- Baking Soda: Acts as a gentle cleanser, aiding in the softening process.
- Lemon Juice: Adds a refreshing touch and helps in cleansing. Use fresh lemon juice for the best results.
- Peppermint Oil: Provides a soothing and cooling sensation. Choose therapeutic-grade Peppermint oil.
- Storage: The ingredients can be stored separately in a cool, dark place, and the soak should be prepared fresh for each use.
- Dosage and Administration: Soak the affected foot once a day, as needed.

- Treatment Duration: Continue treatment until the kernel softens and symptoms subside, typically within a week or two.

Kernel Kicker Foot Soak offers a thoughtful and natural approach to treating bumblefoot with a developed kernel. By understanding the unique properties of each ingredient and adhering to guidelines on quality, consistency, and administration, you can create a nurturing and effective remedy. It's a simple yet powerful way to provide comfort and support, reflecting a deep connection and care for your chickens. Whether used as a standalone treatment or in conjunction with other remedies, Kernel Kicker Foot Soak is a valuable addition to your natural care toolkit. It's a compassionate and convenient solution that aligns with the overall well-being of your feathered friends, offering a gentle and effective way to address bumblefoot and support overall foot health.

Kernel Kicker Poultice

A bumblefoot condition in chickens can lead to the formation of a hard kernel in the foot, causing discomfort and difficulty in walking. The "Kernel Kicker Poultice" is an innovative herbal remedy designed to draw out the kernel, reduce inflammation, and hasten recovery. Made with powerful ingredients like Echinacea root, calendula flowers, and golden seal powder, this poultice brings the benefits of traditional herbal medicine to the aid of your feathered friends.

Ingredients:
• 2 tablespoons Echinacea root (finely powdered)
• 2 tablespoons calendula flowers (dried and crushed)
• 1 tablespoon golden seal powder
• Enough water to create a paste

Directions:
• In a small bowl, combine the Echinacea root, calendula flowers, and golden seal powder.
• Slowly add water while stirring to create a thick paste.
• Apply the paste directly to the affected foot or feet, covering the kernel area thoroughly.
• Wrap the foot with a soft cloth or bandage, ensuring the paste stays in direct contact with the skin.
• Leave the poultice in place for 1 to 2 hours.
• Carefully remove the cloth, and rinse the foot with clean water.
• Repeat daily as needed until the kernel is drawn out and healing is observed.

The Kernel Kicker Poultice is an exceptional treatment in cases where a chicken's bumblefoot has advanced to the point of a kernel forming. The blend of herbs works synergistically to draw out the kernel and soothe the affected area, allowing for faster recovery.

Notes:
- Echinacea Root: Echinacea is renowned for its immune-boosting and anti-inflammatory properties. It helps in the healing process and reduces swelling.
- Calendula Flowers: Known for their healing and antiseptic properties, calendula flowers help soothe the affected area and promote skin regeneration.

- Golden Seal Powder: Golden seal has strong antibacterial properties, aiding in keeping the wound free from infection.
- Storage: Prepare fresh for each use to maintain potency.
- Dosage and Administration: Apply the poultice to the affected foot and allow it to stay in place for 1 to 2 hours. Wrap the foot with a soft cloth or bandage, ensuring the paste stays in direct contact with the skin.
- Treatment Duration: Continue treatment until symptoms subside, typically within a week or two.

The Kernel Kicker Poultice is an excellent addition to your poultry first-aid kit. These natural ingredients combined are gentle yet effective in dealing with bumblefoot cases that have advanced to the kernel stage. Not only does it provide comfort, but it also plays a vital role in the healing process. By understanding the distinct benefits of each herb and implementing them correctly, you can ensure a quick and natural recovery for your clucking companions.

Kernel Ease Ointment

Kernel Ease Ointment is a soothing and healing herbal remedy designed to address bumblefoot in chickens, specifically when a kernel has developed. The combination of Comfrey, Plantain, Calendula, Coconut Oil, and Vitamin E Oil creates a gentle yet effective ointment that targets the kernel, aiding in its softening and removal and promoting overall healing of the affected foot.

Ingredients:
- 1 tablespoon of Comfrey leaves (dried and powdered)
- 1 tablespoon of Plantain leaves (dried and powdered)
- 1 tablespoon of Calendula flowers (dried and powdered)
- 1/2 cup of Coconut Oil
- 1 teaspoon of Vitamin E Oil

Directions:
- In a double boiler, gently heat the Coconut Oil.
- Add the Comfrey, Plantain, and Calendula, allowing them to infuse in the oil for 15-20 minutes.
- Strain the herbs, retaining the infused oil.
- Return the oil to the double boiler, add the Vitamin E Oil, and mix well.
- Pour the mixture into a small jar or tin, allowing it to cool and solidify.
- Apply a small amount to the affected foot, massaging gently once or twice a day.

Kernel Ease Ointment is formulated to address the specific challenges of bumblefoot with a developed kernel. Comfrey promotes tissue repair, Plantain offers anti-inflammatory properties, Calendula aids in wound healing, Coconut Oil nourishes, and Vitamin E Oil adds antioxidant support. Together, these ingredients create a nurturing ointment that can be applied directly to the affected area, providing immediate comfort and ongoing healing support.

Notes:
- Comfrey: Known for its tissue repair properties, Comfrey helps in the healing process. Choose a high-quality, powdered form.
- Plantain: Offers anti-inflammatory benefits and aids in soothing the affected area. Choose a high-quality, powdered form.
- Calendula: Known for its wound-healing properties, Calendula supports recovery. Choose a high-quality, powdered form.
- Coconut Oil: Adds nourishment and helps in infusing the herbs. Choose organic, virgin Coconut Oil for the best quality.
- Vitamin E Oil: Provides antioxidant support and aids in preserving the ointment. Choose natural Vitamin E Oil.
- Storage: Store the ointment in a cool, dark place. It should remain effective for up to a year.
- Dosage and Administration: Apply a small amount to the affected foot once or twice a day, as needed.
- Treatment Duration: Continue treatment until the kernel softens and symptoms subside, typically within a week or two.

Kernel Ease Ointment is a thoughtful and compassionate approach to treating bumblefoot with a developed kernel. By understanding the role of each ingredient and adhering to guidelines on quality, consistency, storage, and administration, you can offer this gentle remedy to your chickens with confidence. It's a natural and nurturing way to address this common issue, reflecting a deep connection and commitment to the well-being of your feathered friends. Whether used as a standalone treatment or in conjunction with other remedies, Kernel Ease Ointment is a valuable addition to your natural care toolkit, providing comfort and support when it's needed most. It's a loving and effective way to address bumblefoot, offering a path to recovery that aligns with a holistic and mindful approach to care.

Happy Cluck Poultice

Happy Cluck Poultice is a specialized herbal remedy crafted to address bumblefoot in chickens, particularly when a kernel has developed. The unique blend of Green Tea, Chamomile, Bentonite Clay, and Aloe Vera Gel creates a soothing and healing poultice that targets the kernel, helping to soften and remove it while providing comfort and support to the affected foot.

Ingredients:
• 1 Green Tea bag or 1 teaspoon of loose Green Tea leaves
• 1 Chamomile Tea bag or 1 teaspoon of loose Chamomile flowers
• 2 tablespoons of Bentonite Clay
• 2 tablespoons of Aloe Vera Gel

Directions:
• Brew the Green Tea and Chamomile in a cup of hot water, allowing them to steep for 5-10 minutes.
• In a small bowl, mix the Bentonite Clay with the brewed tea, creating a smooth paste.
• Add the Aloe Vera Gel to the paste, mixing well.
• Apply the poultice to the affected foot, covering with a bandage or wrap.
• Leave in place for 20-30 minutes, then gently rinse off.
• Repeat daily as needed.

Happy Cluck Poultice is designed to provide targeted support for bumblefoot with a developed kernel. The Green Tea offers antioxidant properties, Chamomile soothes, Bentonite Clay draws out impurities, and Aloe Vera Gel heals and hydrates. Together, these ingredients form a gentle yet effective poultice that can be applied directly to the affected area, providing both immediate relief and ongoing healing support.

Notes:
- Green Tea: Rich in antioxidants, Green Tea helps to protect and heal the affected area. Use a high-quality tea bag or loose leaves.
- Chamomile: Known for its calming properties, Chamomile aids in soothing the affected foot. Use a high-quality tea bag or loose flowers.
- Bentonite Clay: Draws out impurities and helps in the healing process. Choose a high-quality, food-grade Bentonite Clay.
- Aloe Vera Gel: Offers healing and hydrating properties. Choose a pure, organic Aloe Vera Gel.

- Storage: Store any leftover poultice in the refrigerator for up to a week.
- Dosage and Administration: Apply the poultice to the affected foot daily or as needed.
- Treatment Duration: Continue treatment until the kernel softens and symptoms improve, typically within a week or two.

Happy Cluck Poultice is a thoughtful and compassionate approach to treating bumblefoot with a developed kernel. By understanding the role of each ingredient and adhering to guidelines on quality, consistency, storage, and administration, you can offer this gentle remedy to your chickens with confidence. It's a natural and nurturing way to address this common issue, reflecting a deep connection and commitment to the well-being of your feathered friends. Whether used as a standalone treatment or in conjunction with other remedies, Happy Cluck Poultice is a valuable addition to your natural care toolkit, providing comfort and support when it's needed most. It's a loving and effective way to address bumblefoot, offering a path to recovery that aligns with a holistic and mindful approach to care.

Sour Crop & Impacted Crop

Before we jump into the herbal remedies for sour crop and impacted crop let's go over a few practices to safeguard your chickens from the discomforts of developing either. A mindful approach to their environment and diet can make all the difference. Remember the old adage that prevention is the best medicine. Here's how you can create a nurturing space that promotes their well-being:

- Keep Their Foraging Grounds Trimmed: Regularly mowing the area where chickens forage minimizes the risk of them ingesting harmful objects.
- Remove Potential Hazards: Be vigilant in removing strings, twine, and other debris that chickens may accidentally ingest.
- Monitor Their Crop: A routine check for a full crop in the morning can help you catch any issues early.
- Incorporate Probiotics: Providing probiotics in food or water supports a healthy digestive system.
- Ensure Constant Food Availability: Feeding often or keeping food available during the daytime ensures they have a consistent source of nourishment.
- Boost Immunity with Garlic: Feeding garlic not only bolsters their immune systems but also helps in killing harmful bacteria.
- Enhance Water with Oregano Oil: Adding oregano oil to their water can act as a natural antibiotic, promoting overall health.
- Offer Fresh Herbs: Feeding fresh or dried organic oregano and dill leaves can aid digestion and provide essential nutrients.
- Prioritize Fresh Water: ALWAYS provide fresh, clean drinking water DAILY to keep them hydrated and healthy.
- Avoid Spoiled Food: Never give them moldy or rancid food, as it can lead to digestive issues.
- Provide Essential Grit: Always keep crushed granite grit available for your flock, as it aids in digestion.

By embracing these practices, you're not just preventing potential ailments; you're fostering a space where your chickens can thrive. It's a commitment to their health, happiness, and your shared connection with nature.

3. Sour Crop

Sour crop is a digestive issue in chickens that occurs when the crop, a pouch-like organ where food is initially digested, becomes slow-moving or blocked. This can lead to a buildup of fermented food and yeast, giving the crop a sour or unpleasant smell, hence the name "sour crop." Chickens affected by this condition may exhibit symptoms such as a swollen and squishy crop, loss of appetite, lethargy, and regurgitation of foul-smelling fluid. Sour crop can be caused by various factors, including poor diet, ingestion of long or fibrous materials, or underlying health issues. Early intervention with proper care, diet adjustments, and natural remedies can often help in resolving the condition and restoring the chicken's digestive health.

Delightful Digestive Drink

Delightful Digestive Drink is a gentle herbal remedy designed to support digestive health in chickens, specifically targeting the condition known as sour crop. This delightful concoction is designed to aid digestion and help ease the symptoms of sour crop. It's simple to prepare, and chickens generally find it quite palatable.

Ingredients:
• 2 tablespocns of Chamomile flowers
• 1 tablespoon of Peppermint leaves
• 1 tablespoon of Anise seeds
• 4 cups of distilled water

Directions:
• Combine the herbs with the distilled water in a pot.
• Bring the mixture to a boil, then reduce to a simmer for 15-20 minutes.
• Strain the herbs, allowing the liquid to cool to room temperature.
• Offer the cooled infusion to the chickens as their drinking water, refreshing as needed.

Delightful Digestive Drink serves as a calming and supportive remedy for chickens experiencing sour crop. Chamomile is known for its calming effects, peppermint can aid digestion and soothe the digestive tract, and anise has antifungal properties and helps with gas and bloating. Together, these herbs create a balanced blend that targets the root causes of sour crop. Together, these herbs create a balanced infusion that can be easily administered through the drinking water, offering daily support for digestive well-being.

Notes:
- Chamomile: Known for its calming effect, Chamomile can help soothe irritation in the digestive tract. Quality selection is vital, so choose organic or well-sourced dried flowers.
- Peppermint: Peppermint offers a cooling effect to help soothe the digestive tract and can help ease digestive discomfort.
- Anise: Anise has antifungal properties and aids in reducing gas and bloating, contributing to overall digestive comfort.
- Consistency in the application will enhance the benefits.
- Storage: Store any unused portion of the infusion in the refrigerator for up to one week.
- Dosage and Administration: Replace the chickens' regular drinking water with the infusion, providing access throughout the day.
- Treatment Duration: Continue the treatment for 3-5 days or until symptoms subside. Regular monitoring will help you gauge the effectiveness.

Delightful Digestive Drink offers a thoughtful and natural approach to supporting digestive health in chickens. By understanding the unique properties of each herb and adhering to guidelines on quality, consistency, storage, and administration, you can provide this gentle remedy with confidence. It's a compassionate approach to natural care that aligns with the overall well-being of your feathered friends, making it a valuable addition to your chicken care toolkit.

Apple Cider Vinegar & Garlic Tincture

Apple Cider Vinegar & Garlic Tincture is a potent and natural remedy crafted to address sour crop in chickens. Combining the acidic properties of apple cider vinegar with the antibacterial benefits of crushed garlic cloves, this tincture offers a targeted approach to supporting digestive health and alleviating the symptoms of sour crop.

Ingredients:
• 1 cup of Apple Cider Vinegar (organic with the mother)
• 4 crushed Garlic Cloves
• 1 cup of Distilled Water

Directions:
• Combine the apple cider vinegar, crushed garlic cloves, and distilled water in a glass jar.
• Seal the jar and shake well to mix the ingredients.
• Allow the mixture to infuse for 24-48 hours at room temperature, shaking occasionally.
• Strain the garlic, and the tincture is ready to use.
• Add a small amount to the chickens' drinking water as directed.

Apple Cider Vinegar & Garlic Tincture is designed to provide a natural solution to sour crop by harnessing the power of two well-known ingredients. Apple cider vinegar helps balance the pH in the crop, while garlic offers antibacterial properties to combat infection. Together, they create a synergistic effect that can be easily administered through the chickens' drinking water, offering a practical and effective approach to digestive care.

Notes:
- Apple Cider Vinegar: Choose organic with the mother for added health benefits. Its acidity helps balance the crop's environment, making it less hospitable to harmful bacteria.
- Garlic: Known for its antibacterial properties, crushed garlic cloves add potency to the tincture. Fresh, organic garlic is preferred for quality.
- Storage: Store the tincture in a cool, dark place, and it should remain effective for up to one month.
- Dosage and Administration: Add 1 tablespoon of the tincture to 1 gallon of the chickens' drinking water, refreshing daily.
- Treatment Duration: Continue treatment for 5-7 days or until symptoms improve. Regular observation will guide the treatment process.

Apple Cider Vinegar & Garlic Tincture offers a straightforward and natural approach to addressing sour crop in chickens. By understanding the unique properties of each ingredient and adhering to guidelines on quality, consistency, storage, and administration, you can provide this remedy with confidence and care. It's a valuable addition to your natural chicken care repertoire, reflecting a thoughtful and compassionate approach to the well-being of your feathered friends.

Sour Crop Soother

Sour crop, a condition where the crop develops a yeast infection, can leave your chicken feeling quite unwell. Sour Crop Soother is here to lend a helping wing! This natural remedy combines the potent effects of GSE (Grapefruit Seed Extract) oil with select herbs to facilitate digestion, ease discomfort, and support crop health.

Ingredients:
- 10 drops GSE (Grapefruit Seed Extract) oil
- 1 tablespoon Chamomile flowers
- 1 tablespoon Ginger root, grated
- 1 teaspoon Fennel seeds
- 4 cups filtered water

Directions:

- In a small saucepan, combine the Chamomile, Ginger, and Fennel seeds with the filtered water.
- Bring the mixture to a gentle simmer and cook for 15 minutes.
- Remove from heat and allow to cool to room temperature.
- Strain the herbal infusion, discard the solids, and reserve the liquid.
- Stir in the GSE oil and mix well.
- Administer 5 to 10 drops of the mixture to your chicken daily or mix 1 cup with 1 gallon of their drinking water.

The Sour Crop Soother acts as a gentle, supportive elixir that targets the underlying causes of sour crop while providing comfort and relief.

Notes:
- GSE Oil: Recognized for its antimicrobial properties, GSE oil helps in combating the yeast and bacteria often associated with sour crop.
- Chamomile: This calming herb can ease digestive discomfort and inflammation.
- Ginger: With its warming effect, Ginger aids in digestion and can help relieve symptoms of sour crop.
- Fennel Seeds: Fennel seeds are known for their ability to promote healthy digestion and reduce gas, further soothing the crop.
- Quality Matters: Opt for high-quality, organic ingredients, especially the GSE oil, as purity is essential.
- Consistency: Ensure a consistent routine in administering the remedy for best results.
- Compatibility: This remedy can be harmoniously used with a balanced diet and proper hydration.
- Observation: Keep a close eye on your chicken's behavior and crop condition to understand the effectiveness of the remedy.

Sour Crop Soother not only brings together the best of herbal wisdom but also infuses a touch of love and care into every drop. This blend is a delightful concoction, combining the magic of herbs with the essence of nurturing. It's a testament to the connection between nature and our feathered friends, fostering wellness one cluck at a time!

Feathered Friends Recovery Fruity Mash

Feathered Friends Recovery Fruity Mash is a delightful and nourishing herbal remedy designed to address sour crop in chickens. Combining the natural goodness of shredded apple, shredded carrots, cinnamon, apple cider vinegar, and unsweetened Greek yogurt, this fruity mash offers a tasty and supportive approach to digestive health, helping to alleviate the symptoms of sour crop.

Ingredients:
- 1 medium Shredded Apple
- 2 medium Shredded Carrots
- 1 teaspoon of Cinnamon
- 2 tablespoons of Apple Cider Vinegar (organic with the mother)
- 1 cup of Unsweetened Greek Yogurt

Directions:
- Combine the shredded apple, shredded carrots, cinnamon, apple cider vinegar, and Greek yogurt in a bowl.
- Mix well to create a uniform mash.
- Offer the mash to the chickens as a special treat, replacing a portion of their regular feed.

Feathered Friends Recovery Fruity Mash is more than just a tasty treat; it's a carefully crafted remedy to support chickens with sour crop. The apple and carrots provide gentle fiber, while the cinnamon is anti-fungal and antibiotic properties. Apple cider vinegar helps balance the crop's pH, and Greek yogurt introduces beneficial probiotics. Together, these ingredients create a palatable and effective remedy that can be easily integrated into the chickens' daily diet.

Notes:
- Shredded Apple & Carrots: These provide gentle fiber and natural sweetness. Fresh and organic produce is preferred.
- Cinnamon: Adds flavor and has anti-fungal and antibiotic properties.
- Apple Cider Vinegar: Helps balance the Ph of the crop. Choose organic with the mother for added digestive benefits.
- Greek Yogurt: Introduces probiotics to support gut health. Ensure it's unsweetened and unflavored.
- Storage: Store any unused portion in the refrigerator for up to 24 hours.
- Dosage and Administration: Offer the mash during the recovery period after you have withheld feed for 24 hours. Please remember to still offer your chickens their regular feed as well.
- Treatment Duration: Continue offering the mash daily for 3-5 days or until symptoms improve.

Feathered Friends Recovery Fruity Mash offers a creative and compassionate approach to addressing sour crop in chickens. By understanding the unique properties of each ingredient and adhering to guidelines on quality, consistency, storage, and administration, you can provide this delightful remedy with love and care. It's a joyful way to support the well-being of your feathered friends, reflecting a deep connection and thoughtful approach to natural chicken care.

Severe Sour Crop Healing Tincture

Severe Sour Crop Healing Tincture is a potent herbal remedy specifically formulated to address severe cases of sour crop in chickens. By combining the powerful healing properties of Goldenseal, Echinacea, Olive Oil, and Grapefruit Seed Extract, this tincture offers a concentrated approach to digestive care, targeting the underlying causes of sour crop and providing relief for affected chickens.

Ingredients:
- 1 tablespoon of Goldenseal root powder
- 1 tablespoon of Echinacea root powder
- 1 cup of Olive Oil
- 10 drops of Grapefruit Seed Extract

Directions:
- Combine the Goldenseal, Echinacea, Olive Oil, and Grapefruit Seed Extract in a glass jar.
- Seal the jar and shake well to mix the ingredients.
- Allow the mixture to infuse for 1-2 weeks in a cool, dark place, shaking occasionally.
- Strain the herbs, and the tincture is ready to use.
- Administer orally to the affected chickens as directed below in the notes.

Severe Sour Crop Healing Tincture is designed to provide targeted support for chickens experiencing severe sour crop. Goldenseal and Echinacea are known for their antimicrobial and immune-boosting properties, while Olive Oil offers a soothing base, and Grapefruit Seed Extract adds an extra layer of antifungal support. Together, these ingredients create a powerful tincture that can be administered orally, offering a focused and effective approach to digestive healing.

Notes:
- Goldenseal: Known for its antimicrobial properties, Goldenseal is a key ingredient in combating infection. Quality selection is vital, so choose organic or well-sourced root powder.
- Echinacea: Boosts the immune system and aids in recovery. Again, quality matters, so select a reputable source.
- Olive Oil: Acts as a carrier oil, allowing for smooth administration. Extra virgin olive oil is preferred.
- Grapefruit Seed Extract: Adds antifungal properties to the tincture. Ensure it's free from additives or synthetic ingredients.
- Storage: Store the tincture in a cool, dark place, and it should remain effective for up to six months.
- Dosage and Administration: Administer 2-3 drops orally to the affected chickens twice daily.
- Treatment Duration: Continue treatment for 7-10 days or until symptoms resolve. Regular observation will guide the treatment process.

Severe Sour Crop Healing Tincture offers a specialized and natural approach to addressing severe sour crop in chickens. By understanding the unique properties of each ingredient and adhering to guidelines on quality, consistency, storage, and administration, you can provide this remedy with confidence and compassion. It's a valuable addition to your natural chicken care toolkit, reflecting a deep understanding of herbal healing and a commitment to the well-being of your feathered friends.

Intensive Crop Care Water Additive

Intensive Crop Care Water Additive is an herbal remedy designed to provide intensive support for chickens dealing with sour crop. By blending Aloe Vera Juice, Apple Cider Vinegar (with the mother), Cinnamon, and Cayenne Pepper, this water additive offers a multifaceted approach to digestive care. It's meant to be added to the chickens' drinking water, providing a convenient and effective way to address the discomfort and digestive imbalance associated with sour crop.

Ingredients:
- 1 cup of Aloe Vera Juice
- 2 tablespoons of Apple Cider Vinegar (with the mother)
- 1 teaspoon of Cinnamon
- 1/4 teaspoon of Cayenne Pepper

Directions:
- Combine the Aloe Vera Juice, Apple Cider Vinegar, Cinnamon, and Cayenne Pepper in a jug or container.
- Mix well to ensure all ingredients are evenly distributed.
- Add the mixture to the chickens' drinking water, replacing their regular water with this enhanced blend.

Intensive Crop Care Water Additive is formulated to provide targeted relief for sour crop in chickens. Aloe Vera Juice offers soothing properties, while Apple Cider Vinegar helps balance the crop's pH. Cinnamon adds a warming touch, and Cayenne Pepper stimulates digestion. Together, these ingredients create a balanced and supportive remedy that can be easily integrated into the chickens' daily water intake, offering continuous support for digestive health.

Notes:
- Aloe Vera Juice: Known for its soothing and healing properties. Choose a product free from additives or preservatives.
- Apple Cider Vinegar: Balances pH and adds digestive support. Select organic with the mother for maximum benefits.
- Cinnamon: Provides flavor and has anti-fungal and antibacterial properties.
- Cayenne Pepper: Stimulates digestion and adds a gentle kick. Use sparingly, as it's potent.
- Storage: Store any unused portion in the refrigerator for up to 3 days.
- Dosage and Administration: Replace the chickens' regular water with the enhanced water, providing access throughout the day.
- Treatment Duration: Continue offering the enhanced water daily for 5-7 days or until symptoms improve.

Intensive Crop Care Water Additive offers a thoughtful and practical approach to addressing sour crop in chickens. By understanding the unique properties of each ingredient and adhering to guidelines on quality, consistency, storage, and administration, you can provide this remedy with confidence and care. It's a natural and compassionate way to support the well-being of your feathered friends, reflecting a deep connection and thoughtful approach to natural chicken care.

Fennel Tonic

Fennel Tonic is a simple yet effective herbal remedy designed to alleviate symptoms of sour crop in chickens. Utilizing the natural digestive properties of crushed fennel seeds, this tonic helps to ease discomfort, promote healthy digestion, and support the overall well-being of your chickens. It's a gentle and natural approach to addressing a common digestive ailment in poultry. Fennel Tonic is simple, but I have seen it work miracles at curing sour crop! It is fast-acting!

Ingredients:
• 2 tablespoons of crushed fennel seeds (to release the oil)
• 1 cup of distilled Water

Directions:
• Place the crushed fennel seeds in a heat-resistant container.
• Boil the distilled water and pour it over the crushed fennel seeds.
• Cover and allow the mixture to steep for 15-20 minutes.
• Strain the tonic, discard the seeds, and allow it to cool.
• Administer the tonic orally to the affected chickens or add it to their drinking water.

Fennel Tonic is crafted to provide gentle support for chickens experiencing sour crop. Fennel seeds are known for their digestive properties, including easing gastrointestinal spasms and promoting healthy digestion. By creating a simple infusion with distilled water, this tonic offers a natural and soothing remedy that can be easily administered to support digestive health.

Notes:
- Crushed Fennel Seeds: Fennel seeds are known for their digestive benefits. They are anti-fungal and antibacterial, help treat candida yeast infection in the crop, and are full of antioxidants. Choose organic or well-sourced seeds and crush them to release their active compounds.
- Storage: Store any unused portion in the refrigerator for up to 3 days.
- Dosage and Administration: Administer 2 to 3 dropper fulls orally to the affected chickens, 2-3 times daily, or add to their drinking water.
- Treatment Duration: Continue treatment for 3-5 days or until symptoms resolve. Regular observation will guide the treatment process.

Fennel Tonic offers a straightforward, powerful, and compassionate approach to addressing sour crop in chickens. By understanding the unique properties of fennel seeds and adhering to guidelines on quality, consistency, storage, and administration, you can provide this remedy with confidence and care. It's a natural and thoughtful way to support the well-being of your feathered friends, reflecting a deep connection and a holistic approach to chicken care. Whether used as a preventive measure or a targeted treatment, Fennel Tonic is a valuable addition to your natural chicken care toolkit.

4. Impacted Crop

Impacted crop is a common digestive issue in chickens, where the crop, a pouch-like organ that stores food before it enters the digestive tract, becomes obstructed. This obstruction can be caused by the ingestion of long strands of grass, fibrous materials, or other indigestible substances that form a mass, preventing the normal passage of food. As a result, the crop becomes enlarged and hard, leading to discomfort and a lack of appetite in the affected chicken. If left untreated, impacted crop can lead to serious health issues, as the chicken is unable to properly digest food. Natural remedies, proper feeding practices, and careful observation can often help in managing and preventing this condition, supporting the overall health and well-being of the flock.

Crop Comfort Oil Infusion

Crop Comfort Oil Infusion is a specialized herbal remedy designed to address impacted crop in chickens. This oil infusion works by lubricating the digestive tract and aiding in breaking up the impaction in the crop. It's a gentle and natural approach that can be used in conjunction with massaging the crop to help ease the obstruction and restore normal digestion.

Ingredients:
• 2 tablespoons of olive oil or coconut oil
• 1 teaspoon of crushed fennel seeds
• 1 teaspoon of crushed chamomile flowers

Directions:
• In a small saucepan, gently heat the olive or coconut oil.
• Add the crushed fennel seeds and chamomile flowers to the oil.
• Simmer on low heat for 10-15 minutes, allowing the herbs to infuse into the oil.
• Strain the oil, discard the herbs, and allow it to cool to room temperature.
• Administer the oil infusion directly to the side of the chicken's beak using a dropper.

Crop Comfort Oil Infusion is crafted to provide targeted support for chickens experiencing impacted crop. The combination of olive or coconut oil with fennel and chamomile helps to lubricate the digestive tract, while the gentle massaging action aids in breaking up the impaction. This remedy offers a compassionate and natural approach to a common digestive ailment, focusing on gentle intervention and supportive care.

Notes:
- Olive or Coconut Oil: These oils serve as the base for the infusion, providing lubrication to ease the impaction.
- Fennel Seeds and Chamomile Flowers: Known for their digestive properties, these herbs enhance the infusion's effectiveness.
- Storage: Store the oil infusion in a cool, dark place for up to one week.
- Dosage and Administration: Administer 1-2 droppers of the oil infusion, 2-3 times daily, followed by gentle massaging of the crop.
- Treatment Duration: Continue treatment for 3-5 days or until symptoms resolve.

Crop Comfort Oil Infusion reflects a thoughtful and holistic approach to chicken care, utilizing natural ingredients and hands-on intervention to address impacted crop. By understanding the unique properties of each ingredient and adhering to guidelines on quality, consistency, storage, and administration, you can provide this remedy with confidence and compassion. It's a valuable addition to your natural chicken care toolkit, offering support and relief for a common and often distressing condition. Whether used as a targeted treatment or a preventive measure, Crop Comfort Oil Infusion embodies a deep connection to the well-being of your feathered friends, reflecting a commitment to natural and mindful care.

Impaction Intervention Tincture

Impaction Intervention Tincture is a carefully formulated herbal remedy designed to address the challenging issue of impacted crop in chickens. This tincture is composed of specific herbs known to help break up the impaction in the crop, working in harmony with manual massaging of the crop to facilitate the breakdown of the obstruction. It's a natural and compassionate approach to a condition that can cause significant discomfort in your feathered friends.

Ingredients:
• 1 cup of vodka or apple cider vinegar (organic with the mother for an alcohol-free option)
• 2 tablespoons of crushed ginger root
• 2 tablespoons of crushed fennel seeds
• 1 tablespoon of crushed peppermint leaves

Directions:
• Combine the vodka or apple cider vinegar with the crushed ginger, fennel, and peppermint in a glass jar.
• Seal the jar and shake well to mix the ingredients.
• Store in a cool, dark place for 2-4 weeks, shaking the jar daily.
• Strain the tincture, discard the herbs, and transfer to a dropper bottle.
• Administer the tincture directly to the side of the chicken's beak using a dropper, followed by gentle massaging of the crop.

Impaction Intervention Tincture is a targeted herbal solution for impacted crop, a condition where the crop becomes obstructed, preventing normal digestion. By utilizing herbs like ginger, fennel, and peppermint, known for their digestive support properties, this tincture aids in breaking up the impaction. The massaging action further assists in this process, offering a comprehensive and natural approach to this common ailment.

Notes:
− Ginger Root: Aids in digestion and helps break down impactions.
− Fennel Seeds: Known for its ability to support digestive flow.
− Peppermint Leaves: Provides soothing effects to the digestive tract.
− Storage: Store the tincture in a cool, dark place, and it can last up to one year.
− Dosage and Administration: Administer 1-2 droppers of the tincture 2-3 times daily, followed by gentle massaging of the crop.
− Treatment Duration: Continue treatment for 3-5 days or until symptoms resolve.

Impaction Intervention Tincture is more than just a remedy; it's a commitment to natural and mindful care for your chickens. By understanding the unique properties of each ingredient and following the guidelines on quality, consistency, storage, and administration, you can provide this remedy with confidence. It's a valuable tool in your natural chicken care toolkit, offering support and relief for a common and often distressing condition. Whether used as a targeted treatment or a preventive measure, Impaction Intervention Tincture embodies a deep connection to the well-being of your flock, reflecting a commitment to natural and compassionate care.

5. Water Belly (Ascites)

Water belly, also known as ascites or fluid retention in the abdomen, can be an alarming condition in chickens. It's generally a symptom of an underlying issue, such as heart or liver problems. Though the condition can be complex, there are natural ways to support chickens with this condition.

Note from the author: Years ago, I stumbled upon an article detailing the therapeutic benefits of eye bright, milk thistle, dandelion and brewers yeast in treating water belly, an ailment traditionally believed to be incurable. With nothing to lose, I decided to incorporate these healing herbs into the diet of my affected hen. I'm elated to report that dear Betty, a thriving 6-year-old hen, has not required a single draining of her belly since the summer of 2019. She continues to grace me with her lively presence, a testament to the potential power of these natural remedies. Please understand that the effectiveness of these herbs in treating this ailment hinges on both the progression of the disease and your unwavering commitment to administering the herbs.

When we speak of tackling water belly naturally, we focus on herbs that are known for their diuretic properties, supporting liver function, and helping the overall circulatory system. Eye bright, milk thistle, and dandelion are herbs that can be great starting points.

Belly Brew

Water belly, also known as ascites, is a condition that affects the heart and liver function in chickens, leading to the accumulation of fluid in the abdomen. Belly Brew is a specially formulated tincture designed to alleviate symptoms of water belly and support liver and heart health. With the potent healing properties of dandelion root, milk thistle, eye bright, hawthorn berry, and burdock root, this tincture is a loving approach to your feathered friend's well-being.

Ingredients:
- 2 tablespoons dried dandelion root
- 2 tablespoons dried milk thistle seeds
- 1 tablespoon dried eye bright
- 1 tablespoon dried hawthorn berries
- 1 tablespoon dried burdock root
- 2 cups apple cider vinegar (organic with the mother) or vodka (for extraction)

Directions:
- Combine all the dried herbs in a clean glass jar with a lid.
- Pour the apple cider vinegar or vodka over the herbs, making sure they are fully submerged.
- Seal the jar tightly and shake well to mix the ingredients.
- Store the jar in a cool, dark place for 4-6 weeks, shaking it every few days.
- After the steeping period, strain the liquid, discarding the solid herbs.
- Transfer the tincture to a clean glass bottle with a dropper.
- Administer 5-10 drops of the tincture to your chicken orally twice a day.

Together, these herbs create a supportive blend targeting the underlying causes of water belly. The tincture focuses on improving liver and heart function, reducing fluid retention, and promoting overall wellness.

Notes:
- Dandelion Root: Known for its diuretic properties, dandelion root can help reduce fluid accumulation in the abdomen.
- Milk Thistle: A liver tonic that promotes liver function and can assist in detoxifying the liver.
- Eye Bright: Not only does this herb support eye health and overall vitality, but it can also help to detoxify the liver.
- Hawthorn Berries: Known to support heart function, hawthorn berries add an essential component for managing water belly.
- Burdock Root: A natural cleanser that supports both liver and kidney function.
- Storage: Keep the tincture in a cool, dark place. It should last up to a year if properly stored.
- Herb Quality: Always use high-quality, organic dried herbs to ensure efficacy and safety.
- Alcohol vs. Vinegar: Both apple cider vinegar and vodka can be used for extraction. If your chicken is sensitive to alcohol, vinegar might be a better choice.
- Consistency matters to see results!
- Dosage: Administer 5 - 10 drops of the tincture to your chickens twice a day. Continue for 7 days, take 2 days off, and continue for 7 more days. Follow this on - off - on schedule till you see a lack of fluid retention in the belly.
- Storage: Stored in a cool dark place, this tincture should last one year.
- Monitoring: Regularly check your chicken's condition, as water belly can be a complex issue. The tincture is intended as a supportive measure rather than a sole treatment.

Belly Brew offers a compassionate and natural approach to a condition that may otherwise seem daunting. Through the wise selection of herbs known for their beneficial effects on liver and heart health, this tincture provides a gentle yet potent solution. It not only addresses the symptoms but also supports the overall well-being of the chicken, reflecting a deep respect for nature's wisdom and a heartfelt connection to our clucking companions.

Feathered Harmony Water Belly Feed Blend

Water belly, or ascites, is a condition that can cause discomfort in chickens, leading to fluid accumulation in the abdomen. Feathered Harmony Water Belly Feed Blend is a specially crafted feed additive that combines the beneficial properties of eye bright, milk thistle, dandelion, and brewer's yeast. This blend aims to support liver and kidney functions, aiding in the reduction of fluid buildup and promoting overall wellness in your flock.

Ingredients:
• 1 tablespoon of eye bright
• 1 tablespoon of milk thistle
• 1 tablespoon of dandelion
• 2 tablespoons of brewer's yeast
• 1 cup of regular chicken feed

Directions:

- Mix the herbs and brewer's yeast with the chicken feed in a bowl.
- Store the blend in an airtight container.
- Add the blend to your chickens' regular feed as directed.

This feed additive is designed to be a part of your chickens' daily diet, providing a natural approach to managing water belly. The herbs and brewer's yeast work synergistically to support the organs responsible for fluid balance, offering a gentle yet effective solution.

Notes:
- Eye Bright: Known for its supportive properties, eye bright may enhance overall health and aid in detoxification.
- Milk Thistle: This herb is recognized for its liver-supporting functions, aiding in detoxification.
- Dandelion: A natural diuretic, dandelion helps the body manage excess fluids.
- Brewer's Yeast: Rich in B vitamins, brewer's yeast supports digestion and nutrient absorption.
- Quality Matters: Always choose organic and high-quality herbs to ensure the remedy's effectiveness.
- Consistency Matters: Regular feeding, as part of the daily diet, is essential for optimal results.
- Storage: Keep the blend in a cool, dry place, away from direct sunlight.
- Dosage Information: Add 1-2 tablespoons of the blend to the regular feed per chicken daily.
- Treatment Duration: Continue as a regular part of the diet or until symptoms improve.

Feathered Harmony Water Belly Feed Blend is more than just a feed additive; it's a commitment to the well-being of your feathered friends. By incorporating this blend into their daily diet, you're providing them with nature's nurturing touch, helping them thrive and enjoy a happy, healthy life.

6. Egg Binding

Egg binding in chickens is a serious and potentially life-threatening condition where a hen is unable to pass an egg. This can occur for various reasons, including a lack of calcium, obesity, or an egg that's too large. The egg becomes stuck in the oviduct, causing discomfort and distress. If not addressed promptly, egg binding can lead to further complications, such as infection or damage to internal organs and even death. Recognizing the signs of egg binding, such as a hen straining, acting lethargic, or walking abnormally, and implementing appropriate care can be crucial in helping the hen pass the egg and return to normal health.

Soothing Relaxation Soak

Egg binding in hens can be a stressful and painful condition where a hen is unable to lay an egg. The Soothing Relaxation Soak is designed to ease the discomfort and help relax the muscles, facilitating the passage of the egg. This calming soak combines the therapeutic properties of Epsom salt with the calming effects of lavender and chamomile. Be sure to use it in conjunction with the Vent Ease Herbal Ointment

Ingredients:
- 1 cup Epsom Salt
- 5 drops of Lavender Essential Oil
- 1/4 cup Chamomile Flowers
- 1 gallon Warm Water

Directions:
- Fill a basin with 1 gallon of warm water.
- Add the Epsom salt and stir until dissolved.
- Add the lavender essential oil and chamomile flowers.
- Gently place the hen in the basin, ensuring the affected area is submerged.
- Allow the hen to soak for 15-20 minutes, gently massaging the area if needed.
- Remove the hen and pat dry with a clean towel.
- You may have to repeat the above steps 2 to 3 times per day till the egg passes.

The Soothing Relaxation Soak is aimed at relaxing the hen's muscles and providing relief from the discomfort of egg binding. Epsom salt is known for its muscle-relaxing properties, while lavender essential oil adds a calming effect. Chamomile flowers further soothe the hen, making the process of laying the egg smoother and less stressful.

Notes:
- Epsom Salt: Acts as a muscle relaxant, helping to ease the passage of the egg.
- Lavender Essential Oil: Known for its calming properties, it helps in reducing stress.
- Chamomile Flowers: Adds a gentle, soothing effect, further aiding in relaxation.
- Quality Matters: Always use high-quality ingredients to ensure the effectiveness of the remedy.
- Consistency Matters: Regular application may be necessary depending on the severity of the condition.
- Storage: Make a fresh batch every time you soak your hen to ensure potency.

- Correct Dosage Information: Follow the measurements accurately for the best results.
- How to Administer: Gentle handling and a calm environment will make the process easier for the hen. Never leave a hen that is soaking unattended, as this tends to really calm them down to the point of almost sleeping. Their heads could slip under the water.
- How Long Treatment Should Last: Repeat 2 to 3 times per day till the hen passes her egg, monitoring the hen's condition closely.

This remedy is a gentle approach to a common issue in hens, providing comfort and support in a natural and compassionate way.

Vent Ease Herbal Ointment

Egg binding in hens is a condition where an egg gets stuck in the reproductive tract, causing discomfort and potential health risks. The Vent Ease Herbal Ointment is specifically formulated to relax the vent area, easing the passage of the egg. With a blend of soothing and calming ingredients, this ointment can be a gentle aid in a stressful situation. Be sure to use it in conjunction with the Soothing Relaxation Soak.

Ingredients:
• 2 tablespoons Coconut Oil
• 1 tablespoon Aloe Vera Gel
• 5 drops of Calendula Essential Oil
• 5 drops of Lavender Essential Oil

Directions:
In a small bowl, combine the coconut oil, aloe vera gel, calendula essential oil, and lavender essential oil.
Mix well until all ingredients are thoroughly blended.
Gently apply the ointment to the vent area of the hen, massaging it in with soft, circular motions.
Allow the ointment to absorb; do not rinse.
Repeat as needed between soaks and especially before bedtime when the hen is calm and relaxed.

The Vent Ease Herbal Ointment is designed to provide relief and support to hens suffering from egg binding. The combination of coconut oil, aloe vera, calendula, and lavender works together to soothe and relax the muscles around the vent, facilitating the natural process of laying the egg.

Notes:
Coconut Oil: Acts as a moisturizer and carrier oil, allowing other ingredients to penetrate deeply.
Aloe Vera Gel: Known for its soothing properties, it helps reduce irritation.
Calendula Essential Oil: A gentle herb known for its healing and calming effects on the skin.
Lavender Essential Oil: Adds a relaxing scent and has calming properties.
Quality Matters: Selecting high-quality, organic ingredients will enhance the effectiveness of the remedy.

Consistency Matters: Regular application may be necessary, depending on the hen's condition.
Storage: Store the ointment in a cool, dark place in an airtight container.
Correct Dosage Information: Adhering to the measurements ensures the proper balance of ingredients.
How to Administer: Gentle application is key; avoid causing additional stress to the hen.
How Long Treatment Should Last: Monitor the hen's condition and continue treatment as needed.

The Vent Ease Herbal Ointment is a compassionate approach to a delicate issue, providing natural support to ease discomfort and promote well-being in your hens.

Laying Boost Calcium-Enhanced Feed

Egg binding in hens can be a distressing condition where an egg becomes stuck in the reproductive tract. Laying Boost Calcium-Enhanced Feed is a specially formulated feed designed to support hens during this time. By providing essential nutrients and herbs, this feed aims to promote healthy laying and reduce the risk of egg binding.

Ingredients:
• 4 cups Chicken Feed
• 1 cup Crushed Eggshells
• 1/2 cup Flaxseed
• 1/4 cup Dried Nettle
• 1/4 cup Dried Oregano

Directions:
• In a large mixing bowl, combine the chicken feed, crushed eggshells, flaxseed, dried nettle, and dried oregano.
• Mix thoroughly to ensure an even distribution of ingredients.
• Replace the regular feed with this calcium-enhanced feed, providing it to the hens as their main diet.
• Monitor the hens for improvements and continue feeding as part of their regular diet.

Laying Boost Calcium-Enhanced Feed is designed to support hens in laying eggs smoothly. The calcium from the eggshells strengthens the eggshell, while the herbs and flaxseed provide additional nutrients and support for the reproductive system.

Notes:
- Chicken Feed: The base of the feed, providing essential nutrients.
- Crushed Eggshells: A natural source of calcium, vital for strong eggshells. A hen's uterus (aka shell gland) is the muscle responsible for squeezing the egg out of the vent. Since muscles require calcium to contract properly, if a hen has a calcium deficiency, the egg can get stuck in the uterus. The extra calcium can help your hen push the egg out.
- Flaxseed: Rich in Omega-3 fatty acids, supporting overall health.
- Dried Nettle: Known for its nourishing properties, supporting kidney and liver function.
- Dried Oregano: A natural antibiotic supporting the immune system.
- Quality Matters: Use fresh and organic ingredients for the best results.

- Consistency Matters: Feed regularly to maintain the benefits.
- Storage: Store in a cool, dry place in an airtight container.
- Correct Dosage Information: Follow the given measurements to ensure a balanced diet.
- How to Administer: Replace the regular feed with this enhanced feed.
- How Long Treatment Should Last: Can be used as a regular part of the diet or until the issue resolves.

Laying Boost Calcium-Enhanced Feed is a thoughtful approach to supporting your hens during a critical time. By providing essential nutrients and herbs, this feed helps promote healthy laying and offers a natural way to care for your flock.

Preventative Herbal Support Drink

Egg binding in hens is a condition that requires careful attention. The Preventative Herbal Support Drink is a gentle, natural remedy designed to support the overall health of the hen's reproductive system. With the soothing properties of Aloe vera and the supportive nature of comfrey, this drink aims to prevent egg binding and promote smooth laying.

Ingredients:
- 2 cups Distilled Water
- 1/2 cup Aloe Vera Gel (freshly extracted)
- 1/4 cup Comfrey Leaves (dried or fresh)

Directions:
- In a small saucepan, bring the distilled water to a gentle boil.
- Add the comfrey leaves and simmer for 10 minutes.
- Remove from heat and allow to cool to room temperature.
- Strain the comfrey leaves and mix in the Aloe vera gel.
- Serve to the hens in a clean waterer, replacing their regular drinking water.

The Preventative Herbal Support Drink is formulated to provide gentle support to the hen's reproductive system. Aloe vera's soothing properties help relax the muscles, while comfrey's historical use in supporting muscle and bone health adds an extra layer of care. Together, these ingredients work to prevent egg binding and promote healthy laying.

Notes:
- Aloe Vera: Known for its soothing and hydrating properties, supports the digestive system.
- Comfrey: Historically used for muscle and bone health, supports the reproductive system.
- Distilled Water: Ensures a pure and clean base for the remedy.
- Quality Matters: Use fresh and organic Aloe vera and comfrey for optimal results.
- Consistency Matters: Regular administration is key to maintaining benefits.
- Storage: Store any unused portion in the refrigerator for up to 3 days.
- Correct Dosage Information: Replace regular drinking water with this herbal drink as needed.
- How to Administer: Serve in a clean dish, observing the hens for acceptance.
- How Long Treatment Should Last: Can be used as a regular part of the diet or as a preventative measure during known risk periods. Aim to provide this support drink at least once per week.

The Preventative Herbal Support Drink is a thoughtful and natural way to care for your hens, providing them with the support they need to lay eggs smoothly. By understanding the properties of each ingredient and administering with care, you can offer a loving and natural approach to hen care.

7. External Parasites

External parasites on chickens are a common concern for poultry keepers, as they can lead to discomfort, stress, and health issues within the flock. Various types of external pests can affect chickens, including mites, lice, fleas, and ticks. Mites are tiny arachnids that can infest the feathers, skin, and even the respiratory tract, leading to itching and irritation. Lice are insects that feed on dead skin and feathers, causing similar discomfort. Fleas can jump from host to host, biting and feeding on the chickens' blood, while ticks can attach themselves to the skin, leading to localized swelling and potential transmission of diseases. These parasites can multiply quickly if left unchecked, making regular inspection and proper care essential to maintain the health and well-being of the flock. Natural remedies, proper hygiene, and environmental management can often effectively control and prevent these infestations.

Feathered Friend Anti-Parasite Powder

Introducing Feathered Friend Anti-Parasite Powder, a natural remedy formulated to combat external parasites that may affect your beloved chickens. Crafted with care, this blend contains Diatomaceous Earth, Peppermint, Thyme, Rosemary, and Garlic Powder, each chosen for their potent anti-parasitic properties. By using this powder, you're taking proactive steps to help keep your chickens comfortable and free from the discomfort caused by these pesky intruders.

Ingredients:
- 1/2 cup of Diatomaceous Earth
- 2 tablespoons of Peppermint leaves
- 1 tablespoon of Thyme leaves
- 1 tablespoon of Rosemary leaves
- 1 tablespoon of Garlic powder

Directions:
- Combine all the dry ingredients in a bowl.
- Thoroughly mix the ingredients to ensure an even blend.
- Gently dust the powder onto your chickens' feathers, under their wings, and around their vent area. While applying the powder to your chicken, be sure to avoid the eyes and nostrils. Apply around their coop, in their nesting boxes, and in their dust bath area, focusing on areas prone to infestation.
- Reapply as needed, especially after rainy weather or when you notice signs of infestation.

Feathered Friend Anti-Parasite Powder serves as a proactive defense against external parasites that can affect your chickens' well-being. Diatomaceous Earth acts as a mechanical pest deterrent, while Peppermint, Thyme, Rosemary, and Garlic contribute natural compounds that pests find uninviting. By applying this powder regularly, you create an environment that discourages these unwelcome visitors, promoting your chickens' comfort and health.

Notes:
- Diatomaceous Earth: Known for its abrasive texture, it helps deter pests by dehydrating them upon contact.

- Peppermint: The strong scent of peppermint oil is known to repel various pests, including mites and lice.
- Thyme: Contains thymol, which has natural insecticidal properties and aids in repelling parasites.
- Rosemary: Its aromatic compounds deter pests and have additional benefits for overall chicken health.
- Garlic: Contains allicin, a compound known for its antimicrobial and insect-repelling properties.
- Quality Matters: Choose high-quality, food-grade Diatomaceous Earth and herbs to ensure effectiveness.
- Consistency: Regular application is key to maintaining a deterrent effect against parasites.
- Storage: Keep the powder in a dry, airtight container away from moisture and sunlight.
- Dosage: Gently dust the powder onto your chickens' feathers, under their wings, and around their vent area. While applying the powder to your chicken, be sure to avoid the eyes and nostrils. Apply around their coop, in their nesting boxes, and in their dust bath area, focusing on areas prone to infestation.
- Treatment Duration: Apply as part of your regular chicken care routine, especially during peak parasite seasons.

Feathered Friend Anti-Parasite Powder provides a natural and effective means to support your chickens' comfort and well-being by addressing external parasites. By understanding the role of each ingredient and following guidelines on quality, consistency, and administration, you're taking a thoughtful approach to promoting a harmonious and pest-free environment for your feathered companions.

Preen Queen (or King) Parasite Spray

Introducing Preen Queen (or King) Parasite Spray, a soothing and aromatic remedy designed to help protect your cherished chickens from the discomfort of external parasites. Crafted with care, this blend features Apple Cider Vinegar, Lavender Oil, Neem Oil, Rosemary Oil, and Distilled Water, each contributing their unique properties to create a potent and refreshing spray. By using this spray, you're pampering your feathered friends while helping to keep them free from the irritation caused by unwanted pests.

Ingredients:
- 1/2 cup of Apple Cider Vinegar
- 10 drops of Lavender Oil
- 5 drops of Neem Oil
- 5 drops of Rosemary Oil
- 1 cup of Distilled Water

Directions:
- In a spray bottle, combine the Apple Cider Vinegar, Lavender Oil, Neem Oil, and Rosemary Oil.
- Add the Distilled Water to the mixture and close the spray bottle.
- Shake well to ensure thorough blending of the ingredients.
- Gently mist the spray onto your chickens' feathers, avoiding their eyes and sensitive areas.

- Apply as needed, especially after rain or during peak pest seasons.

Preen Queen (or King) Parasite Spray offers a dual-purpose remedy that not only helps repel external parasites but also provides a calming and aromatic experience for your cherished chickens. Apple Cider Vinegar acts as a mild disinfectant and can help deter pests. Lavender Oil and Rosemary Oil contribute aromatic compounds that pests find unpleasant while also providing a soothing atmosphere for the chickens. Neem Oil, known for its natural insect-repelling properties, further enhances the protective benefits of this spray.

Notes:
- Apple Cider Vinegar: Offers mild disinfection properties and helps create an environment less attractive to pests.
- Lavender Oil: Known for its soothing aroma, it also helps discourage parasites.
- Neem Oil: Contains azadirachtin, a natural insect repellent, and contributes to the spray's effectiveness.
- Rosemary Oil: Adds an aromatic element and provides additional pest-repelling benefits.
- Distilled Water: Use distilled water to maintain the spray's freshness and quality.
- Quality Matters: Choose high-quality essential oils and apple cider vinegar for the best results.
- Consistency: Apply the spray regularly to help maintain its protective effect.
- Storage: Store the spray bottle in a cool, dry place away from direct sunlight.
- Dosage: Gently mist the chickens' feathers, avoiding their eyes and sensitive areas.
- Treatment Duration: Incorporate into your regular chicken care routine, especially during peak pest seasons.

Preen Queen (or King) Parasite Spray offers a delightful and practical way to support your chickens' comfort and well-being. By understanding the role of each ingredient and following guidelines on quality, consistency, and administration, you're providing your feathered companions with a refreshing and protective experience that enhances their quality of life.

Happy Hen & Roo Herbal Water Additive

The Happy Hen & Roo Herbal Water Additive is a refreshing and proactive remedy designed to support your chickens' well-being by naturally addressing external parasites from the inside out. Carefully crafted with Garlic Cloves, Oregano Leaves, Lemon Balm, this additive offers a simple and effective way to enhance your chickens' environment while helping to repel unwanted pests. By incorporating this additive into their water supply, you're contributing to your chickens' comfort and overall health.

Ingredients:
- 2-3 Garlic Cloves (crushed)
- 1 tablespoon of Oregano Leaves
- 1 tablespoon of Lemon Balm Leaves
- 1 gallon of Filtered Water

Directions:
- In a container, combine the crushed Garlic Cloves, Oregano Leaves, and Lemon Balm Leaves.

- Boil the filtered water and pour it over the herbal mixture.
- Allow the mixture to steep and cool down to room temperature.
- Strain the mixture to remove the herbal leaves and cloves.
- Pour the herbal-infused water into your chickens' water dispenser.

Happy Hen & Roo Herbal Water Additive offers a proactive approach to promoting your chickens' comfort and repelling external parasites naturally. Garlic is well-known for its repelling properties against various pests, while Oregano Leaves and Lemon Balm contribute aromatic compounds that pests find uninviting. By incorporating this additive into your chickens' water supply, you're providing them with a refreshing and protective drink that contributes to their overall well-being.

Notes:
Garlic Cloves: Contains allicin, a natural pest repellent, and contributes to your chickens' health.
Oregano Leaves: Known for its antimicrobial properties, oregano helps deter parasites.
Lemon Balm Leaves: The lemony aroma of this herb is disliked by pests, enhancing the repellent effect.
Filtered Water: Ensure the water quality is good for your chickens' consumption.
Quality Matters: Use fresh, high-quality herbs and garlic cloves for optimal results.
Consistency: Provide the herbal water additive regularly to maintain its pest-repelling benefits.
Storage: Store any leftover herbal water in a cool, dark place to maintain freshness.
Dosage: Add the herbal water additive to your chickens' water dispenser at each refill.
Treatment Duration: Incorporate into your regular chicken care routine, especially during peak pest seasons.

Happy Hen & Roo Herbal Water Additive contributes to a harmonious and pest-resistant environment for your feathered companions. By understanding the benefits of each ingredient and following guidelines on quality, consistency, and administration, you're taking steps to provide your chickens with a refreshing and protective drink that enhances their overall quality of life.

Nest Comfort Parasite-Repelling Powder

Introducing Nest Comfort Parasite-Repelling Powder, a thoughtful and aromatic remedy designed to create a soothing and pest-resistant nesting environment for your cherished chickens. Crafted with Peppermint Leaves, Eucalyptus Leaves, Neem Powder, and Diatomaceous Earth, this powder offers a natural way to help protect your chickens from the irritation caused by external parasites. By applying this powder to their nesting area, you're providing a comfortable and protective space that enhances their well-being.

Ingredients:
- 1 tablespoon of Peppermint Leaves
- 1 tablespoon of Eucalyptus Leaves
- 1 tablespoon of Neem Powder
- 1/4 cup of Diatomaceous Earth

Directions:
- In a container, combine the Peppermint Leaves, Eucalyptus Leaves, Neem Powder, and Diatomaceous Earth.
- Gently mix the ingredients to ensure even distribution.
- Sprinkle a thin layer of the powder in the nesting area, focusing on areas where parasites are likely to reside.
- Reapply as needed, especially after cleaning or when you notice signs of infestation.

Nest Comfort Parasite-Repelling Powder offers a thoughtful approach to promoting a safe and pest-resistant nesting space for your chickens. Peppermint Leaves and Eucalyptus Leaves contribute aromatic compounds that pests find uninviting, creating an environment that discourages their presence. Neem Powder, known for its natural insect-repelling properties, further enhances the protective benefits of this powder. Diatomaceous Earth acts as a mechanical deterrent, helping to keep the nesting area free from unwanted pests.

Notes:
- Peppermint Leaves: The strong aroma of peppermint is disliked by pests, enhancing the powder's repellent effect.
- Eucalyptus Leaves: Known for their aromatic compounds, eucalyptus leaves help to create an uninviting nesting environment for parasites.
- Neem Powder: Contains azadirachtin, a natural insect repellent, and contributes to the powder's effectiveness.
- Diatomaceous Earth: Known for its abrasive texture, it helps deter pests by dehydrating them upon contact.
- Quality Matters: Use high-quality herbs and neem powder for optimal results.
- Consistency: Regular application helps maintain a pest-resistant nesting space.
- Storage: Store the powder in a dry, airtight container away from moisture and sunlight.
- Dosage: Sprinkle a thin layer in the nesting area.
- Treatment Duration: Apply as part of your regular chicken care routine, especially during peak parasite seasons.

Nest Comfort Parasite-Repelling Powder contributes to a cozy and pest-free nesting environment for your feathered companions. By understanding the benefits of each ingredient and following guidelines on quality, consistency, and administration, you're taking steps to create a space that promotes your chickens' comfort and well-being.

Flock Guard Parasite Spray

Introducing Flock Guard Parasite Spray, a powerful and versatile remedy designed to provide your flock of chickens with a protective shield against external parasites. Formulated with Witch Hazel, Tea Tree Oil, Lemongrass Oil, Neem Oil, Clove Oil, this spray offers a comprehensive approach to keeping unwanted pests at bay. By applying this spray to your chickens' feathers, nesting boxes or roosting areas, you're contributing to their comfort and overall health in a natural and effective way.

Ingredients:
- 1/4 cup of Witch Hazel

- 10 drops of Tea Tree Oil
- 10 drops of Lemongrass Oil
- 5 drops of Neem Oil
- 5 drops of Clove Oil
- 1 cup of Distilled Water

Directions:
- In a spray bottle, combine the Witch Hazel, Tea Tree Oil, Lemongrass Oil, Neem Oil, and Clove Oil.
- Add the Distilled Water to the mixture and close the spray bottle.
- Shake well to ensure thorough blending of the ingredients.
- Gently mist the spray onto your chickens' feathers, avoiding their eyes and sensitive areas. You can also use this spray in nesting boxes and roosting areas. Pay special attention to the cracks and crevices in these areas.
- Apply as needed, especially during peak pest seasons or after rain.

Flock Guard Parasite Spray offers a potent and multi-faceted approach to supporting your chickens' well-being by repelling external parasites. Witch Hazel acts as a mild astringent and carrier for the essential oils, while Tea Tree Oil, Lemongrass Oil, and Clove Oil contribute their natural pest-repelling properties. Neem Oil further enhances the spray's effectiveness, creating a comprehensive barrier against unwanted pests. By using this spray, you're providing your chickens with a protective shield that enhances their quality of life.

Notes:
- Witch Hazel: Acts as a carrier for essential oils and provides mild astringent properties.
- Tea Tree Oil* Known for its natural pest-repelling properties, it contributes to the spray's effectiveness.
- Lemongrass Oil: The citrusy aroma is disliked by pests, enhancing the repellent effect.
- Neem Oil: Contains azadirachtin, a natural insect repellent, and contributes to the spray's potency.
- Clove Oil: Adds an aromatic element and enhances the overall repellent properties.
- Distilled Water: Use clean and distilled water to ensure the spray's freshness.
- Quality Matters: Use high-quality essential oils and ingredients for the best results.
- Consistency: Apply the spray regularly, especially during peak pest seasons.
- Storage: Store the spray bottle in a cool, dry place away from direct sunlight.
- Dosage: Gently mist the chickens' feathers, avoiding their eyes and sensitive areas. You can also use this spray in nesting boxes and roosting areas. Pay special attention to the cracks and crevices in these areas
- Treatment Duration: Incorporate into your regular chicken care routine, as needed.

Flock Guard Parasite Spray offers a comprehensive and effective way to protect your flock from external pests. By understanding the role of each ingredient and following guidelines on quality, consistency, and administration, you're contributing to your chickens' overall comfort and health in a natural and proactive manner.

Feather Shield Parasite Defense Dip

Introducing Feather Shield Parasite Defense Dip, a robust and holistic remedy designed to shield your chickens' feathers from the intrusion of external parasites. Crafted with a blend of Neem Leaves, Eucalyptus Leaves, Lavender Flowers, Garlic Cloves, Apple Cider Vinegar, this dip offers a natural and protective solution that helps maintain your chickens' comfort and well-being. By immersing your chickens in this nourishing dip, you're actively supporting their defense against unwanted pests.

Ingredients:
- 1 cup of Neem Leaves
- 1/2 cup of Eucalyptus Leaves
- 1/4 cup of Lavender Flowers
- 4-5 Garlic Cloves
- 1 cup of Apple Cider Vinegar
- 2 cups of Distilled Water

Directions:
- In a large container, combine the Neem Leaves, Eucalyptus Leaves, Lavender Flowers, and Garlic Cloves.
- Boil the Apple Cider Vinegar and Distilled Water, and then pour the hot mixture over the herbs and garlic.
- Allow the mixture to steep and cool to room temperature.
- Strain the liquid to remove the herb and garlic remnants, leaving only the infused liquid.
- Place the liquid in a large basin or container suitable for dipping your chickens.
- Gently dip each chicken in the solution, ensuring the feathers are thoroughly soaked.
- Allow the chickens to air dry in a warm and protected area.

Feather Shield Parasite Defense Dip offers a comprehensive and effective approach to protecting your chickens from the discomfort caused by external parasites. Neem Leaves and Eucalyptus Leaves contribute natural pest-repelling properties, while Lavender Flowers add a soothing and aromatic element. Garlic Cloves contain natural compounds that deter pests. Apple Cider Vinegar acts as a carrier, allowing the herbs' beneficial properties to infuse the dip. By using this dip, you're actively enhancing your chickens' resilience against pests.

Notes:
- Neem Leaves: Known for their insect-repelling properties, neem leaves contribute to the dip's effectiveness.
- Eucalyptus Leaves: The aromatic compounds in eucalyptus leaves help create an unwelcome environment for pests.
- Lavender Flowers: Lavender's soothing aroma adds a calming touch to the dip.
- Garlic Cloves: Garlic contains natural compounds that pests find uninviting.
- Apple Cider Vinegar: Acts as a carrier, allowing the herbs' properties to infuse the dip.
- Distilled Water: Use clean and distilled water to ensure the dip's freshness.
- Quality Matters: Choose high-quality ingredients for optimal results.
- Consistency: Administer the dip as needed, especially during peak pest seasons.
- Storage: Store any unused dip in a cool, dark place.
- Dosage: Ensure feathers are thoroughly soaked during the dip.
- Treatment Duration: Incorporate into your regular chicken care routine for best results.

Feather Shield Parasite Defense Dip provides your chickens with a protective barrier against external parasites. By understanding the purpose of each ingredient and following guidelines on quality, consistency, and administration, you're taking steps to ensure your chickens' comfort and overall well-being in a natural and thoughtful manner.

Mite-B-Gone Spray

Introducing Mite-B-Gone Spray, a potent and effective remedy crafted to banish external parasites from your beloved chickens. This spray, formulated with a blend of cedarwood oil, clove oil, lemongrass oil, neem oil, lavender oil, geranium oil, and cottonseed oil, is designed to offer your flock relief from the discomfort caused by these pests. By using this spray, you're taking proactive steps to ensure your chickens' comfort and well-being.

Ingredients:
- 10 drops of Cedarwood Oil
- 5 drops of Clove Oil
- 5 drops of Lemongrass Oil
- 5 drops of Neem Oil
- 5 drops of Lavender Oil
- 5 drops of Geranium Oil
- 1 teaspoon of Cottonseed Oil
- 1 cup of Distilled Water

Directions:
- In a spray bottle, combine the Cedarwood Oil, Clove Oil, Lemongrass Oil, Neem Oil, Lavender Oil, Geranium Oil, and Cottonseed Oil.
- Add the Distilled Water to the mixture, close the spray bottle, and shake well to ensure thorough blending.
- Lightly mist your chickens' feathers, paying attention to areas where pests may congregate.
- Avoid spraying directly on their eyes and sensitive areas.
- Apply as needed, especially during peak pest seasons or when signs of infestation arise.

Mite-B-Gone Spray offers an efficient and natural approach to addressing the presence of external parasites on your chickens. Cedarwood Oil, Clove Oil, Lemongrass Oil, Neem Oil, Lavender Oil, and Geranium Oil contribute their pest-repelling properties, creating an unwelcome environment for pests. Cottonseed Oil acts as a carrier for the essential oils, ensuring proper application. By using this spray, you're providing your chickens with a layer of protection that enhances their quality of life.

Notes:
- Cedarwood Oil: Known for its pest-repelling properties, cedarwood oil adds an aromatic touch to the spray.
- Clove Oil: Clove oil contains natural compounds that pests find uninviting.
- Lemongrass Oil: The citrusy aroma of lemongrass deters pests from approaching.
- Neem Oil Neem oil contributes to the spray's potency due to its pest-repelling attributes.
- Lavender Oil: Lavender adds a soothing and aromatic element to the spray.

- Geranium Oil: Geranium oil enhances the spray's effectiveness by creating an unwelcome environment for pests.
- Cottonseed Oil: Acts as a carrier for the essential oils, ensuring even distribution.
- Distilled Water: Use clean and distilled water to maintain the spray's freshness.
- Quality Matters: Choose high-quality essential oils and ingredients for optimal results.
- Consistency: Apply the spray regularly, especially during peak pest seasons.
- Storage: Store the spray bottle in a cool, dark place.
- Dosage: Lightly mist the chickens' feathers, avoiding eyes and sensitive areas.
- Treatment Duration: Incorporate the spray into your regular chicken care routine for ongoing protection.

Mite-B-Gone Spray empowers you to actively address the presence of external parasites on your chickens. By understanding the purpose of each ingredient and following guidelines on quality, consistency, and administration, you're contributing to your chickens' overall comfort and well-being in a natural and effective manner.

Mite Smothering Leg Salve (Scaly Leg Mites)

Introducing Mite Smothering Leg Salve, a natural remedy designed to provide comfort and relief to your chickens suffering from scaly leg mites. Crafted with care using Coconut Oil, Beeswax, Neem Oil, Calendula Extract, and Eucalyptus Oil, this salve is a soothing solution to help alleviate the discomfort caused by leg mites. By using this salve, you're taking a proactive approach to ensure your chickens' leg health and overall well-being.

Ingredients:
- 2 tablespoons of Coconut Oil
- 1 tablespoon of Beeswax
- 10 drops of Neem Oil
- 1 teaspoon of Calendula Extract
- 5 drops of Eucalyptus Oil

Directions:
- In a double boiler, melt the Coconut Oil and Beeswax together until fully combined.
- Remove from heat and allow the mixture to cool slightly.
- Add the Neem Oil, Calendula Extract, and Eucalyptus Oil to the mixture, stirring well to ensure even distribution.
- Transfer the salve to a clean, airtight container for storage.
- Gently apply the salve to the affected areas on your chickens' legs, ensuring thorough coverage.
- Use as needed to provide relief and support for your chickens' leg health.

Mite Smothering Leg Salve is specifically formulated to address the discomfort caused by scale leg mites on chickens' legs. Coconut Oil and Beeswax create a soothing base for the salve, providing a protective barrier for the skin. Neem Oil is known for its pest-repelling properties, while Calendula Extract and Eucalyptus Oil contribute to soothing and calming the affected areas. All of these ingredients work together to smother the leg mites and restore health to your chicken's legs. By applying this salve, you're supporting your chickens' leg health and helping them feel more comfortable.

Notes:
- Coconut Oil: Coconut oil acts as a moisturizing base for the salve, aiding in the application and soothing of the skin.
- Beeswax: Beeswax helps solidify the salve, ensuring easy application and providing a protective barrier.
- Neem Oil: Neem oil adds its natural pest-repelling qualities to the salve.
- Calendula Extract: Calendula is known for its soothing properties, promoting comfort for irritated skin.
- Eucalyptus Oil: Eucalyptus oil contributes a calming effect to the salve and supports skin health.
- Quality Matters: Use high-quality ingredients to ensure the efficacy of the salve.
- Consistency: Apply the salve as needed, focusing on affected leg areas.
- Storage: Store the salve in a cool, dry place to maintain its integrity. Stored properly it should last 6 months.
- Dosage: Gently apply the salve to affected areas, avoiding contact with eyes and sensitive areas.
- Treatment Duration: Continue applying the salve until the chickens' leg health improves.

Mite Smothering Leg Salve offers a gentle and natural approach to addressing leg discomfort caused by external parasites. By understanding the purpose of each ingredient and following guidelines on quality, consistency, and administration, you're providing your chickens with a solution that promotes their well-being and overall comfort.

8. Internal Parasites

Internal parasites are a prevalent concern among chickens that can lead to discomfort and compromised health. Chickens can be affected by various types of internal parasites, including roundworms, tapeworms, coccidia, and gapeworms. Roundworms are intestinal worms that can lead to poor growth and nutrient absorption. Tapeworms attach to the intestinal lining, potentially causing weight loss and weakness. Coccidia are protozoan parasites that can impact the digestive tract and lead to diarrhea. Gapeworms can lodge in the trachea, causing respiratory distress. These parasites are often contracted through contaminated environments or contact with infected birds, making regular deworming and proper management essential to maintaining the overall well-being of the flock. Natural remedies and preventative measures can help manage internal parasites and promote a healthier environment for chickens.

Wormwood Wonder Tonic

This natural herbal remedy is designed to support your chickens' internal health by addressing the presence of internal parasites. This tonic is a blend of potent herbs including Wormwood, Chamomile, Fennel Seeds, and Ginger Root, known for their potential to help expel unwanted parasites from your chickens' system.

Ingredients:
- 1 tablespoon Wormwood
- 2 tablespoons Chamomile
- 1 tablespoon Fennel Seeds
- 1 teaspoon Ginger Root
- 2 cups of Distilled Water

Directions:
- In a small pot, bring 2 cups of water to a gentle simmer.
- Add the Wormwood, Chamomile, Fennel Seeds, and Ginger Root to the simmering water.
- Let the herbs steep for 15 minutes, then remove from heat.
- Allow the mixture to cool to room temperature.
- Strain the mixture to remove the herb solids, leaving only the liquid.

The Wormwood Wonder Tonic harnesses the natural properties of its herbal ingredients to provide a gentle yet effective way to address internal parasites in chickens. Wormwood is known for its potential to expel parasites from the digestive tract, while Chamomile soothes the gastrointestinal system. Fennel Seeds offer digestive support, and Ginger Root aids in maintaining a healthy intestinal environment. When combined, these herbs create a powerful tonic to promote your chickens' overall health and vitality.

Notes:
- Wormwood: Wormwood is known for its potential to help expel intestinal parasites. It contains compounds that are thought to discourage the growth and survival of parasites.
- Chamomile: Chamomile offers soothing properties to the digestive system and supports overall gastrointestinal health. It also aids in reducing inflammation.

- Fennel Seeds: Fennel Seeds are believed to possess anti-parasitic properties and can help ease digestive discomfort in chickens.
- Ginger Root: Ginger Root aids in digestion and helps to maintain a healthy gut environment, which is essential for preventing and managing parasites.
- Quality Matters: When selecting herbs, opt for organic options to ensure the absence of harmful chemicals or pesticides.
- Consistency Matters: Administer the tonic regularly as a preventive measure or during parasite outbreaks. It's important to establish a routine for the best results.
- Dosage and Administration: Add 1 tablespoon of the Wormwood Wonder Tonic to 1 gallon of your chickens' water source. Use once a week for maintenance or during episodes of concern.
- Duration of Treatment: For infestations, administer the tonic for at least 7 days or until the presence of internal parasites is no longer observed.

By incorporating the Wormwood Wonder Tonic into your chickens' care routine, you're taking a natural approach to promoting their internal health and well-being. Remember that consistency and proper care play a significant role in maintaining a healthy flock.

Poultry Parasite Prowess Tincture

This herbal remedy is designed to help your chickens combat internal parasites from within. This tincture is a blend of potent ingredients, including Black Walnut Hull, Pumpkin Seeds, Thyme, and Clover, carefully chosen for their potential to support your chickens' overall well-being.

Ingredients:
• 1 tablespoon Black Walnut Hull
• 1 tablespoon Pumpkin Seeds
• 1 tablespoon Thyme
• 1 tablespoon Clover
• Enough Alcohol (vodka) or Apple Cider Vinegar (organic with the mother) to fully cover the herbs

Directions:
• In a glass jar, combine the Black Walnut Hull, Pumpkin Seeds, Thyme, and Clover.
• Fill the jar with alcohol (vodka) or Apple Cider Vinegar, ensuring that the herbs are fully covered.
• Seal the jar tightly and store it in a cool, dark place for at least two weeks.
• Shake the jar daily to help infuse the tincture.
• After two weeks, strain the tincture through a fine mesh strainer or cheesecloth into a clean glass bottle.

The Poultry Parasite Prowess Tincture is formulated to naturally assist in combating internal parasites that may affect your chickens. Each ingredient contributes to the remedy's potential effectiveness.

Notes:

- Black Walnut Hull: Known for its potential to expel parasites, Black Walnut Hull is a powerful ally in maintaining intestinal health.
- Pumpkin Seeds: Pumpkin Seeds contain compounds that may help support digestive wellness and discourage parasites.
- Thyme: Thyme is believed to have antimicrobial properties that could contribute to the chickens' overall well-being.
- Clover: Clover is rich in nutrients and may offer support for the digestive system.
- Quality Matters: Choose high-quality herbs and alcohol (vodka) or Apple Cider Vinegar for optimal results.
- Consistency is Key: Administer the tincture consistently to support your chickens' health.
- Dosage: Add approximately 1 tablespoon of the Poultry Parasite Prowess Tincture to every gallon of your chickens' drinking water.
- Storage: Store the tincture in a cool, dark place to preserve its potency. Stored correctly, it should last 1 year.
- Duration: Administer the tincture in their drinking water for 7 consecutive days. After the initial 7-day treatment, give your chickens a break from the tincture for about 2 weeks. If needed, you can repeat the 7-day treatment followed by the 2-week break for up to 3 cycles.

By incorporating the Poultry Parasite Prowess Tincture into your chickens' routine, you're embracing a natural approach to internal parasite management. As with any herbal remedy, closely observe your chickens' behavior and consult a professional if necessary. The power of natural ingredients can contribute to the vitality of your flock. By harnessing the benefits of this tincture, you're taking a proactive step in supporting your chickens' health and happiness.

Cluck Cleanse Elixir

This is a natural and effective herbal remedy designed to support your chickens in their battle against internal parasites. This decoction is a powerful blend of Turmeric, Garlic, Papaya Seeds, and Cinnamon, carefully selected to provide a holistic approach to maintaining your chickens' intestinal health.

Ingredients:
- 1 tablespoon Turmeric
- 3 cloves Garlic, crushed
- 1 teaspoon Papaya Seeds, crushed
- 1 small Cinnamon stick
- 4 cups water

Directions:
- In a small pot, bring 4 cups of water to a gentle simmer.
- Add the Turmeric, crushed Garlic, Papaya Seeds, and Cinnamon stick to the simmering water.
- Allow the mixture to simmer on low heat for about 20-25 minutes, stirring occasionally.
- Remove the pot from the heat and let the decoction cool down to room temperature.
- Strain the mixture to remove the solid particles, leaving you with the liquid elixir.
- Pour the Cluck Cleanse Elixir into a clean container for storage.

Notes:

- Turmeric: Known for its anti-inflammatory and antioxidant properties, Turmeric supports overall digestive health and helps manage internal parasites.
- Garlic: Garlic has natural anti-parasitic properties that can help expel worms and other parasites from the digestive system.
- Papaya Seeds: Papaya Seeds contain enzymes that have been traditionally used to eliminate parasites from the intestines.
- Cinnamon: Cinnamon is believed to help regulate digestive processes and create an environment less favorable for parasites.
- Quality Matters: Select fresh, high-quality herbs and ingredients for optimal effectiveness. Organic options are preferred.
- Consistency Matters: Administer the Cluck Cleanse Elixir as a decoction to your chickens every other day for a period of 10 days. Observe their response and adjust the treatment schedule if needed.
- Dosage and Administration: Mix 1/4 cup of the Cluck Cleanse Elixir with 1 gallon of clean water. Make sure your chickens have access to this mixture for the specified 10-day period.
- Storage: Store any remaining elixir in a cool, dark place. Discard if any signs of spoilage appear.

Keep in mind that prevention is key to maintaining your chickens' health. Regular cleaning of their environment, maintaining good hygiene, and providing a balanced diet can significantly contribute to parasite prevention.

Worm-B-Gone

Introducing Worm-B-Gone, an all-natural herbal remedy designed to support your chickens in their battle against internal parasites. This potent decoction combines the power of Marigold, Pumpkin Seeds, Fenugreek, and Cumin, offering a holistic approach to maintaining your chickens' digestive health.

Ingredients:
- 2 tablespoons Marigold petals
- 1/4 cup Pumpkin Seeds
- 1 tablespoon Fenugreek seeds
- 1 teaspoon Cumin seeds
- 4 cups water

Directions:
- In a small pot, bring 4 cups of water to a gentle simmer.
- Add Marigold petals, Pumpkin Seeds, Fenugreek seeds, and Cumin seeds to the simmering water.
- Allow the mixture to simmer on low heat for about 20-25 minutes, stirring occasionally.
- Remove the pot from the heat and let the decoction cool down to room temperature.
- Strain the mixture to remove any solid particles, leaving you with the liquid Worm-B-Gone decoction.
- Transfer the decoction to a clean container for storage.

Notes:

- Marigold: Marigold is known for its anti-inflammatory and antimicrobial properties, which can help combat digestive issues and support overall gut health.
- Pumpkin Seeds: Pumpkin Seeds contain an amino acid called cucurbitacin, which is believed to paralyze and eliminate worms from the digestive system.
- Fenugreek: Fenugreek seeds are known for their antiparasitic properties and can help expel worms from the intestines.
- Cumin: Cumin seeds can support digestion and help create an environment less favorable for the survival of parasites.
- Quality Matters: Opt for fresh, high-quality herbs and ingredients for maximum effectiveness. Organic options are preferable.
- Consistency Matters: Administer the Worm-B-Gone decoction to your chickens every other day for a period of 7-10 days. Monitor their response and adjust the treatment schedule if necessary.
-
- Dosage and Administration: Mix 1/4 cup of the Worm-B-Gone decoction with 1 gallon of clean water. Make sure your chickens have access to this mixture for the specified treatment period.
- Storage: Store any remaining decoction in a cool, dark place. Discard if any signs of spoilage arise.

Consistency is key in ensuring the effectiveness of herbal remedies. While this remedy is designed to support your chickens' digestive health, it's important to remember that maintaining good hygiene, proper nutrition, and a clean living environment are also crucial for preventing internal parasites.

Parasite Pursuit Decoction

Introducing Parasite Pursuit Decoction, a natural and effective herbal remedy to aid your chickens in their quest to fend off internal parasites. This decoction combines the power of Rosemary, Oregano, Spearmint, and Lemon Balm, providing a comprehensive approach to maintaining your flock's overall well-being.

Ingredients:
• 2 sprigs of fresh Rosemary
• 2 tablespoons Oregano leaves
• 1 handful of fresh Spearmint leaves
• 1 handful of Lemon Balm leaves
• 4 cups water

Directions:
• In a pot, bring 4 cups of water to a gentle simmer.
• Add the Rosemary sprigs, Oregano leaves, Spearmint leaves, and Lemon Balm leaves to the simmering water.
• Allow the mixture to simmer on low heat for about 15-20 minutes, stirring occasionally.
• Remove the pot from the heat and let the decoction cool down to room temperature.
• Strain the mixture to separate the liquid decoction from the herbal solids.
• Transfer the Parasite Pursuit Decoction to a clean container for storage.

Notes:
- Rosemary: Rosemary is known for its antimicrobial and antioxidant properties, which can support the immune system and help fight off parasites.
- Oregano: Oregano leaves contain compounds such as thymol and carvacrol, which possess antiparasitic and antibacterial properties.
- Spearmint: Spearmint leaves offer digestive support and can help create an environment less conducive to parasites.
- Lemon Balm: Lemon Balm is believed to have calming effects on the digestive system and may help maintain overall gut health.
- Quality Matters: Choose fresh, high-quality herbs for optimal results. If using dried herbs, use about half the amount listed.
- Consistency Matters: Administer the Parasite Pursuit Decoction to your chickens for 7 consecutive days. Observe their response and adjust the treatment plan if needed.
- Dosage and Administration: Mix 1/4 cup of the Parasite Pursuit Decoction with 1 gallon of clean water. Make sure your chickens have access to this mixture throughout the day.
- Storage: Store any remaining decoction in a cool, dark place. Discard if any signs of spoilage are detected.

Remember, while herbal remedies can play a supportive role in maintaining your chickens' health, good husbandry practices, clean living conditions, and proper nutrition are vital components of overall parasite prevention.

9. Coccidiosis

Coccidiosis is a common and highly contagious intestinal disease that affects chickens and other poultry. It is caused by protozoa of the Eimeria genus, which can multiply in the intestinal lining, leading to inflammation, damage, and sometimes death. Chickens with coccidiosis often exhibit symptoms such as diarrhea, weight loss, decreased appetite, and lethargy. The disease spreads through contaminated water, feed, and living environments, making prevention and treatment crucial for maintaining a healthy flock. Implementing good hygiene practices, providing a clean and dry environment, and incorporating herbal remedies can help support the flock's immune system and reduce the impact of coccidiosis.

As we delve into the remedies for coccidiosis, I will furnish two distinct sets of instructions. The initial set of guidelines pertains to chicks, while the subsequent set is tailored for adult chickens. Although coccidiosis can impact poultry of any age, its prevalence is particularly pronounced in chicks.

(A)Silver Shield Solution for Chicks

Silver Shield Solution is an herbal remedy tailored for baby chicks, aiming to rid them of the coccidia parasite. Utilizing Colloidal Silver's potent properties, this solution is designed to cleanse the chicks' systems of unwanted organisms, fostering healthy growth and development.

Ingredients:
• 1 tablespoon of Colloidal Silver

Directions:
• Combine 1 tablespoon of Colloidal Silver with 1 gallon of fresh water.
• Replace the baby chicks' regular drinking water with the Silver Shield Solution.
• Continue this treatment for a period of 5 days, making sure the baby chicks consume the solution as their main water source.

Colloidal Silver, a suspension of silver particles in liquid, is renowned for its antimicrobial attributes. In baby chicks, it can be instrumental in eradicating intestinal parasites by targeting the enzymes these organisms depend on, thus promoting a healthy start to life.

Notes:
- Colloidal Silver: Selecting a high-quality Colloidal Silver is vital. Opt for a trusted brand that guarantees the proper concentration of silver particles. Its antibacterial, antiviral, and antifungal properties make it a versatile ingredient.
- Consistency Matters: Maintaining a consistent treatment schedule is essential for the remedy's success. Ensure that the baby chicks are consuming the solution throughout the entire 5-day treatment.
- Storage: Keep the Colloidal Silver in a cool, dark place to preserve its effectiveness.
- Correct Dosage Information and How to Administer: The dosage for baby chicks is 1 tablespoon of Colloidal Silver mixed with 1 gallon of water. Providing it through their drinking water allows for a stress-free administration.

- How Long Treatment Should Last: A 5-day treatment duration is recommended to ensure the comprehensive elimination of all parasites.

(B)Silver Shield Solution for Adult Chickens

Silver Shield Solution is an herbal remedy specifically designed to combat intestinal parasites in adult chickens. Utilizing the powerful properties of Colloidal Silver, this solution aims to cleanse the system of unwanted organisms, promoting overall health and well-being.

Ingredients:
• 2 tablespoons of Colloidal Silver

Directions:
• Mix the Colloidal Silver with 1 gallon of fresh water.
• Administer the solution to the chickens by replacing their regular drinking water with the Silver Shield Solution.
• Continue this treatment for a period of 7 days, ensuring that the chickens consume the solution as their primary source of water.

Colloidal Silver is a suspension of tiny silver particles in a liquid base. It has been used historically for its antimicrobial properties. In the context of chickens, it may help eliminate internal parasites by attacking and disabling the enzymes that these organisms rely on for survival.

Notes:
- Colloidal Silver: Quality matters when selecting Colloidal Silver. Look for a reputable brand that ensures a proper concentration of silver particles. Colloidal Silver is known for its antibacterial, antiviral, and antifungal properties.
- Consistency Matters: Consistency in treating with the remedy is key to its effectiveness. Ensure that the chickens are consuming the solution throughout the entire 7-day treatment period.
- Storage: Store the Colloidal Silver in a cool, dark place to maintain its efficacy.
- Correct Dosage Information and How to Administer:** The correct dosage is 2 tablespoons of Colloidal Silver mixed with 1 gallon of water. Administering through the drinking water ensures that the chickens receive the treatment in a non-stressful manner.
- How Long Treatment Should Last: The treatment should last for 7 days to ensure that all parasites are effectively eradicated.

(A)GSE Guard Tonic for Chicks

GSE Guard Tonic is a specialized herbal remedy formulated to address Coccidiosis in baby chicks. Comprising a blend of Grapefruit Seed Extract, Oregano Oil, Garlic Powder, Apple Cider Vinegar, and distilled Water, this tonic aims to fortify the chicks' immune system and combat the Coccidia parasites.

Ingredients:
• 1 teaspoon of Grapefruit Seed Extract

- 1 teaspoon of Oregano Oil
- 1 teaspoon of Garlic Powder
- 2 tablespoons of Apple Cider Vinegar (organic with the mother)
- 1 gallon of distilled Water

Directions:
- Mix all the ingredients in a large container.
- Replace the baby chicks' regular drinking water with the GSE Guard Tonic.
- Administer this tonic for a period of 10 days, ensuring that the baby chicks consume it as their primary water source.

GSE Guard Tonic is a synergistic blend of natural ingredients known for their antimicrobial and immune-boosting properties. Together, they work to strengthen the chicks' immune system and directly combat the Coccidia parasites, which can cause severe digestive issues in young poultry.

Notes:
- Grapefruit Seed Extract: Known for its antimicrobial effects, it helps in fighting off various pathogens, including Coccidia.
- Oregano Oil: Rich in antioxidants, it supports the immune system and has antibacterial properties.
- Garlic Powder: Acts as a natural antibiotic, enhancing the body's ability to fight infections.
- Apple Cider Vinegar: Helps in digestion and boosts the immune system. Ensure it's organic and contains the mother for maximum benefits.
- Consistency Matters: Consistent administration over the 10-day period is crucial for the remedy's effectiveness.
- Storage: Store the tonic in a cool, dark place, and shake well before each use.
- Correct Dosage Information and How to Administer: Administer this tonic for a period of 10 days, ensuring that the baby chicks consume it as their primary water source. Administer through the drinking water for stress-free consumption.
- How Long Treatment Should Last: A 10-day treatment period is advised to ensure complete eradication of the Coccidia parasites.

(B)GSE Guard Tonic for Adult Chickens

GSE Guard Tonic is an innovative herbal remedy designed specifically for adult chickens suffering from Coccidiosis. Composed of Grapefruit Seed Extract, Oregano Oil, Garlic Powder, Apple Cider Vinegar, and distilled Water, this tonic aims to target and eliminate the Coccidia parasites, thereby restoring the health and vitality of the affected chickens.

Ingredients:
- 2 teaspoons of Grapefruit Seed Extract
- 2 teaspoons of Oregano Oil
- 2 teaspoons of Garlic Powder
- 4 tablespoons of Apple Cider Vinegar (organic with the mother)
- 1 gallon of distilled Water

Directions:

- Combine all the ingredients in a large container, ensuring thorough mixing.
- Substitute the adult chickens' regular drinking water with the GSE Guard Tonic.
- Administer this tonic consistently for a period of 14 days, making sure the chickens consume it as their main water source.

GSE Guard Tonic leverages the natural antimicrobial and immune-enhancing properties of its ingredients to combat Coccidiosis in adult chickens. This condition, caused by Coccidia parasites, can lead to digestive disturbances and overall weakness. The tonic's unique blend works synergistically to both attack the parasites and bolster the chickens' immune response.

Notes:
- Grapefruit Seed Extract: Renowned for its antimicrobial action, it's instrumental in targeting Coccidia.
- Oregano Oil: A powerful antioxidant that supports the immune system and offers antibacterial benefits.
- Garlic Powder: Functions as a natural antibiotic, aiding the body in warding off infections.
- Apple Cider Vinegar: Facilitates digestion and immune support. Ensure to use organic and with the mother for optimal results.
- Quality Matters: Selecting high-quality ingredients is essential for the remedy's effectiveness.
- Consistency Matters: Adhering to the 14-day treatment schedule is vital for complete eradication of the parasites.
- Storage: Keep the tonic in a cool, dark place, and shake well before each use.
- Correct Administer this tonic consistently for a period of 14 days, making sure the chickens consume it as their main water source.It's best administered through their drinking water.
- How Long Treatment Should Last: A 14-day treatment duration is recommended to ensure comprehensive elimination of the Coccidia parasites.

(A)Cocci-Free Elixir for Chicks

Cocci-Free Elixir is a natural herbal remedy crafted to address Coccidiosis in chicks. Comprising a blend of Wormwood, Thyme, Chamomile, Pumpkin Seeds, and Water, this elixir aims to target and neutralize the Coccidia parasites, fostering healthy growth and development in the young birds.

Ingredients:
- 1 teaspoon of Wormwood
- 1 teaspoon of Thyme
- 1 teaspoon of Chamomile
- 1 tablespoon of Pumpkin Seeds
- 1 gallon of Water

Directions:
- Crush the Pumpkin Seeds and combine them with Wormwood, Thyme, and Chamomile.
- Boil the herbs in 1 gallon of Water for 20 minutes.
- Strain the mixture and allow it to cool.
- Replace the baby chicks' regular drinking water with the Cocci-Free Elixir.
- Continue administering this elixir for a period of 7 days.

Cocci-Free Elixir is a synergistic blend of herbs known for their anti-parasitic and immune-boosting properties. Together, they work to strengthen the chicks' immune system and directly combat the Coccidia parasites, which can cause severe digestive issues in young poultry.

Notes:
- Wormwood: Known for its anti-parasitic properties, Wormwood helps fight off Coccidia.
- Thyme: Rich in antioxidants, Thyme supports the immune system and has antibacterial properties.
- Chamomile: Acts as a gentle digestive aid, soothing the digestive tract.
- Pumpkin Seeds: Contain compounds that can paralyze and eliminate parasites.
- Quality Matters: Selecting high-quality, organic herbs is essential for the remedy's effectiveness.
- Consistency Matters: Consistent administration over the 7-day period is crucial for the remedy's success.
- Storage: Store any unused elixir in the refrigerator and use it within 3 days.
- Correct Dosage Information and How to Administer: The dosage for baby chicks is as listed in the ingredients, administered through their drinking water. Please adhere to the measurements of the herbs. Replace their drinking water with 1 gallon of the elixir for the 7-day period. Make a fresh batch each day to retain potency.
- How Long Treatment Should Last: A 7-day treatment period is advised to ensure complete eradication of the Coccidia parasites.

(B)Cocci-Free Elixir for Adult Chickens

Cocci-Free Elixir is an herbal remedy formulated specifically for adult chickens to combat Coccidiosis. This condition, caused by Coccidia parasites, can lead to digestive disturbances and overall weakness. The elixir's unique blend of Wormwood, Thyme, Chamomile, Pumpkin Seeds, and Water works synergistically to both attack the parasites and bolster the chickens' immune response.

Ingredients:
- 2 teaspoons of Wormwood
- 2 teaspoons of Thyme
- 2 teaspoons of Chamomile
- 2 tablespoons of Pumpkin Seeds
- 1 gallon of Water

Directions:
- Crush the Pumpkin Seeds and mix them with Wormwood, Thyme, and Chamomile.
- Boil the mixture in 1 gallon of Water for 30 minutes.
- Strain the concoction and allow it to cool to room temperature.
- Substitute the adult chickens' regular drinking water with the Cocci-Free Elixir.
- Administer this elixir consistently for a period of 10 days.

Cocci-Free Elixir leverages the natural anti-parasitic and immune-enhancing properties of its ingredients to combat Coccidiosis in adult chickens. Wormwood, Thyme, Chamomile, and

Pumpkin Seeds each play a vital role in targeting the Coccidia parasites and strengthening the chickens' ability to fight off the infection.

Notes:
- Wormwood: Renowned for its anti-parasitic action, it's instrumental in targeting Coccidia.
- Thyme: A powerful antioxidant that supports the immune system and offers antibacterial benefits.
- Chamomile: Functions as a gentle digestive aid, soothing the digestive tract.
- Pumpkin Seeds: Contain compounds that can paralyze and eliminate parasites.
- Quality Matters: Selecting high-quality, organic herbs is essential for the remedy's effectiveness.
- Consistency Matters: Adhering to the 10-day treatment schedule is vital for the complete eradication of the parasites.
- Storage: Keep the elixir in a cool, dark place, and shake well before each use.
- Correct Dosage Information and How to Administer: The dosage for adult chickens is as listed in the ingredients, administered through their drinking water. Please adhere to the measurements of the herbs. Replace their drinking water with 1 gallon of the elixir for the 7-day period. Make a fresh batch each day to retain potency.
- How Long Treatment Should Last: A 10-day treatment duration is recommended to ensure comprehensive elimination of the Coccidia parasites.

(A)Coccidiosis Control Mix for Chicks

Coccidiosis Control Mix is a specially crafted herbal remedy designed to address Coccidiosis in baby chicks. Utilizing a blend of Turmeric, Ginger Root, Cinnamon, Coconut Oil, Fenugreek Seeds, and Water, this mix aims to fortify the chicks' immune system and combat the Coccidia parasites, promoting healthy growth and development.

Ingredients:
- 1 teaspoon of Turmeric
- 1 teaspoon of Ginger Root (finely grated)
- 1 teaspoon of Cinnamon
- 1 tablespoon of Coconut Oil
- 1 teaspoon of Fenugreek Seeds
- 1 gallon of Water

Directions:
- Crush the Fenugreek Seeds and combine them with Turmeric, Ginger Root, Cinnamon, and Coconut Oil.
- Boil the mixture in 1 gallon of Water for 20 minutes.
- Strain the concoction and allow it to cool.
- Replace the baby chicks' regular drinking water with the Coccidiosis Control Mix.
- Continue administering this mix for a period of 7 days.

Coccidiosis Control Mix is a synergistic blend of herbs and spices known for their anti-parasitic and immune-boosting properties. Together, they work to strengthen the chicks' immune system and directly combat the Coccidia parasites, which can cause severe digestive issues in young poultry.

Notes:
- Turmeric: Known for its anti-inflammatory and antioxidant properties, Turmeric helps boost the immune system.
- Ginger Root: Acts as a digestive aid and has antibacterial properties.
- Cinnamon: Rich in antioxidants, Cinnamon supports the immune system.
- Coconut Oil: Contains fatty acids that have antimicrobial effects.
- Fenugreek Seeds: Known for their anti-inflammatory and digestive benefits.
- Quality Matters: Selecting high-quality, organic ingredients is essential for the remedy's effectiveness.
- Consistency Matters: Consistent administration over the 7-day period is crucial for the remedy's success.
- Storage: Store any unused mix in the refrigerator and use it within 3 days.
- Correct Dosage Information and How to Administer: The dosage for baby chicks is listed in the ingredients and administered through their drinking water.
- How Long Treatment Should Last: A 7-day treatment period is advised to ensure complete eradication of the Coccidia parasites.

(B) Coccidiosis Control Mix for Adult Chickens

Coccidiosis Control Mix is an herbal remedy formulated specifically for adult chickens to combat Coccidiosis. This condition, caused by Coccidia parasites, can lead to digestive disturbances and overall weakness. The mix's unique blend of Turmeric, Ginger Root, Cinnamon, Coconut Oil, Fenugreek Seeds, and Water works synergistically to both attack the parasites and bolster the chickens' immune response.

Ingredients:
- 2 teaspoons of Turmeric
- 2 teaspoons of Ginger Root (finely grated)
- 2 teaspoons of Cinnamon
- 2 tablespoons of Coconut Oil
- 2 teaspoons of Fenugreek Seeds
- 1 gallon of Water

Directions:
- Crush the Fenugreek Seeds and mix with Turmeric, Ginger Root, Cinnamon, and Coconut Oil.
- Boil the mixture in 1 gallon of Water for 30 minutes.
- Strain the concoction and allow it to cool to room temperature.
- Substitute the adult chickens' regular drinking water with the Coccidiosis Control Mix.
- Administer this mix consistently for a period of 10 days.

Coccidiosis Control Mix leverages the natural anti-parasitic and immune-enhancing properties of its ingredients to combat Coccidiosis in adult chickens. Turmeric, Ginger Root, Cinnamon, Coconut Oil, and Fenugreek Seeds each play a vital role in targeting the Coccidia parasites and strengthening the chickens' ability to fight off the infection.

Notes:
- Turmeric: Renowned for its anti-inflammatory and antioxidant properties, it's instrumental in boosting the immune system.
- Ginger Root: A powerful digestive aid that offers antibacterial benefits.
- Cinnamon* Functions as an antioxidant, supporting the immune system.
- Coconut Oil: Contains fatty acids that have antimicrobial effects.
- Fenugreek Seeds: Known for their anti-inflammatory and digestive benefits.
- Quality Matters: Selecting high-quality, organic herbs is essential for the remedy's effectiveness.
- Consistency Matters: Adhering to the 10-day treatment schedule is vital for the complete eradication of the parasites.
- Storage: Keep the mix in a cool, dark place, and shake well before each use.
- Correct Dosage Information and How to Administer: The dosage for adult chickens is as listed in the ingredients, and it's best administered through their drinking water.
- How Long Should Treatment Last? To ensure comprehensive elimination of the coccidia parasites, a 10-day treatment duration is recommended.

(A)Herbal Defense Blend for Chicks

Herbal Defense Blend is a natural herbal remedy crafted to address Coccidiosis in baby chicks. Utilizing a blend of Echinacea, Goldenseal, Marshmallow Root, Lemon Balm, and Water, this mix aims to fortify the chicks' immune system and combat the Coccidia parasites, promoting healthy growth and development.

Ingredients:
• 1 teaspoon of Echinacea
• 1 teaspoon of Goldenseal
• 1 teaspoon of Marshmallow Root
• 1 teaspoon of Lemon Balm
• 1 gallon of Water

Directions:
• Combine Echinacea, Goldenseal, Marshmallow Root, and Lemon Balm.
• Boil the mixture in 1 gallon of Water for 20 minutes.
• Strain the concoction and allow it to cool.
• Replace the baby chicks' regular drinking water with the Herbal Defense Blend.
• Continue administering this blend for a period of 7 days.

Herbal Defense Blend is a synergistic blend of herbs known for their anti-parasitic and immune-boosting properties. Together, they work to strengthen the chicks' immune system and directly combat the Coccidia parasites, which can cause severe digestive issues in young poultry.

Notes:
• Echinacea: Known for its immune-boosting properties, Echinacea helps in enhancing the body's ability to fight infections.
• Goldenseal: Acts as a natural antibiotic and has antibacterial properties.

- Marshmallow Root: Functions as a gentle digestive aid, soothing the digestive tract.
- Lemon Balm: Rich in antioxidants, Lemon Balm supports the immune system.
- Quality Matters: Selecting high-quality, organic herbs is essential for the remedy's effectiveness.
- Consistency Matters: Consistent administration over the 7-day period is crucial for the remedy's success.
- Storage: Store any unused blend in the refrigerator and use it within 3 days.
- Correct Dosage Information and How to Administer: The dosage for baby chicks is as listed in the ingredients, administered through their drinking water.
- How Long Treatment Should Last: A 7-day treatment period is advised to ensure complete eradication of the Coccidia parasites.

(B) Herbal Defense Blend for Adult Chickens

Herbal Defense Blend is an herbal remedy formulated specifically for adult chickens to combat Coccidiosis. This condition, caused by Coccidia parasites, can lead to digestive disturbances and overall weakness. The blend's unique combination of Echinacea, Goldenseal, Marshmallow Root, Lemon Balm, and Water works synergistically to both attack the parasites and bolster the chickens' immune response.

Ingredients:
- 2 teaspoons of Echinacea
- 2 teaspoons of Goldenseal
- 2 teaspoons of Marshmallow Root
- 2 teaspoons of Lemon Balm
- 1 gallon of Water

Directions:
- Combine Echinacea, Goldenseal, Marshmallow Root, and Lemon Balm.
- Boil the mixture in 1 gallon of Water for 30 minutes.
- Strain the concoction and allow it to cool to room temperature.
- Substitute the adult chickens' regular drinking water with the Herbal Defense Blend.
- Administer this blend consistently for a period of 10 days.

Herbal Defense Blend leverages the natural antiparasitic and immune-enhancing properties of its ingredients to combat Coccidiosis in adult chickens. Echinacea, Goldenseal, Marshmallow Root, and Lemon Balm each play a vital role in targeting the Coccidia parasites and strengthening the chickens' ability to fight off the infection.

Notes:
Echinacea: Renowned for its immune-boosting properties, it's instrumental in enhancing the body's ability to fight infections.
Goldenseal: A powerful natural antibiotic that offers antibacterial benefits.
Marshmallow Root: Functions as a gentle digestive aid, soothing the digestive tract.
Lemon Balm: Contains antioxidants that support the immune system.
Quality Matters: Selecting high-quality, organic herbs is essential for the remedy's effectiveness.

Consistency Matters: Adhering to the 10-day treatment schedule is vital for complete eradication of the parasites.

Storage: Keep the blend in a cool, dark place, and shake well before each use.

Correct Dosage Information and How to Administer: The dosage for adult chickens is as listed in the ingredients, and it's best administered through their drinking water.

How Long Should Treatment Last? To ensure comprehensive elimination of the coccidia parasites, a 10-day treatment duration is recommended.

10. Gapeworm

Gapeworm, a common affliction in chickens, is caused by the parasitic nematode Syngamus trachea. These thread-like worms inhabit the trachea and bronchi, causing respiratory distress as they obstruct the airways. Infected chickens often display signs of gasping for breath, head shaking, and neck stretching in an attempt to alleviate their discomfort. Gapeworms can spread through contaminated water, grass, and soil, posing a threat to poultry health. Addressing this issue promptly with effective herbal remedies is crucial to ensuring the well-being of the flock.

GapeGuard Tincture

GapeGuard Tincture is an herbal remedy specifically crafted to combat Gapeworm in chickens. Gapeworm is a parasitic infection that can cause severe respiratory distress in poultry. The tincture's unique blend of Wormwood, Thyme, Black Walnut Hull, and Alcohol (vodka) or Apple Cider Vinegar works synergistically to attack the Gapeworm and bolster the chickens' immune response.

Ingredients:
• 2 teaspoons of Wormwood
• 2 teaspoons of Thyme
• 2 teaspoons of Black Walnut Hull
• 1 cup of Alcohol (vodka) or Apple Cider Vinegar (organic with the mother)

Directions:
• Combine Wormwood, Thyme, and Black Walnut Hull in a glass jar.
• Pour Alcohol (vodka) or Apple Cider Vinegar over the herbs until fully submerged.
• Seal the jar and shake well.
• Allow the mixture to steep for 4 weeks, shaking daily.
• Strain the tincture and store it in a dark glass bottle.
• Administer 5 drops of the tincture in 1 gallon of the chickens' drinking water daily for 14 days.

GapeGuard Tincture leverages the natural anti-parasitic properties of its ingredients to combat Gapeworm in chickens. Wormwood, Thyme, and Black Walnut Hull each play a vital role in targeting the Gapeworm, while the Alcohol or Apple Cider Vinegar acts as a preservative and enhances the extraction of the beneficial compounds.

Notes:
- Wormwood: Known for its strong anti-parasitic properties, Wormwood is instrumental in eliminating Gapeworm.
- Thyme: A powerful herb that supports the immune system and offers antibacterial benefits.
- Black Walnut Hull: Contains compounds that can paralyze and eliminate parasites.
- Alcohol (vodka) or Apple Cider Vinegar: Acts as a solvent to extract the beneficial compounds from the herbs.
- Quality Matters: Selecting high-quality, organic herbs and solvents is essential for the remedy's effectiveness.
- Consistency Matters: Adhering to the 14-day treatment schedule is vital for completely eradicating the parasites.

- Storage: Store the tincture in a cool, dark place, away from sunlight.
- Correct Dosage Information and How to Administer: The dosage for chickens is 5 drops per 1 gallon of water daily, administered through their drinking water.
- How Long Treatment Should Last: A 14-day treatment duration is recommended to ensure comprehensive elimination of the Gapeworm.

Parasite Purge Potion

This herbal remedy, the Parasite Purge Potion, is crafted to target and alleviate the symptoms of gapeworm in chickens. Harnessing the power of nature, each ingredient has been chosen for its traditional use in combating internal parasites, promoting respiratory health, and supporting the overall well-being of your feathered friends.

Ingredients:
- 2 tablespoons of Wormwood
- 5 fresh Garlic cloves, crushed
- 1 tablespoon of Black walnut hulls, finely crushed
- 2 teaspoons of Thyme, dried or fresh
- 1 liter of Filtered water

Directions:
- In a large pot, bring the filtered water to a boil.
- Once boiling, reduce the heat to a simmer and add the wormwood, garlic, black walnut hulls, and thyme.
- Let the mixture simmer for about 20 minutes, allowing the herbs to release their beneficial properties.
- Remove from heat and let it cool to room temperature.
- Strain the mixture to remove the solid herbs, retaining the liquid.
- Store the potion in a clean, airtight container.

The Parasite Purge Potion is a blend of herbs traditionally believed to possess anthelmintic properties, meaning they can help expel parasitic worms. The combination of these specific ingredients aims to create an environment within the chicken's system that's inhospitable to parasites like the gapeworm, while also providing supportive benefits to the respiratory and digestive systems.

Notes:
- Wormwood (Artemisia absinthium): This herb has been used for centuries for its potential anthelmintic properties. It's believed to create an environment that's unwelcoming to parasites, helping to expel them from the host's system.
- Garlic: Beyond its culinary uses, garlic has been revered for its potential medicinal properties. It's believed to have antiparasitic effects, and its strong aroma can also help in clearing respiratory passages.
- Black Walnut Hulls: Black walnut hulls have traditionally been used in herbal worming mixtures. They contain juglone, tannins, and iodine, compounds believed to have antiparasitic effects.

- Thyme: This aromatic herb isn't just for cooking. It has been used for its potential antiparasitic and antimicrobial properties, and it can also soothe the respiratory system.
- Quality Matters: When selecting ingredients, always opt for organic or wild-crafted herbs free from pesticides and other chemicals. The potency and efficacy of the remedy can be influenced by the quality of the ingredients.
- Consistency in Treatment: For best results, administer the remedy consistently. Inconsistencies can reduce its effectiveness.
- Storage: Store the Parasite Purge Potion in a cool, dark place. If refrigerated, it can last up to a week. Always ensure the container is sealed tightly to maintain its potency.
- Dosage and Administration: For a standard-sized chicken, administer 10ml of the potion daily, either directly using a dropper or mixed in with their water. Adjust the dosage proportionally for larger or smaller birds.
- Duration of Treatment: To ensure all parasites are eradicated, continue the treatment for at least 7 days, even if symptoms improve.

FeatherGuard Worm Elixir

FeatherGuard Worm Elixir is a specially crafted herbal blend designed to address the challenges of gapeworm in chickens. By combining potent herbs and the acidity of apple cider vinegar, this elixir aims to create an environment that's unwelcoming to internal parasites while supporting the overall vitality of your flock.

Ingredients:
• 10 Clove buds, whole
• 1/4 cup Pumpkin seeds, crushed
• 2 tablespoons Fennel seeds
• 1 tablespoon Oregon grape root, finely chopped
• 2 cups Apple cider vinegar

Directions:
• In a glass jar, combine the clove buds, crushed pumpkin seeds, fennel seeds, and Oregon grape root.
• Pour the apple cider vinegar over the herbal mixture, ensuring all ingredients are submerged.
• Seal the jar tightly and shake well.
• Allow the mixture to infuse in a cool, dark place for 2-3 weeks, shaking the jar every couple of days.
• After the infusion period, strain the elixir to remove the solid herbs, retaining the liquid.
• Store the elixir in a clean, airtight container.

FeatherGuard Worm Elixir combines the traditional antiparasitic properties of its herbal ingredients with the acidic environment created by apple cider vinegar. This dual-action approach aims to both directly target the gapeworm and support the chicken's natural defenses against such parasites.

Notes:

- Clove Buds: Cloves have been historically prized for their potential antiparasitic and antimicrobial properties. Their active compound, eugenol, is believed to be responsible for these effects.
- Pumpkin Seeds: These seeds have been traditionally used as a natural dewormer. They contain a compound called cucurbitacin, which is believed to paralyze and expel worms from the digestive tract.
- Fennel Seeds: Fennel is not only aromatic but has also been used for its potential antiparasitic properties. Additionally, it can soothe the digestive system.
- Oregon Grape Root: This root contains berberine, a compound believed to have antiparasitic and antimicrobial effects. It's traditionally used to combat a variety of internal and external pathogens.
- Apple Cider Vinegar: Its acidic nature can create an inhospitable environment for parasites. Additionally, it's believed to support digestive health and boost the immune system.
- Quality Matters: Always prioritize high-quality, organic, or wild-crafted ingredients. The purity and potency of the ingredients can influence the effectiveness of the elixir.
- Consistency in Treatment: Regular and consistent administration is key to maximizing the potential benefits of the elixir.
- Storage: Store the FeatherGuard Elixir in a cool, dark place, away from direct sunlight. If stored correctly, it can last for several months.
- Dosage and Administration: For a standard-sized chicken, administer 5ml of the elixir daily, either directly using a dropper or mixed in with their feed. Adjust the dosage proportionally for larger or smaller birds.
- Duration of Treatment: A consistent treatment of at least 10 days is recommended, even if symptoms seem to improve, to ensure a comprehensive approach to potential parasites.

BreatheEasy Brew

BreatheEasy Brew is a harmonious blend of herbs, each chosen for their traditional properties that support respiratory health and combat internal parasites. This brew aims to provide relief to chickens affected by gapeworm, ensuring they breathe easier and feel more comfortable.

Ingredients:
- 2 tablespoons Tansy , dried
- 1 tablespoon Hyssop, dried
- 1-inch piece of Ginger root, sliced
- 1 teaspoon Cayenne pepper
- 1 liter of Filtered water

Directions:
- In a large pot, bring the filtered water to a boil.
- Add the tansy, hyssop, ginger root, and cayenne pepper to the boiling water.
- Reduce the heat and let the mixture simmer for about 25 minutes, allowing the herbs to infuse their properties into the water.
- After simmering, remove the pot from the heat and allow the brew to cool to room temperature.
- Strain the liquid, discard the solid herbs, and store the brew in a clean, airtight container.

BreatheEasy Brew is formulated to address the discomfort and respiratory distress caused by gapeworm in chickens. The combination of these specific herbs not only targets the parasites but also soothes the respiratory tract, reduces inflammation, and boosts the chicken's natural defenses.

Notes:
- Tansy (Tanacetum vulgare): Tansy has been traditionally used for its potential anthelmintic properties, meaning it can help expel parasitic worms. It's also known to have a calming effect on the digestive system.
- Hyssop: This herb is often used for respiratory conditions due to its potential expectorant properties. It can help clear mucus and soothe respiratory distress.
- Ginger Root: Ginger is renowned for its anti-inflammatory properties. It can help reduce swelling in the respiratory tract and boost the immune system, making it harder for parasites to thrive.
- Cayenne Pepper: Cayenne can stimulate circulation and create an environment that's less hospitable to parasites. Its spicy nature can also help clear respiratory passages.
- Quality Matters: When sourcing ingredients, it's crucial to opt for organic or wild-crafted herbs. The potency and overall effectiveness of the brew can be influenced by the quality and purity of the ingredients.
- Consistency in Treatment: To achieve the best results, the brew must be administered consistently. Skipping doses or being irregular can reduce its potential benefits.
- Storage: BreatheEasy Brew should be stored in a cool, dark place. If refrigerated, it can last up to a week. Ensure the container is sealed tightly to maintain its potency.
- Dosage and Administration: For a standard-sized chicken, administer 15ml of the brew daily, either directly using a dropper or mixed in with their water. Adjust the dosage based on the size of the bird.
- Duration of Treatment: A treatment period of at least 10 days is recommended to ensure a comprehensive approach to potential parasites and to provide ongoing respiratory support.

WingGuard Wellness Tincture

WingGuard Wellness Tincture is a potent blend of herbs, each selected for their traditional properties in supporting respiratory health, combating internal parasites, and enhancing overall vitality. This tincture is designed to offer a holistic approach to the challenges posed by gapeworm in chickens, ensuring they remain lively and in high spirits.

Ingredients:
- 1/4 cup Yarrow, dried
- 1/4 cup Neem leaves, dried
- 2 tablespoons Peppermint, dried
- 1/2 cup Olive oil
- 1 cup Vodka or Apple Cider Vinegar

Directions:
- In a glass jar, combine the yarrow, neem leaves, and peppermint.
- Pour in the olive oil, ensuring the herbs are well-coated.
- Add the vodka or apple cider vinegar to the jar, ensuring all ingredients are submerged.

- Seal the jar tightly and shake well.
- Store the jar in a cool, dark place, allowing the mixture to infuse for 3-4 weeks. Shake the jar every few days.
- After the infusion period, strain the tincture to remove the solid herbs, retaining the liquid.
- Transfer the tincture to a clean, airtight container, preferably a dropper bottle for easy administration.

WingGuard Wellness Tincture is a harmonious blend of herbs known for their potential antiparasitic and respiratory-supporting properties. The combination aims to directly target the gapeworm while also providing a soothing effect on the respiratory tract and boosting the chicken's natural defenses against such challenges.

Notes:
- Yarrow (Achillea millefolium): Yarrow has been traditionally used for its potential antiparasitic properties and its ability to support the respiratory system. It's also known to be beneficial for the digestive system.
- Neem Leaves: Neem is renowned for its potential antiparasitic and antimicrobial properties. It's been used in various cultures to combat a range of internal and external pathogens.
- Peppermint: Beyond its refreshing aroma, peppermint is believed to have antiparasitic properties. It can also be soothing to the respiratory and digestive systems.
- Olive Oil: This acts as a carrier oil, enhancing the absorption of the herbal properties. It's also nourishing and can help in delivering the benefits of the herbs more effectively.
- Vodka or Apple Cider Vinegar: These act as solvents, extracting the beneficial compounds from the herbs. They also serve as preservatives, ensuring the tincture remains potent for longer.
- Quality Matters: When sourcing ingredients, prioritize high-quality, organic, or wild-crafted herbs. The purity and potency of the ingredients can influence the effectiveness of the tincture.
- Consistency in Treatment: Regular and consistent administration is key. Inconsistencies can reduce the tincture's potential benefits.
- Storage: Store the WingGuard Wellness Tincture in a cool, dark place, away from direct sunlight. If stored correctly, it can last for several months to a year.
- Dosage and Administration: For a standard-sized chicken, administer 1/2 teaspoon of the tincture daily, either directly using a dropper or mixed in with their feed. Adjust the dosage based on the bird's size.
- Duration of Treatment: A consistent treatment period of at least 14 days is recommended to ensure a comprehensive approach to potential parasites and to provide ongoing respiratory support.

11. Drawing Salve

HerbaDraw Healing Salve

HerbaDraw Healing Salve is a potent blend of herbs and natural ingredients, meticulously chosen for their traditional properties in supporting skin health, drawing out impurities, and promoting healing. This salve is designed to address skin irritations and minor wounds and help draw out foreign objects or toxins, making it an essential addition to any natural first-aid kit.

Ingredients:
- 2 tablespoons Comfrey root, dried and finely ground
- 2 tablespoons Plantain leaf, dried and finely ground
- 2 tablespoons Calendula flowers, dried and finely ground
- 1 tablespoon Echinacea root, dried and finely ground
- 1/2 cup Olive oil
- 1/4 cup Beeswax pellets
- 1 tablespoon Activated charcoal powder
- 1 tablespoon Bentonite clay
- 10 drops Lavender essential oil
- 8 drops Tea tree essential oil

Directions:
- In a double boiler, combine the olive oil, comfrey root, plantain leaf, calendula flowers, and echinacea root. Allow the mixture to simmer gently for 1-2 hours, ensuring the herbs infuse their properties into the oil.
- Strain the oil through a fine mesh strainer or cheesecloth, discarding the solid herbs.
- Return the infused oil to the double boiler and add the beeswax pellets. Heat until the beeswax is fully melted.
- Remove from heat and stir in the activated charcoal and bentonite clay until fully incorporated.
- Once the mixture is slightly cooled but still liquid, add the lavender and tea tree essential oils.
- Pour the mixture into a clean tin or glass jar and allow it to cool and solidify.

HerbaDraw Healing Salve is a multi-purpose herbal remedy designed to draw out impurities, soothe irritated skin, and promote faster healing. The combination of herbs and essential oils not only provides drawing properties but also offers antiseptic, anti-inflammatory, and skin-nourishing benefits.

Notes:
- Comfrey Root: Traditionally used for its skin-healing properties, comfrey is believed to promote faster cell growth and repair.
- Plantain Leaf: This common weed is renowned for its anti-inflammatory and wound-healing properties, making it a staple in many herbal salves.
- Calendula Flowers: Calendula is known for its skin-soothing and anti-inflammatory effects, helping to reduce redness and irritation.

- Echinacea Root: Often associated with immune support, echinacea also offers antimicrobial properties, which can help prevent infections in minor wounds.
- Olive Oil: A nourishing carrier oil that helps in the absorption of herbal properties and moisturizes the skin.
- Beeswax: Provides structure to the salve, ensuring it remains solid at room temperature but melts upon skin contact.
- Activated Charcoal & Bentonite Clay: Both known for their drawing properties, they help pull out toxins, foreign objects, or impurities from the skin.
- Lavender & Tea Tree Essential Oils: Both essential oils offer antiseptic properties, with lavender adding a calming scent and tea tree providing additional antimicrobial benefits.
- Quality Matters: Always prioritize high-quality, organic, or wild-crafted ingredients. The salve's effectiveness can be influenced by the purity and potency of the ingredients.
- Consistency in Treatment: For best results, apply the salve consistently to the affected area, covering it with a bandage if necessary.
- Storage: Store the HerbaDraw Healing Salve in a cool, dark place, away from direct sunlight. Properly stored, it can last up to a year.
- Dosage and Administration: Apply a generous amount to the affected area 2-3 times daily or as needed. Ensure the area is clean before application.
- Duration of Treatment: Continue application until the skin irritation subsides or the foreign object is drawn out. For persistent issues, consider seeking additional remedies or treatments.

12. Anti-Peck Spray

AzureGuard Anti-Pecking Spray

AzureGuard Anti-Pecking Spray is a natural blend explicitly crafted for chickens to deter pecking behavior. Infused with lavender's calming properties and the healing touch of aloe vera and calendula, this spray not only discourages pecking but also promotes skin healing and wellness.

Ingredients:
- 1/2 teaspoon Blue Spirulina Powder (adjust as needed for desired color)
- 1/4 cup Aloe Vera Gel
- 1/4 cup Witch Hazel
- 2 tablespoons Calendula Extract
- 10 drops Lavender Essential Oil
- 1 tablespoon Yarrow Tincture (recipe below)
- 1/2 cup Distilled Water

Directions:
- Start by dissolving the blue spirulina powder in a small amount of warm distilled water to create a concentrated blue solution. Adjust the amount of spirulina to achieve the desired shade of blue.
- In a mixing bowl, combine the aloe vera gel, witch hazel, and calendula extract.
- Slowly add the blue spirulina, stirring continuously to ensure an even distribution of color.
- Incorporate the lavender essential oil and yarrow tincture into the mixture.
- Gradually add the distilled water, stirring until all ingredients are well combined.
- Using a funnel, transfer the mixture to a spray bottle.

AzureGuard Anti-Pecking Spray serves a dual purpose. The blue spirulina provides a visible deterrent, signaling to other chickens that the sprayed area is off-limits. Meanwhile, the combination of aloe vera, calendula, and lavender works to soothe any irritated skin, reduce inflammation, and promote healing. The yarrow tincture adds an extra layer of protection, aiding in stopping any bleeding from peck-induced wounds.

Notes:
- Blue Spirulina: Beyond its vibrant color it provides a natural, non-toxic blue pigment that helps mask the appearance of wounds, reducing pecking attraction. Additionally, its antimicrobial properties aid in protecting the wound from infection, supporting the healing process.
- Aloe Vera Gel: Renowned for its skin-soothing properties, aloe vera provides immediate relief to irritated skin and accelerates healing.
- Witch Hazel: Acts as an astringent, reducing skin inflammation and providing a cooling effect.
- Calendula Extract: Known for its anti-inflammatory and wound-healing properties, calendula helps in skin regeneration.
- Lavender Essential Oil: Its calming scent can deter pecking, and its antiseptic properties help prevent infections.

- Yarrow Tincture: Yarrow is traditionally used to stop bleeding and promote healing, making it a valuable addition to this spray.
- Quality Matters: Always opt for high-quality, preferably organic ingredients. The purity and potency of the ingredients can influence the spray's effectiveness.
- Consistency in Treatment: Regular application is key, especially in the early stages of introducing the spray to the flock.
- Storage: Store the AzureGuard Anti-Pecking Spray in a cool, dark place. If stored correctly, it can last for several months.
- Dosage and Administration: Spray the affected area of the chicken lightly, ensuring even coverage. Reapply as needed, especially if you notice continued pecking.
- Duration of Treatment: Continue application until pecking behavior subsides. For persistent issues, consider re-evaluating the environment or potential stressors for the chickens.

Yarrow Tincture Recipe

Ingredients:
- Fresh Yarrow flowers and leaves
- High-proof alcohol (like vodka) or Apple Cider Vinegar

Directions:
- Fill a jar halfway with fresh yarrow flowers and leaves.
- Pour the alcohol over the yarrow until the jar is full, ensuring the plant material is completely submerged.
- Seal the jar and store it in a cool, dark place for 4-6 weeks, shaking it every few days.
- After the infusion period, strain out the plant material, retaining the liquid.
- Store the yarrow tincture in a dark glass dropper bottle for easy administration.

13. Year Round Respiratory Health

HerbalFowl Vitality Drops

HerbalFowl Vitality Drops is a carefully crafted blend of natural ingredients, designed to bolster the overall health and vitality of chickens. This herbal concoction harnesses the power of nature's finest to promote a robust immune system, support digestive health, and ensure your flock remains lively and thriving.

Ingredients:
- 10 drops Oregano Essential Oil
- 8 drops Thyme Essential Oil
- 1 tablespoon Garlic (finely minced or crushed)
- 1 tablespoon Echinacea (either as a tincture or finely ground dried root)
- 1/2 cup Apple Cider Vinegar
- 1 teaspoon Rosemary (finely chopped or crushed)

Directions:
- In a mixing bowl, combine the apple cider vinegar, oregano essential oil, and thyme essential oil.
- Add the finely minced garlic and echinacea, ensuring they are well dispersed throughout the mixture.
- Stir in the rosemary, blending all ingredients thoroughly.
- Transfer the mixture to a glass bottle with a tight-sealing lid.
- Store in a cool, dark place, shaking well before each use.

HerbalFowl Vitality Drops is more than just a supplement; it's a natural wellness booster for your chickens. The combination of oregano and thyme essential oils offers potent antimicrobial properties, ensuring your flock's internal systems remain free from unwanted invaders. Garlic, a known natural antibiotic, further enhances this protective shield. Echinacea, often dubbed the "immune system herb," works to fortify your chickens' natural defenses, while apple cider vinegar ensures a balanced gut environment. Lastly, rosemary not only imparts a pleasant aroma but also provides valuable antioxidants that support overall health.

Notes:
- Oregano Essential Oil: Renowned for its antimicrobial properties, oregano oil can help in warding off various pathogens, ensuring your chickens remain healthy.
- Thyme Essential Oil: Beyond its aromatic appeal, thyme has antiseptic properties, further bolstering the protective nature of this remedy.
- Garlic: A natural powerhouse, garlic has been used for centuries for its antibiotic properties, ensuring internal health.
- Echinacea: This herb is a staple in many natural remedies, known for its ability to boost the immune system and combat infections.
- Apple Cider Vinegar: A balanced gut is crucial for overall health. Apple cider vinegar promotes a healthy pH level, ensuring optimal digestion and nutrient absorption.
- Rosemary: This aromatic herb is not just for flavor; it's packed with antioxidants that support cellular health and vitality.

- Quality Matters: Always opt for high-quality, preferably organic ingredients. The remedy's effectiveness can be influenced by the purity and potency of the ingredients.
- Consistency in Treatment: For best results, administer the HerbalFowl Vitality Drops consistently, ensuring your flock gets a regular dose of wellness.
- Storage: Store the HerbalFowl Vitality Drops in a cool, dark place, away from direct sunlight. Properly stored, it can last for several months.
- Dosage and Administration: Add 1 tablespoon of the HerbalFowl Vitality Drops to every gallon of your chickens' drinking water. Ensure the water container is shaken or stirred well to disperse the drops evenly.
- Duration of Treatment: Administer as a regular supplement, at least once per week, to ensure ongoing health benefits for your flock. Adjust or pause administration based on the specific needs and observations of your chickens.

14. First Aid Salve

NatureSoothe Herbal Healing Salve

NatureSoothe Herbal Healing Salve is a handcrafted blend designed especially for chickens, aiming to address common skin issues they might face. From minor cuts and pecks to skin irritations, this salve harnesses the power of nature to provide relief and promote healing, ensuring your flock remains in top condition.

Ingredients:
- 1/4 cup Calendula Flowers (dried and finely ground)
- 1/4 cup Plantain Leaves (dried and finely ground)
- 1/4 cup Comfrey Leaves (dried and finely ground)
- 1/4 cup Yarrow Flowers (dried and finely ground)
- 15 drops Lavender Essential Oil
- 1/4 cup Chamomile Flowers (dried and finely ground)
- 1/2 cup Beeswax pellets
- 1 cup Olive Oil
- 1 teaspoon Vitamin E Oil

Directions:
- In a double boiler, combine the olive oil, calendula flowers, plantain leaves, comfrey leaves, yarrow flowers, and chamomile flowers. Allow the mixture to simmer gently for 1-2 hours, ensuring the herbs infuse their properties into the oil.
- Strain the oil through a fine mesh strainer or cheesecloth, discarding the solid herbs.
- Return the infused oil to the double boiler and add the beeswax pellets. Heat until the beeswax is fully melted.
- Remove from heat and stir in the lavender essential oil and vitamin E oil.
- Pour the mixture into clean tins or glass jars and allow it to cool and solidify.

NatureSoothe Herbal Healing Salve is a guardian for your chickens' skin health. The blend of calendula, plantain, and chamomile offers a trifecta of soothing properties, reducing redness and irritation. Comfrey, often dubbed the "knit-bone," aids in rapid cell growth, mending minor cuts or abrasions swiftly. Yarrow steps in with its ability to halt bleeding, while lavender essential oil not only imparts a calming aroma but also brings its antiseptic properties to the table. The olive oil acts as a carrier, ensuring all these herbal benefits penetrate deeply, while beeswax seals in the moisture and provides a protective barrier. Vitamin E is the final touch, known for its skin-rejuvenating properties and acting as a natural preservative.

Notes:
- Calendula Flowers: These bright blooms are not just for show; they're packed with skin-soothing properties, making them a staple in herbal skin remedies.
- Plantain Leaves: Often considered a common weed, plantain leaves are a hidden gem in the world of herbal remedies, known for their wound-healing prowess.
- Comfrey Leaves: With a longstanding reputation for promoting cell growth, comfrey ensures rapid healing of minor skin issues.

- Yarrow Flowers: Beyond its beautiful appearance, yarrow is a powerhouse in stopping bleeding and reducing inflammation.
- Lavender Essential Oil: A dual-purpose ingredient, lavender offers antiseptic properties and a calming scent.
- Chamomile Flowers: Renowned for their calming properties, chamomile also soothes the skin, reducing redness and irritation.
- Olive Oil: A nourishing carrier oil that ensures deep penetration of the herbal benefits.
- Beeswax: Beyond providing structure, beeswax offers a protective barrier, sealing in moisture and the salve's beneficial properties.
- Vitamin E Oil: A skin-rejuvenating agent that also acts as a natural preservative, extending the salve's shelf life.
- Quality Matters: Always prioritize high-quality, organic, or wild-crafted ingredients. The salve's effectiveness can be influenced by the purity and potency of the ingredients.
- Consistency in Treatment: For best results, apply the salve consistently to the affected area, ensuring the skin fully absorbs it.
- Storage: Store the NatureSoothe Herbal Healing Salve in a cool, dark place, away from direct sunlight. Properly stored, it can last up to a year.
- Dosage and Administration: Apply a pea-sized amount to the affected area 2-3 times daily or as needed. Ensure the area is clean before application.
- Duration of Treatment: Continue application until the skin issue subsides. For persistent issues, consider seeking additional remedies or treatments.

15. Natural Antibiotic Eye Ointment

HerbaSight Soothing Eye Salve

Introducing HerbaSight Soothing Eye Salve, a gentle yet potent herbal blend designed specifically for the delicate eyes of chickens. Crafted with nature's finest, this salve aims to address eye irritations and infections, ensuring your flock's eyes remain clear and healthy.

Ingredients:
- 1/4 cup Calendula Flowers (dried and finely ground)
- 1/4 cup Chamomile Flowers (dried and finely ground)
- 1/4 cup Eyebright Herb (dried and finely ground)
- 2 tablespoons Honey (preferably raw and organic)
- 1/2 cup Coconut Oil
- 10 drops Lavender Essential Oil
- 1/4 cup Beeswax pellets

Directions:
- In a double boiler, melt the coconut oil and beeswax together until fully liquefied.
- Add the calendula, chamomile, and eyebright herbs to the oil and wax mixture, allowing them to infuse on low heat for about an hour.
- Strain the oil through a fine mesh strainer or cheesecloth, discarding the solid herbs.
- While the oil is still warm, stir in the honey until it's fully incorporated.
- Add the lavender essential oil to the mixture and stir well.
- Pour the liquid salve into small glass jars or tins and allow it to cool and solidify.

HerbaSight Soothing Eye Salve is a harmonious blend of nature's finest, tailored to address the unique needs of chicken eyes. The combination of calendula, chamomile, and eyebright offers a trifecta of soothing and healing properties, targeting inflammation, irritation, and potential infections. Honey, nature's liquid gold, brings its renowned antibacterial properties to the table, ensuring a protective shield against harmful microbes. Coconut oil acts as a gentle carrier, ensuring deep penetration of the herbal benefits, while lavender essential oil not only imparts a calming aroma but also brings its antiseptic properties into play. The result? A salve that not only soothes but also promotes the healing of your chickens' eyes.

Notes:
- Calendula Flowers: These vibrant blooms are revered for their skin-soothing properties, making them an ideal choice for delicate eye areas.
- Chamomile Flowers: Beyond their calming aroma, chamomile flowers are known for their anti-inflammatory effects, reducing redness and irritation.
- Eyebright Herb: A traditional remedy for eye ailments, eyebright is aptly named, offering relief from irritations and infections.
- Honey: A natural antibacterial, honey promotes healing and offers a protective barrier against potential infections.
- Coconut Oil: A gentle carrier that ensures the deep penetration of herbal benefits while also offering mild antimicrobial properties.

- Lavender Essential Oil: Renowned for its calming scent, lavender also possesses antiseptic properties beneficial for eye health.
- Beeswax: Beyond providing structure, beeswax offers a protective barrier, sealing in the salve's beneficial properties.
- Quality Matters: Always opt for high-quality, preferably organic ingredients. The purity and potency of the ingredients can influence the remedy's effectiveness.
- Consistency in Treatment: For optimal results, apply the salve consistently to the affected eye area, ensuring it's fully absorbed.
- Storage: Store the HerbaSight Soothing Eye Salve in a cool, dark place, away from direct sunlight. Properly stored, it can last up to a year.
- Dosage and Administration: Using a clean fingertip or cotton swab, apply a pea-sized amount to the affected eye area 2-3 times daily or as needed. Ensure the area is clean before application.
- Duration of Treatment: Continue application until the eye issue subsides. For persistent issues, consider seeking additional remedies or treatments.

16. Botulism

Botulism is a form of poisoning caused by toxins produced by the bacterium *Clostridium botulinum*. This bacterium thrives in low-oxygen environments and produces spores that can survive in the environment for years. When conditions are right (anaerobic, moist, and at a certain pH level), these spores can germinate and produce the botulinum toxin, which is one of the most potent toxins known. Botulism in chickens, often referred to as "limberneck", can occur when they ingest the toxin, usually by consuming a decaying carcass, contaminated water, or feed. The toxin affects the nervous system and leads to muscle paralysis.

Symptoms in Chickens Include:
• Progressive muscular paralysis starting with the legs and wings.
• The neck becomes limp, which is why it's often called "limberneck".
• Difficulty breathing due to paralysis of respiratory muscles.
• The bird may appear to be drowsy or drunk.
• In severe cases, death can occur, especially if the respiratory muscles are affected.

BotuGuard Herbal Flush

Introducing BotuGuard Herbal Flush, a nature-inspired concoction crafted specifically for chickens facing the challenges of botulism. This blend harnesses the detoxifying powers of select herbs and activated charcoal, aiming to flush out toxins and support the overall well-being of your flock.

Ingredients:
• 2 tablespoons Dandelion Root (finely ground)
• 2 tablespoons Milk Thistle Seeds (crushed)
• 1 tablespoon Activated Charcoal
• 16 ounces Filtered Water

Directions:
• In a pot, bring the filtered water to a boil.
• Add the dandelion root and milk thistle seeds to the boiling water.
• Reduce the heat and let it simmer for about 20 minutes.
• Remove from heat and allow it to cool to room temperature.
• Once cooled, strain out the herbs, retaining the liquid.
• Mix in the activated charcoal until it's fully dissolved.
• Store the mixture in a clean bottle or container.

BotuGuard Herbal Flush is a thoughtfully curated blend, designed to address the toxin challenges that botulism presents in chickens. The dandelion root, renowned for its detoxifying properties, aids in flushing out toxins from the system. Milk thistle seeds, on the other hand, are champions in supporting liver function, ensuring that the primary detoxifying organ is in optimal shape. The star player, activated charcoal, is a potent binder to toxins, ensuring they are safely escorted out of the body. Together, these ingredients form a potent defense against the debilitating effects of botulism, aiming to restore vitality and health to your chickens.

Notes:
- Dandelion Root: This humble plant is more than just a garden weed. Its roots are packed with compounds that aid in detoxification, making it a staple in many herbal detox remedies.
- Milk Thistle Seeds: A renowned liver supporter, milk thistle seeds contain silymarin, a compound known to aid liver function and detoxification.
- Activated Charcoal: Not your regular BBQ charcoal, activated charcoal has an incredible surface area that binds to toxins, ensuring they don't get absorbed into the body but are instead excreted.
- Quality Matters: Always ensure you're sourcing high-quality ingredients. The potency and purity of the ingredients can significantly influence the remedy's effectiveness.
- Consistency in Treatment: For optimal results, administer the BotuGuard Herbal Flush consistently, ensuring your chickens receive the full course of the remedy.
- Storage: Store the BotuGuard Herbal Flush in a cool, dark place, preferably in a glass container to maintain its potency.
- Dosage and Administration: Administer 1 teaspoon of the BotuGuard Herbal Flush in your chicken's drinking water daily for a week. Ensure they have access to fresh, untreated water as well.
- Duration of Treatment: A week-long treatment is typically recommended, but it is key to observe your chickens and adjust based on their condition.

ToxiCleanse Herbal Elixir

Introducing the ToxiCleanse Herbal Elixir, a potent blend designed to combat the challenges of botulism in chickens. This elixir combines the detoxifying properties of select herbs with the acidic nature of apple cider vinegar to create a powerful solution that aims to cleanse and rejuvenate your flock from the inside out.

Ingredients:
- 2 tablespoons Burdock Root (finely chopped)
- 1 tablespoon Cilantro Leaves (freshly chopped)
- 1 teaspoon Ginger Root (grated)
- 8 ounces Apple Cider Vinegar

Directions:
- In a glass jar, combine the burdock root, cilantro leaves, and grated ginger root.
- Pour the apple cider vinegar over the herbs, ensuring they are fully submerged.
- Seal the jar and allow the mixture to infuse in a cool, dark place for about 2 weeks, shaking it gently every day.
- After 2 weeks, strain out the herbs, retaining the liquid elixir.
- Store the elixir in a clean, airtight bottle.

ToxiCleanse Herbal Elixir is a synergistic blend of herbs and apple cider vinegar, each chosen for their unique properties in detoxification and overall health promotion. Burdock root, a renowned detoxifier, works diligently to cleanse the system of unwanted toxins. Cilantro, often used in culinary dishes, has a lesser-known talent for aiding in the removal of heavy metals. Ginger root, with its warming properties, supports digestion and enhances the body's natural detox processes. Lastly, apple cider vinegar, with its acidic nature, creates an environment where harmful bacteria struggle to thrive while also aiding in digestion. Together, these ingredients form a formidable defense against the toxins introduced by botulism, striving to restore health and vitality to your chickens.

Notes:
- Burdock Root: This root is a powerhouse when it comes to detoxification. It's known to support liver function and help cleanse the blood.
- Cilantro Leaves: Beyond their culinary appeal, cilantro leaves have been suggested to help in the removal of heavy metals from the body.
- Ginger Root: A common kitchen ingredient with powerful properties. Ginger not only aids digestion but also supports the body's natural detoxification processes.
- Apple Cider Vinegar: A versatile ingredient, apple cider vinegar aids digestion, supports a healthy gut environment, and provides a host of beneficial enzymes and acids.
- Quality Matters: Always prioritize high-quality, organic ingredients. The effectiveness of the elixir is directly tied to the purity and potency of its components.
- Consistency in Treatment: Regular and consistent administration of ToxiCleanse Herbal Elixir ensures optimal results.
- Storage: Store the elixir in a cool, dark place. Using a glass container helps maintain its potency and purity.
- Dosage and Administration: Add 1 teaspoon of the ToxiCleanse Herbal Elixir to your chicken's drinking water daily for a week. Always ensure they have access to fresh, untreated water alongside.
- Duration of Treatment: A week-long treatment is typically recommended. However, observing your chickens and adjusting based on their condition is always beneficial.

Molasses Toxin Purge

Introducing the Molasses Toxin Purge, a specialized blend crafted to address the challenges of botulism in chickens. This remedy combines the natural detoxifying properties of blackstrap molasses with the potent benefits of select herbs to create a solution that aims to cleanse and fortify your flock from within.

Ingredients:
- 4 tablespoons Blackstrap Molasses
- 2 tablespoons Echinacea Root (finely chopped)
- 1 tablespoon Turmeric Root (grated)
- 16 ounces Filtered Water

Directions:
- In a pot, bring the filtered water to a gentle boil.
- Add the echinacea root and turmeric root to the boiling water.
- Reduce the heat and let it simmer for about 15 minutes.
- Remove from heat and allow it to cool to room temperature.
- Once cooled, strain out the herbs, retaining the liquid.
- Stir in the blackstrap molasses until it's fully dissolved.
- Store the mixture in a clean bottle or container.

Molasses Toxin Purge is a unique concoction designed to harness the detoxifying power of blackstrap molasses, combined with the immune-boosting properties of echinacea and the anti-inflammatory benefits of turmeric. Blackstrap molasses, rich in essential minerals, aids in flushing out toxins from the system. Echinacea, a well-known immune system booster, supports the body's natural defenses, while turmeric, with its curcumin content, provides anti-inflammatory benefits and supports liver function. Together, these ingredients form a potent blend that aims to cleanse the system, bolster immunity, and promote the overall well-being of your chickens in the face of botulism challenges.

Notes:
- Blackstrap Molasses: This is the dark, viscous molasses remaining after maximum extraction of sugar from raw sugar cane. It's rich in minerals like iron, magnesium, and calcium, making it a nutritious choice for detoxification.
- Echinacea Root: Renowned for its immune-boosting properties, echinacea has been used for centuries to fortify the body's natural defenses against various ailments.
- Turmeric Root: A golden-hued root known for its anti-inflammatory properties, largely due to its active compound, curcumin. Turmeric also supports liver function, a crucial organ in detoxification.
- Quality Matters: Always opt for high-quality, preferably organic ingredients. The remedy's effectiveness is closely tied to the purity and potency of its components.
- Consistency in Treatment: For best results, it's essential to administer the Molasses Toxin Purge consistently, ensuring your chickens receive the full course of the remedy.
- Storage: Store the mixture in a cool, dark place, preferably in a glass container to maintain its potency.
- Dosage and Administration: Add 2 teaspoons of the Molasses Toxin Purge to your chicken's drinking water daily for a week. Always ensure they also have access to fresh, untreated water.
- Duration of Treatment: Typically, a week-long treatment is recommended. However, always observe your chickens and adjust based on their condition.

HerbaDetox Soothing Blend

Introducing the HerbaDetox Soothing Blend, a meticulously crafted herbal concoction designed to address the challenges of botulism in chickens. This blend combines the soothing properties of slippery elm bark with the detoxifying abilities of bentonite clay, complemented by the digestive benefits of fennel seeds and the calming effects of chamomile flowers.

Ingredients:
• 3 tablespoons Slippery Elm Bark (powdered)
• 2 tablespoons Fennel Seeds (crushed)
• 1 tablespoon Bentonite Clay
• 2 tablespoons Chamomile Flowers (dried)

Directions:
• In a mixing bowl, combine the powdered slippery elm bark and bentonite clay.
• Add the crushed fennel seeds and dried chamomile flowers to the mixture.
• Mix the ingredients thoroughly until they are well-blended.

• Store the blend in an airtight container away from direct sunlight.

HerbaDetox Soothing Blend is a harmonious combination of herbs and clay, each chosen for their unique therapeutic properties. Slippery elm bark, known for its mucilaginous content, forms a protective layer on the digestive tract, aiding in the soothing of inflammation and irritation. Bentonite clay, a natural detoxifier, binds to toxins, helping in their removal from the body. Fennel seeds, with their carminative properties, aid in digestion and reduce gas, while chamomile flowers, renowned for their calming effects, help in reducing stress and inflammation. Together, these ingredients aim to provide a holistic approach to combat the effects of botulism, promoting digestive health and overall well-being in your chickens.

Notes:
- Slippery Elm Bark: This bark is rich in mucilage, a sticky substance that becomes a slick gel when mixed with water. It coats and soothes the mouth, throat, stomach, and intestines, making it ideal for digestive issues.
- Fennel Seeds: Often used as a culinary spice, fennel seeds have carminative properties, meaning they help expel gas from the intestines and provide relief from bloating.
- Bentonite Clay: This clay has been used for centuries as a natural detoxifier. It has the ability to bind to toxins and help in their excretion from the body.
- Chamomile Flowers: Recognized for their calming effects, chamomile flowers can help reduce stress, which is essential for chickens combating illness.
- Quality Matters: Always prioritize high-quality, organic ingredients. The effectiveness of the blend is directly tied to the purity and potency of its components.
- Consistency in Treatment: Regular and consistent administration of HerbaDetox Soothing Blend ensures optimal results.
- Storage: Store the blend in a cool, dark place. Using a glass or ceramic container helps maintain its potency and purity.
- Dosage and Administration: Sprinkle 1 teaspoon of the HerbaDetox Soothing Blend over your chicken's feed daily for a week.
- Duration of Treatment: A week-long treatment is typically recommended. However, observing your chickens and adjusting based on their condition is always beneficial.

17. Aspergillosis (Brooder Pneumonia)

Aspergillosis, commonly referred to as Brooder Pneumonia when it affects young poultry, is a respiratory disease caused by the fungus *Aspergillus*. The *Aspergillus* species, especially *Aspergillus fumigatus*, are ubiquitous in the environment and can be found in soil, decaying vegetation, and organic debris. While the fungus is widespread, it becomes problematic when birds inhale large amounts of the fungal spores. It primarily affects the lungs and air sacs and can lead to symptoms such as gasping, coughing, and general weakness.

LungClear Herbal Tonic

Introducing the LungClear Herbal Tonic, a specialized blend crafted to support respiratory health in chickens, particularly those facing challenges like Aspergillosis (Brooder Pneumonia). This tonic harnesses the power of select herbs known for their respiratory and immune-boosting properties.

Ingredients:
- 2 tablespoons Mullein leaves (dried)
- 1 tablespoon Echinacea root (dried and crushed)
- 1 tablespoon Oregano leaves (dried)
- 1 teaspoon Thyme (dried)
- 1 tablespoon Licorice root (dried and crushed)
- 16 ounces Filtered water

Directions:
- Combine all the dried herbs in a pot.
- Pour the filtered water over the herbs.
- Bring the mixture to a boil, then reduce to a simmer.
- Let it simmer for about 20-25 minutes.
- Strain the herbs, collecting the liquid in a clean container.
- Allow the tonic to cool before use.

LungClear Herbal Tonic is a thoughtfully curated blend aiming to bolster respiratory health in chickens. Mullein is renowned for its ability to soothe the respiratory tract and reduce inflammation. Echinacea, a well-known immune booster, helps the body's natural defense against infections. Oregano and thyme, both packed with antifungal and antibacterial properties, work in tandem to combat the fungal agents of Aspergillosis. Lastly, licorice root acts as an expectorant, aiding in the removal of mucus and easing respiratory discomfort.

Notes:
- Mullein Leaves: These leaves have been traditionally used for respiratory issues due to their anti-inflammatory properties. They can soothe irritated respiratory tracts and help reduce mucus production.
- Echinacea Root: A staple in herbal medicine, echinacea is known to boost the immune system, helping the body fight off infections more effectively.
- Oregano Leaves: Beyond its culinary uses, oregano has potent antifungal and antibacterial properties, making it a valuable ally against respiratory infections.

- Thyme: This aromatic herb is not just for cooking. It's packed with compounds that have antifungal and antibacterial effects.
- Licorice Root: Licorice is an adaptogenic herb that can help soothe the respiratory system and also acts as an expectorant, helping to clear mucus.
- Quality Matters: Always opt for high-quality, preferably organic herbs. The potency and purity of your ingredients directly influence the remedy's effectiveness.
- Consistency in Treatment: For best results, administer the tonic consistently, as per the recommended dosage.
- Storage: Store the tonic in a cool, dark place, preferably in a glass container. Use within 5-7 days for maximum potency.
- Dosage and Administration: Administer 1 teaspoon of the cooled tonic to your chickens daily, directly or mixed with their feed.
- Duration of Treatment: A consistent 7-day treatment is recommended, but always observe your chickens and adjust based on their condition.

Garlic-y Respiratory Flush

Introducing the Garlick-y Respiratory Flush, a potent concoction designed to aid chickens in their battle against Aspergillosis (Brooder Pneumonia). This remedy combines the antifungal and antibacterial properties of ginger, garlic, and cayenne pepper, aiming to cleanse the system and support respiratory health.

Ingredients:
- 1 inch Ginger root (finely grated)
- 5 Garlic cloves (crushed)
- 1/4 teaspoon Cayenne pepper
- 32 ounces Filtered water

Directions:
- In a pot, combine the filtered water, grated ginger, crushed garlic, and cayenne pepper.
- Bring the mixture to a boil, then reduce to a simmer for 15 minutes.
- Remove from heat and let it cool down to room temperature.
- Strain the mixture to remove solid particles, collecting the liquid in a clean container.

The Garlic-y Respiratory Flush is a holistic approach to addressing respiratory challenges in chickens. Ginger, with its anti-inflammatory properties, soothes the respiratory tract, while garlic's potent antifungal and antibacterial properties help combat the fungal agents causing Aspergillosis. Cayenne pepper, a circulatory stimulant, ensures these beneficial ingredients are effectively distributed throughout the body.

Notes:
- Ginger Root: Ginger is a powerful anti-inflammatory and can help soothe irritated respiratory tracts. It also possesses antifungal properties.
- Garlic Cloves: Garlic is a natural antifungal and antibacterial agent. It's been used for centuries to combat various infections.
- Cayenne Pepper: This spicy pepper is known to boost circulation, ensuring that the beneficial properties of the other ingredients are effectively distributed throughout the chicken's body.

- Quality Matters: Always choose high-quality ingredients. The effectiveness of the remedy is directly tied to the purity and potency of the ingredients used.
- Consistency in Treatment: Administer the flush consistently for best results.
- Storage: Store the flush in a cool, dark place. To ensure maximum potency, use within 3-5 days.
- Dosage and Administration: Provide 1 to 2 tablespoons of the flush mixed with their regular drinking water daily.
- Duration of Treatment: A consistent 7-day treatment is recommended. However, always monitor the condition of your chickens and adjust based on their needs.

BreathEase Herbal Blend

Introducing the BreathEase Herbal Blend, a carefully crafted mixture designed to support respiratory health in chickens battling Aspergillosis (Brooder Pneumonia). This blend harnesses the power of nature, combining herbs known for their respiratory benefits with the nourishing properties of olive oil.

Ingredients:
- 2 tablespoons Elecampane root (finely chopped)
- 1 tablespoon Peppermint leaves (crushed)
- 2 tablespoons Marshmallow root (finely chopped)
- 1 tablespoon Eucalyptus leaves (crushed)
- 8 ounces Olive oil (as a base)

Directions:
- In a glass jar, combine the finely chopped Elecampane root, crushed Peppermint leaves, finely chopped Marshmallow root, and crushed Eucalyptus leaves.
- Pour the olive oil over the herbs, ensuring they are fully submerged.
- Seal the jar tightly and place it in a sunny spot for 2-3 weeks, shaking it gently every day.
- After the infusion period, strain the oil through a fine mesh strainer or cheesecloth, discarding the herbs and retaining the oil.
- Store the oil in a dark, cool place.

BreathEase Herbal Blend is a natural approach to supporting respiratory health in chickens. Elecampane root is traditionally used for its expectorant properties, aiding in clearing mucus from the respiratory system. Peppermint leaves provide a cooling sensation, helping to soothe irritated airways. Marshmallow root offers a protective layer on the mucous membranes, while Eucalyptus leaves are known for their antiseptic properties and ability to promote clearer breathing. The olive oil acts as a carrier, ensuring the beneficial properties of the herbs are effectively delivered.

Notes:
- Elecampane Root: This root has been traditionally used for respiratory ailments due to its expectorant properties, helping to clear mucus and soothe irritation.
- Peppermint Leaves: Known for its cooling and soothing effects, peppermint can help reduce inflammation in the respiratory tract.

- Marshmallow Root: This herb provides a protective layer on the mucous membranes, aiding in reducing irritation.
- Eucalyptus Leaves: With antiseptic properties, eucalyptus can help clear congestion and promote easier breathing.
- Olive Oil: Acts as a carrier oil, ensuring the beneficial properties of the herbs are effectively absorbed.
- Quality Matters: Always opt for high-quality, organic herbs and cold-pressed olive oil to ensure the potency and purity of the remedy.
- Consistency in Treatment: For best results, apply the oil blend consistently to the affected areas.
- Storage: Store the blend in a cool, dark place. Use within 6 months for maximum effectiveness.
- Dosage and Administration: Apply a few drops of the oil blend to the affected areas, gently massaging it in. Avoid contact with eyes.
- Duration of Treatment: Continue treatment for 7-10 days or until symptoms improve, always monitoring the condition of your chickens.

FungalFighter Herbal Elixir

Meet the FungalFighter Herbal Elixir, a potent blend crafted to support chickens in their battle against Aspergillosis (Brooder Pneumonia). This elixir combines the antifungal properties of select herbs with the acidity of apple cider vinegar to create a powerful natural remedy.

Ingredients:
- 2 tablespoons Pau d'arco bark (finely chopped)
- 1 tablespoon Olive leaf (crushed)
- 2 tablespoons Astragalus root (finely chopped)
- 1 tablespoon Goldenseal root (finely chopped)
- 8 ounces Apple cider vinegar

Directions:
- Combine Pau d'arco bark, Olive leaf, Astragalus root, and Goldenseal root in a glass jar.
- Pour apple cider vinegar over the herbs, ensuring they are fully submerged.
- Seal the jar tightly and let it sit in a cool, dark place for 3-4 weeks, shaking it gently every day.
- After the infusion period, strain the mixture through a fine mesh strainer or cheesecloth, discarding the herbs and retaining the liquid.
- Store the elixir in a cool, dark place.

The FungalFighter Herbal Elixir is designed to harness the antifungal and immune-boosting properties of its ingredients. Pau d'arco bark and Olive leaf are renowned for their antifungal attributes, making them essential in combating Aspergillosis. Astragalus root is a potent immune booster, helping the body's natural defenses, while Goldenseal root offers antimicrobial benefits. The apple cider vinegar acts not only as a preservative but also aids in the absorption of the herbal benefits.

Notes:
- Pau d'arco Bark: Known for its antifungal properties, this bark has been traditionally used to combat various fungal infections.
- Olive Leaf: Contains oleuropein, a compound known for its antimicrobial and antifungal effects.
- Astragalus Root: A powerful adaptogen, it helps boost the immune system, making it easier for the body to fight off infections.
- Goldenseal Root: Offers antimicrobial properties and has been traditionally used to combat infections.
- Apple Cider Vinegar: Its acidic nature helps preserve the elixir and aids in the absorption of the herbal benefits.
- Quality Matters: Always choose high-quality, organic ingredients to ensure the remedy's effectiveness and purity.
- Consistency in Treatment: For optimal results, administer the elixir consistently.
- Storage: Keep the elixir in a cool, dark place. Use within 6 months for best results.
- Dosage and Administration: Add a few drops of the elixir to the chicken's water or food daily. Monitor for any adverse reactions.
- Duration of Treatment: Continue treatment for 10-14 days or until symptoms improve, always observing the condition of your chickens.

Appendix 4

Let's unravel the the miraculous Powers of Colloidal Silver and Grapefruit Seed Extract Colloidal Silver and Grapefruit Seed Extract may not be herbs, but they have many uses to help your flock flourish!

The Magic of Colloidal Silver: Uses and Benefits for Your Flock

Dive into the shimmering world of colloidal silver, a solution that contains tiny silver particles suspended in liquid. This magical elixir has been used in various forms for centuries for its health benefits, and it's not just for people - it can work wonders for your chickens, too.

- ## Boosting Immune System

Colloidal silver is recognized for its immune-supporting properties. Regular but moderated use can help keep your chicken's immune system robust, enabling them to resist infections and diseases more effectively. A few drops in their drinking water can work as a preventative measure.

- ## Wound Care

Colloidal silver can be used topically on cuts, wounds, or abrasions. It's known for its antimicrobial properties, which can help prevent infection and speed up healing. To apply, gently dab the solution on the affected area using a clean cloth or spray directly.

- ## Eye and Beak Care

Issues with eyes or beaks, like eye infections or sinus problems, can be soothed with colloidal silver. Using a dropper, you can apply a few drops into your chicken's eyes or nostrils. Its soothing properties can provide relief and contribute to faster recovery.

- ## Water Purifier

Adding colloidal silver to your chicken's water can help keep it free from bacteria, algae, and viruses. It's an easy way to ensure your flock has access to clean drinking water, contributing to overall health.

- ## Parasite Control

While it's not a cure-all, some chicken keepers have found that colloidal silver can help control parasites. Regular use can deter external parasites like mites and lice and help manage internal parasites as well.

Now, remember, while colloidal silver has many potential benefits, it's essential to use it wisely. Here are some tips:

- ## Moderation is Key

Like with most things, excessive amounts of colloidal silver can be harmful to chickens. It's always best to use it in moderation. Typically, a few drops in the water or directly on the affected area are enough.

- Quality Matters

Not all colloidal silver products are created equal. Look for high-quality options, ideally those with a high concentration of silver particles (10-30 ppm, or parts per million, is a common range).

- Observe Your Chickens

As you start using colloidal silver, pay attention to your chickens. Notice any changes in their behavior, appetite, or general health. This will help you understand whether the treatment is working or if adjustments are needed.

Feathered Friend Dosage: Administering Colloidal Silver Safely

The silver speckles floating in a bottle of colloidal silver might look benign, but it's critical to remember that even the most natural solutions must be administered properly to ensure safety and effectiveness. Therefore, this section will shed light on how to safely provide your feathered friends with colloidal silver.

- Start With a Lower Dosage

If you're introducing colloidal silver to your chickens for the first time, it's a good idea to start with a lower dosage to see how they react. Observe their behavior, energy levels, and overall health. Any adverse reactions should become evident within a few days. If everything seems normal, you can gradually increase the dosage.

- Know the Concentration

Before you can determine the appropriate dosage, you need to know the concentration of your colloidal silver solution. This is usually measured in parts per million (ppm). A standard concentration is between 10 and 30 ppm. A higher ppm means more silver particles in the solution, so a lower dosage is necessary.

- Calculating Dosage for Water

A common way to administer colloidal silver to chickens is through their drinking water. Add approximately one tablespoon of colloidal silver (10-30 ppm) per gallon of water. This concentration provides a general immune support level and can help keep the water clean. If dealing with a specific health issue, you might consider increasing the dosage to two tablespoons per gallon, but not for extended periods.

- Direct Application

When dealing with wounds, eye infections, or beak problems, direct application of colloidal silver can be beneficial. Using a dropper or spray bottle, apply the solution directly to the affected area. For minor issues, one or two applications per day should suffice. For more severe problems, you might need to apply the solution more frequently.

- Internal Use

If a chicken is sick and you're using colloidal silver as part of their treatment plan, you can administer it directly. Use a dropper to give your chicken around 1/4 to 1/2 a teaspoon of colloidal silver once or twice a day. Please be sure that you know how to administer liquid to chickens without causing them to aspirate.

- Prolonged Use

While colloidal silver can be a great support for your chicken's health, it's not meant for prolonged use at high dosages. Extended exposure to large amounts of silver can lead to a condition known as argyria, which causes a blue-gray discoloration of the skin. This is extremely rare but worth keeping in mind.

Notes:
- Administering colloidal silver to your flock is a responsibility that should not be taken lightly. You're dealing with the health of living creatures, so always err on the side of caution.
- Always keep a close eye on your chickens, especially when introducing new elements like colloidal silver into their routine. Your careful observation is often the first line of defense in noticing any health issues.
- Finally, enjoy the process of caring for your flock. Chickens are wonderful creatures, and the chance to enhance their health and happiness with natural remedies like colloidal silver is part of the joy of keeping them. Happy clucking!

Grapefruit Seed Extract: A Zesty Solution for Poultry Health

When it comes to the health of your poultry flock, few natural remedies pack as much punch as grapefruit seed extract (GSE). This zesty solution offers an array of benefits that can contribute to the overall well-being of your chickens.

So, what's the deal with grapefruit seed extract?

- What is Grapefruit Seed Extract?

Grapefruit seed extract is a potent liquid derived from the seeds, pulp, and white membranes of grapefruit. The extract is rich in beneficial plant compounds, including flavonoids and vitamin C. These properties give GSE its antimicrobial, antiviral, and antioxidant qualities.

- Antibacterial Properties

One of the primary benefits of GSE is its antibacterial properties. It's been found to be effective against a wide range of bacteria, which makes it a versatile tool in your poultry health kit. Whether it's combatting harmful bacteria in the coop or preventing the spread of infection in a wound, GSE could lend a helping hand.

- Antifungal and Anti-parasitic Actions

In addition to fighting bacteria, GSE also has antifungal and anti-parasitic properties. For instance, it can help combat yeast and fungal infections. If your chickens suffer from parasites like mites or lice, a GSE solution could also serve as a useful deterrent.

- ## Immune System Boost
Thanks to its rich array of antioxidants, GSE can help support your chickens' immune systems. Regularly incorporating it into their routine could help your flock fight off illness and stay in top form.

- ## Cleaning and Disinfecting Coops
GSE isn't just for the chickens - it can also come in handy around the coop. Its antimicrobial properties make it an excellent natural choice for cleaning and disinfecting the coop without resorting to harsh chemicals.

- ## How to Use GSE for Your Chickens
Using GSE for your chickens is relatively straightforward. You can add it to their drinking water, apply it topically for skin issues, or use it to clean and disinfect your coop. When adding it to water, a ratio of 10 drops per gallon is a good starting point.

Now, let's explore the specifics of using grapefruit seed extract for various health and maintenance purposes.

- ## Using GSE in Drinking Water
Adding GSE to your chickens' drinking water can help keep them in good health. The antimicrobial properties of GSE can help keep the water fresh and free from harmful bacteria, which could otherwise multiply rapidly, especially in warm weather.

- ## Topical Applications
For skin conditions, wounds, or external parasites, GSE can be applied topically. You can dilute it with water (10 drops per cup of water) and use a clean cloth or a spray bottle to apply it to the affected area.

- ## Coop Cleaning
To clean and disinfect your coop naturally, mix one teaspoon of GSE with one gallon of water. This solution can be used to scrub down surfaces, clean feeders and waterers, and freshen up nest boxes. Remember, a clean coop is a crucial step in maintaining a healthy flock.

Notes:
- As you can see, grapefruit seed extract is a versatile addition to your poultry health toolkit. It can help combat bacteria, fungi, and parasites, and it supports the immune system. Plus, it can be used to clean your coop naturally.
- Remember to always dilute GSE appropriately, as it's highly concentrated. Start with smaller amounts and increase as needed, monitoring your flock for any changes or adverse reactions.

- Incorporating natural solutions like GSE can contribute to your holistic poultry care practices. By understanding and utilizing the power of natural substances, you're taking an active role in supporting the health and happiness of your feathered friends.
- A happy, healthy flock is a joy to behold, and with tools like grapefruit seed extract, you're well on your way to achieving that goal. May your coop be filled with clucks of contentment and the soft rustle of feathers!

Peck the Right Dose: Guidelines for Grapefruit Seed Extract Usage

Navigating the world of natural remedies for your chicken flock might seem a bit daunting at first. Yet, with the right knowledge, you'll find that it can be as easy as pie. One of the important aspects of implementing natural treatments like Grapefruit Seed Extract (GSE) is determining the correct dosage.

- ### Start Small
When starting out with GSE, it's best to begin with a smaller dosage. This is simply because GSE is incredibly potent. Although it's a natural product, it can still cause adverse reactions if it's administered in large quantities right off the bat.

- ### A Drop in the Bucket
For daily maintenance and immune support, adding GSE to your chickens' drinking water can be beneficial. It's generally suggested to add about 10 drops of GSE per gallon of water. This creates a solution that's potent enough to provide health benefits but not so strong as to risk upsetting your chickens' systems.

- ### Topical Talk
If you're dealing with external issues like wounds or skin irritations, a more concentrated application might be in order. In such cases, it's recommended to use about 10 drops of GSE per cup of water. This solution can be gently applied to the affected area with a clean cloth or a spray bottle.

- ### Coop Cleaning
As for cleaning the coop, a stronger solution is usually more effective. Mixing one teaspoon of GSE with one gallon of water is typically recommended. This solution is powerful enough to tackle most common coop messes, and it's safe for your chickens.

- ### Proactive Parasite Control
If your flock is struggling with parasites, a slightly higher dosage can be beneficial. In this case, using about 15 drops of GSE per gallon of water can help to deter pests and keep your chickens comfortable.

- ### A Word on Consistency
Consistency is key when it comes to using GSE. Regular, steady usage yields better results than sporadic, high-dose applications. Therefore, aim to incorporate GSE into your flock's routine in a balanced, consistent manner.

Notes:
- Choosing the correct dosage of GSE for your chickens isn't rocket science, but it does require attention and care. Always keep in mind that the potency of GSE can vary from brand to brand, so it's crucial to adjust the dosage according to the specific product you're using.
- Moreover, while GSE is generally safe for chickens, it's still crucial to monitor your flock closely, especially when you first introduce this new substance into their regimen. Pay attention to their behavior, appetite, and general demeanor. If you notice any significant changes, it may be necessary to adjust the dosage or stop using GSE altogether.
- GSE offers an array of health benefits and can be a valuable addition to your poultry care arsenal. With the right knowledge and careful application, you can utilize this natural powerhouse to support the health and well-being of your feathered friends. Your herbal journey with your chickens will not only deepen your connection with nature but also foster a sustainable and harmonious living environment. We've explored the bountiful benefits of integrating herbs into your flock's routine, from enhancing their immune system to creating a serene habitat for them to thrive.

As you step forward, armed with the knowledge and insights from this book, remember that the true essence of herbal care lies in the balance and natural rhythm of life. Each herb, with its unique properties, contributes to a symphony of wellness that resonates through your flock, echoing the age-old wisdom of nature's healing powers.

Embrace the role of a mindful steward, nurturing your chickens with the wholesome goodness of herbs, and witness the transformation in their health, vitality, and joy. Let your herb garden be a testament to the harmonious coexistence of human care and nature's bounty.

May your journey through the Herbal Henhouse not only lead to healthier, happier chickens but also inspire a greater appreciation for the simple yet profound connections between all living things. Here's to the flourishing of your feathered friends under the nurturing canopy of nature's remedies.

Happy herbing, and may your coop always be a haven of health and happiness!

About the Author

Mary Butler's heart has always had room for the love of animals. For the past ten years, she has nurtured a growing flock of chickens, becoming more than just their caretaker—they have become her cherished companions. A committed vegetarian, Mary's journey into chicken rearing began when her husband, a non-vegetarian, introduced some chicks into their lives. From that moment, those chicks became much more than poultry; they became pets, friends, and a part of Mary's very soul.

Seven years ago, Mary took a leap into holistic aviculture, treating her feathered friends with herbs and witnessing transformative effects on their health and behavior. She became a haven for those in need, rescuing ex-battery hens, roosters, and special needs chickens, each with their own story of resilience and recovery.

At home, Mary's diverse pet family—a blend of chickens, dogs, cats, and even a turtle—exemplifies her all-encompassing love for creatures great and small, reflecting a life filled with interspecies harmony.

Beyond the coop and her animal adventures, Mary is set to release a cozy mystery series, "The Hen House Mysteries," infused with the same warmth and spirited energy that she brings to her daily life. Readers can look forward to an enchanting mix of intrigue and homely charm as each mystery unfolds against the backdrop of rural bliss.

For the latest updates on Mary Butler's books — including release dates for The Hen House Mysteries — follow her on Facebook, visit her author page on Amazon, or explore her website at www.authormarybutler.com. For inquiries, contact: hello@authormarybutler.com.

📣 A Note from the Author

Dear Reader,

If you've made it this far, thank you. Truly. Writing *The Herbal Henhouse* was a labor of love — full of early mornings, late nights, muddy boots, herbal trials, and lots (and lots) of chicken watching. It's incredibly meaningful to know the words I've poured onto these pages are now in your hands.

As a self-published author, I don't have a big team or a marketing budget. What I *do* have is **you** — and readers like you make all the difference.

If you enjoyed this book, I would be so grateful if you took just a moment to leave an **honest and kind review**. Reviews help other readers find my work and help me keep creating more books like this one. Even a few thoughtful sentences can go a long way.

Yes, I read every single review — and your words matter to me more than you know. Whether you share what you loved, what you learned, or even what you'd like to see more of, your feedback helps me grow as a writer and a chicken keeper.

You can leave a review by scanning the QR code or visiting my Amazon author page:

🔗 https://Amazon.com/review/create-review?&asin=B0CYR3CJFK

From the bottom of my heart (and on behalf of my happy hens), thank you for your support. I wouldn't be here without you.

Warmly,
Mary Butler *and her feathered editorial team* 🐔

Please Scan This QR Code To Leave Your Review

www.ingramcontent.com/pod-product-compliance
Lightning Source LLC
Chambersburg PA
CBHW081144270326
41930CB00014B/3030